Clinics in Developmental Medicine

COGNITION AND BEHAVIOUR IN CHILDHOOD
EPILEPSY

Clinics in Developmental Medicine

Cognition and Behaviour in Childhood Epilepsy

Edited by

LIEVEN LAGAE
University Hospitals KU Leuven,
Leuven, Belgium

2017
Mac Keith Press

© 2017 Mac Keith Press 6 Market Road,
London, N7 9PW

Managing Director: Ann-Marie Halligan
Production Manager and Commissioning Editor: Udoka Ohuonu
Project Management: Lumina Datamatics

First published in this edition in 2017

British Library Cataloguing-in-Publication data A catalogue record for this book is
available from the British Library

Cover design: Hannah Rogers

ISBN: 978-1-909962-87-3

Typeset by Lumina Datamatics, Chennai, India

Printing managed by Jellyfish Solutions Ltd

Mac Keith Press is supported by Scope

CONTENTS

AUTHORS' APPOINTMENTS

Albert P Aldenkamp Professor, Academic Center for Epileptology Kempenhaeghe/Maastricht UMC; Eindhoven University of Technology, the Netherlands; Ghent University Hospital, Belgium

Alexis Arzimanoglou Director, Department of Paediatric Clinical Epileptology, Sleep Disorders and Functional Neurology, University Hospitals of Lyon (HCL), France; Epilepsy Programme, Paediatric Neurology Department, Hospital San Juan de Dios, Barcelona, Spain

Stéphane Auvin Professor, Epilepsy & Child Neurology, Paris Diderot University; Robert-Debré Hospital & INSERM U1141, Paris, France

Anne T Berg Research Professor, Ann & Robert H. Lurie Children's Hospital of Chicago, Northwestern University Feinberg School of Medicine, Chicago, IL, USA

Madison M Berl Director of Research, Division of Pediatric Neuropsychology; Pediatric Neuropsychologist, Comprehensive Pediatric Epilepsy Program (CPEP); Associate Director T32 Fellowship Program, Children's National Medical Center; Associate Professor, Departments of Psychiatry and Behavioral Sciences, George Washington University School of Medicine, Washington, DC, USA

Kees P J Braun Professor of Child Neurology, Brain Center Rudolf Magnus, University Medical Center Utrecht, the Netherlands

Carol Camfield Department of Pediatrics, Dalhousie University and the IWK Health Centre, Halifax, Nova Scotia, Canada

Peter Camfield Department of Pediatrics, Dalhousie University and the IWK Health Centre, Halifax, Nova Scotia, Canada

J Helen Cross	Professor, Clinical Neurosciences Unit, UCL Institute of Child Health & Great Ormond Street Hospital for Children, London, UK
Xavier De Tiège	Professor, Department of Functional Neuroimaging, Service of Nuclear Medicine, ULB-Hôpital Erasme, Brussels, Belgium
Melissa Filippini	Child Neurology Unit, IRCCS Istituto delle Scienze Neurologiche, Bologna, Italy
Giuseppe Gobbi	Child Neurology Unit, ISNB IRCCS Istituto delle Scienze Neurologiche, Bologna, Italy
Gregory L Holmes	Chair, Department of Neurological Sciences; Professor of Neurological Sciences and Pediatrics, The Robert Larner, M.D. College of Medicine, University of Vermont, Burlington, VT, USA
Dominique Ijff	Academic Center for Epileptology, Kempenhaeghe/Maastricht UMC, the Netherlands
Faustine Ilski-Lecoanet	Neurpsychologist Epilepsy, Sleep and Paediatric Neurophysiology Department, HFME, University Hospitals of Lyon (HCL), France
Jonathan K Kleen	Chief Resident, Department of Neurology, University of California, San Francisco Medical Center, CA, USA
Agathe Laurent	Neuropsychologist, Epilepsy, Sleep and Paediatric Neurophysiology Department, HFME, University Hospitals of Lyon, France
Willem Lavrijssen	Medical Psychologist, Kempenhaeghe Expertise Centre for Epileptology, Heeze, the Netherlands
Emma Losito	Pediatric Neuropsychiatrist, Centre de référence épilepsies rares (CReER), Service de Neurologie Pédiatrique, Hôpital Necker-Enfants Malades, Université Paris Descartes, Paris, France
Andrew Lux	Consultant Paediatric Neurologist, Department of Paediatric Neurology, Bristol Royal Hospital for Children, Bristol, UK
Romina Moavero	Research Fellow, Child Neurology Unit, Neuroscience and Neurorehabilitation Department, Bambino Gesù Children's Hospital, IRCCS; Researcher, Child Neurology and Psychiatry Unit, Systems Medicine Department, Tor Vergata University of Rome, Italy

Rima Nabbout Professor, Department of Paediatric Neurology, Necker-Enfants Malades, APHP, University hospital of Paris Descartes University, Paris, France

Eleni Panagiotakaki Senior Consultant, Department of Clinical Epileptology, Sleep Disorders and Functional Neurology in Children, HFME, University Hospitals of Lyon (HCL), France

Alia Ramirez Camacho Paediatric Neurologist, Epilepsy Programme, Paediatric Neurology Department, Hospital San Juan de Dios, Barcelona, Spain

Leigh N Sepeta Pediatric Neuropsychologist, Comprehensive Pediatric Epilepsy Program (CPEP); Assistant Professor, Departments of Psychiatry and Behavioral Sciences, George Washington University School of Medicine, Washington, DC, USA

Renée A Shellhaas Clinical Associate Professor, Division of Pediatric Neurology, Department of Pediatrics & Communicable Diseases, University of Michigan, Ann Arbor, MI, USA

Patrick Van Bogaert Department of Pediatric Neurology, ULB-Hôpital Erasme, Brussels, Belgium

Monique M J van Schooneveld Clinical Neuropsychologist, Department of Pediatric Psychology, Sector of Neuropsychology, Wilhelmina Children's Hospital, University Medical Center Utrecht, the Netherlands

Federico Vigevano Child Neurology Unit, Neuroscience and Neurorehabilitation Department, Bambino Gesù Children's Hospital, IRCCS, Rome, Italy

Courtney J Wusthoff Assistant Professor, Division of Pediatric Neurology, Department of Neurology, Stanford University, Palo Alto, CA, USA

ACKNOWLEDGEMENT

Chapter 6. The work was supported by the National Institutes of Health grants NS074450, NS074450, and NS073083, and the Emmory R. Shapses Research Fund and Michael J. Pietroniro Research Fund.

FOREWORD

Childhood epilepsy is a multi-dimensional phenomenon that does not end with seizure control. To understand this complex medical issue, each of these dimensions must be considered alongside the other, especially in relation to the effects of epilepsy on cognition and behaviour.

In line with the modern approach to medicine, this disorder requires differentiation and personalization. Understanding the brain function and its development should be combined with recognizing the patient as an individual.

In this regard, *Cognition and Behaviour in Childhood Epilepsy* is a milestone in the field.

The opening chapter draws the link between genetics, biology, physiology, antiepileptic drugs and the social context of the child and his or her family. Other chapters emphasise the crucial lesson learned for testing and treatment, especially for epilepsy surgery: be early!

This book also discusses the relation between epilepsy and cognition and behaviour within the clinical spectrum of benign childhood epilepsy with centrotemporal spikes, continous spikes and waves during slow wave sleep (including Lennox – Gastaut syndrome): no syndromology, no epilepsy. A highlight is the chapter on modern technologies and the new perspectives they offer on brain imaging.

Cognition and Behaviour in Childhood Epilepsy is clinical neuroscience at its best and reflects the intellectual rigour, depth of scientific knowledge and patient care for which the editor, Lieven Lagae, is known. It will serve as both an introduction to this fascinating field and a tool for even the most experienced clinical neuroscientist. It provides practical guidance for bedside paediatric neurology decision-making and a roadmap for cognitive neuroscience in epileptology.

I hope this book will be widely used by all those who love both cognitive neuroscience and the children with epilepsy whom they care for on a daily basis.

Prof Florian Heinen
Head of Paediatric Neurology and Developmental Medicine
Hauner Children's Hospital, University of Munich
Germany

PREFACE

For many parents of children with epilepsy, not only are the unpredictable seizures a major concern, but equally so are the frequently associated cognitive and behavioural problems. As clinicians, we often do not pay enough attention to these comorbidities, perhaps because we do not have a full understanding of their aetiology and treatment possibilities. Cognitive and behavioural comorbidities in childhood epilepsies are multifactorial: aetiology, seizure type and frequency, syndromic classification, age at onset of the epilepsy, EEG abnormalities and treatment (failure). The challenge is that we need to understand the exact burden of each individual factor.

I was, therefore, very happy that many influential authors agreed to contribute to this unique book on cognition and behaviour in childhood epilepsy. This book is unique in that it focuses on the most frequent childhood epilepsy syndromes separately and describes the specific cognitive and behavioural issues associated with them. The primary aim is to give a state-of-the-art description of contemporary clinical research in this area.

This book has become an interesting anthology of the many different aspects of the comorbidities associated with the disorder. The first seven chapters deal with the importance of the diverse contributing factors, and make reference to the ongoing clinical and translational research.

What is required now is the prevention of cognitive decline and the development of specific treatment paradigms for the behavioural problems associated with childhood epilepsy.

I hope this book will be a valuable support for all professionals dealing with childhood epilepsy in their search for these desperately needed treatments.

Lieven Lagae
Leuven, Belgium,
March 2017

1
COGNITIVE DIFFICULTIES IN CHILDREN WITH EPILEPSY: SOURCES AND IMPLICATIONS

Anne T Berg

The general population of all children with epilepsy, between a fifth and a quarter, have developmental or intellectual impairment severe enough to qualify as intellectual disability (formerly mental retardation) (Ellenberg et al. 1984; Camfield and Camfield 2007; Berg et al. 2008; Geerts et al. 2011). Even in children whose overall cognitive function falls within the "normal" range, there is overwhelming evidence of subtle or selective deficits in various cognitive behavioral domains that may impact school performance. Understanding the reasons for these findings has implications for prevention, treatment, management, and anticipatory guidance.

The sources of cognitive comorbidity associated with epilepsy can be broken down into at least the following categories: (1) shared underlying causes for epilepsy and cognitive or behavior disorders; (2) the impact of seizures and of abnormal electrographic activity on cognitive function and on brain development; (3) effects of drugs used to treat seizures; (4) misdiagnosis; and (5) parental influences on proxy reports. There is good evidence that each of these plays a role. Understanding these roles can implicitly pave the way for specific preventive and interventional strategies.

Shared underlying causes
The most common, known causes of epilepsy in children are malformations of brain development, intraventricular hemorrhage and other complications of preterm birth, central nervous system infections, and neurocutaneous disorders (Berg et al. 2009; Wirrell et al. 2011). Cognition and behavior are brain functions, so it is no surprise that insults to or disorders of the brain of the kind that can cause epilepsy are frequently accompanied by alterations or impairments in cognition and behavior (Washburn et al. 2007; Lucas et al. 2011; Kihara et al. 2012; Als et al. 2013). In children with epilepsy who have an identified congenital or acquired lesion, only about 35% fall in the overall "normal" range for cognitive function, and almost 45% have moderate to severe intellectual disability (Berg et al. 2008). This contrasts with 85% of children with no recognized cause for their epilepsy being in the normal range and only 2.5% being moderately to severely impaired (Berg et al. 2008). Of course, among those with no identified cause when these studies were carried

out, there are likely to be many who, with advances made in genetic testing, would now be considered to have a specific genetic disorder.

With the recent advances in genetic testing and the knowledge afforded by molecular genetics, many forms of epilepsy, especially those beginning in early life and associated with the worst outcomes, are now being linked to a host of genetic errors in genes and systems involved in brain development (Paciorkowski et al. 2011; Mastrangelo and Leuzzi 2012). In fact, most malformations of cortical development are genetic (Barkovich et al. 2012). Somatic mutations in many of these same genes, however, can still be associated with epilepsy and intellectual disability and autism even in the absence of obvious malformations (Gleeson et al. 2000; Matsumoto et al. 2001; Guerrini et al. 2004; Qin et al. 2010; Riviere et al. 2012; Mirzaa et al. 2013). Any single genetic disorder is likely to be rare and accounts for only a tiny fraction of all epilepsy. For example, one recent study estimated GLUT-1 deficiency syndrome to be present in 2.6/1 000 000 population (Ramm-Pettersen et al. 2013). The number of genes involved in epilepsy associated with intellectual disability is rapidly expanding, and the proportion of epilepsies, especially those occurring in young children, that are now associated with specific genetic factors is increasing as testing is more available and acceptable (Paciorkowski et al. 2011; Lemke et al. 2012; Mastrangelo and Leuzzi 2012). In addition to point mutations, larger deletions and duplications of a wide variety of genes are commonly associated with intellectual disability syndromes (Mefford et al. 2012). Currently in the United States, the American Academy of Neurology and Child Neurology Society recommend that a chromosome array be performed in children presenting with moderate to severe developmental delay or intellectual disability (Michelson et al. 2011). It is perhaps not surprising that many of the genes associated with intellectual disability and epilepsy are also associated with autism as well as early life epilepsy (Mefford et al. 2012).

Although a substantial proportion of children have frank intellectual disability, the vast majority do not. In fact, most children are in the normal intellectual range, have normal brain imaging, normal neurological examinations, and no obvious past insult that might explain their epilepsy. Of children with initial onset under the age of 15 or 16, roughly 20–25% have forms of epilepsy that, in the past, were presumed to be "genetic" (Callenbach et al. 1998; Berg et al. 1999), the so-called "idiopathic" epilepsies. These epilepsies occur in otherwise "normal" children (Berg et al. 2010). For the generalized genetic epilepsies (GGEs), long before genetic testing was available, strong family histories provided the evidence for a genetic-familial basis for these disorders (Marini et al. 2004; Vadlamudi et al. 2004a). For benign epilepsy with central-temporal spikes (BECTS), the evidence has been more elusive (Vadlamudi et al. 2004b). Our understanding of the genetic basis of these epilepsies is rapidly changing. For the moment, however, it is important to realize that these epilepsies were often considered "benign" because they responded well to medication and, in many instances, resolved after a few years, approximately 100% for BECTS and up to 70% for childhood absence epilepsy (CAE), the most common of the GGEs.

These epilepsies are associated with subtle but potentially important decrements in specific cognitive functions. BECTS and CAE are two of the best studied of these epilepsies. Specific language impairment has been found in children with BECTS (Lundberg et al. 2005;

Northcott et al. 2005; Danielsson and Petermann 2009; Lillywhite et al. 2009). Not surprisingly, with advances in neuroimaging, both the structural (Pardoe et al. 2013) and functional (Lillywhite et al. 2009; Oser et al. 2014) correlates of this disruption are increasingly being revealed. Further, genetic studies are making inroads into identifying genetic bases for BECTS. Also not surprising are the findings that, even when the epilepsy itself is not found in other family members, the language disruption can be demonstrated in siblings (Smith et al. 2012; Verrotti et al. 2013), suggesting that this serves as an endophenotype for BECTS.

A similar sequence of findings is reported in children with CAE. Genetic associations are being established, specific cognitive disturbances are documented, particularly in attention (D'Agati et al. 2012; Masur et al. 2013), and the structural (Chan et al. 2006; Pardoe et al. 2008) as well as functional (Bai et al. 2011; Carney et al. 2012; Carney and Jackson 2014) correlates of these disturbances are increasingly being uncovered. As with BECTS, there is evidence for cognitive endophenotypes that may be found in relatives who do not have epilepsy (Chowdhury et al. 2014). Such findings in unaffected family members suggest that the complex underlying genetic predisposition involves more than seizures and that the cognitive elements may be a partial expression of the disorder.

Many epilepsies in "neurotypical" or "typically developing" children do not fit neatly into any of the well-defined syndromic categories. Yet all, to some degree, seem to be associated with an increased level of more subtle impairments in broad ranges of cognitive function with the greatest difference found for processing speed, a nonspecific marker of many disorders of the brain (Hermann et al. 2006; Zelko et al. 2014).

The onset of these relative cognitive impairments is key to understanding their nature. Good evidence suggests that they are present prior to or by the time epilepsy is diagnosed and before medications are initiated. Therefore, they do not appear to be a consequence of either uncontrolled seizures or medications used to suppress seizures. Three studies independently found that, compared to same-aged controls, neurotypical cases were more likely already to be receiving special education services before ever being diagnosed with epilepsy (Oostrom et al. 2003; Hermann et al. 2006; Berg et al. 2011). A few studies have also been able to perform detailed neurocognitive testing immediately following diagnosis and before the initiation of medications. In a large randomized trial of children with newly diagnosed CAE, evidence of attentional deficits was already present in a third of the children prior to initiation of medication (Masur et al. 2013). These deficits persisted despite treatment and despite seizure freedom. In another randomized trial, albeit of adults, a detailed analysis of new-onset patients with epilepsy compared cognitive test performance with healthy controls without epilepsy (Taylor et al. 2010). The affected adults scored lower (worse) on 11 of 14 measures, most particularly those related to memory and processing speed. Two pediatric studies documented similar patterns of results in children with newly or recently diagnosed epilepsy, although many of the children had already initiated mediations to control seizures (Hermann et al. 2006; Fastenau et al. 2009). On the whole, these data suggest that subtle cognitive impairments may be part of the expression of the underlying disorder, that is, they may share the same underpinnings or be somehow related to the same factors that cause the brain to produce seizures.

3

Whether the cognitive variants normalize in time if and when the epilepsy resolves is not fully clear (Northcott et al. 2006).

The impact of seizures and electrical brain storms

The notion of epileptic encephalopathy has been around for many years. It was formally defined by DuLac in reference to a group of epilepsy syndromes in which cognitive declines seem to occur in association with and perhaps secondary to uncontrolled seizures and prolonged abnormal electrographic brain activity (Dulac 2001). These epilepsies, as a group, begin in infancy or very early childhood and most are highly drug resistant and include diagnoses such as West, Dravet, and Lennox-Gastaut syndromes. In 2010, the concept was redefined as a process and not a group of diagnostic entities: "the epileptic activity itself may contribute to severe cognitive and behavioral impairments above and beyond what might be expected from the underlying pathology alone (e.g. cortical malformation), and that these can worsen over time" (Berg et al. 2010). This shift reflected the developing understanding of the cellular basis of learning, long-term potentiation (Lamprecht and LeDoux 2004). In essence, learning occurs when cells fire. Seizures and other abnormal activities in the brain occur as a result of the same firing of cells. In the developing brain, cells are rapidly growing processes, creating synapses, and organizing into networks. Some cells, processes, and synapses are pruned; in fact, programed cell death is a normal part of development. The process follows a pattern set up by a predetermined program interacting with environmental factors (experiential and others) and unfolds over many years, arguably throughout the lifespan. It is most active, however, and sensitive to disruption early in life during the critical period or periods of development.

The role of development and critical periods in brain development comes with several predictions concerning cognition. First, cognition should be more severely and globally affected the earlier in life seizures begin. In addition, more severe presentations (more seizures, worse EEG) should be associated with poorer cognitive outcomes. The longer seizures and severe electrographic abnormalities persist, the greater the impact should be on development. Finally, because seizures can, in theory, interfere with normal developmental processes during critical periods in development, there is also the concern that their impacts on cognition will be to some degree irreversible.

The data supporting each of these predictions are substantial. In children with refractory epilepsy, those with the youngest age at onset tend to have worse cognitive performance than those at older onset (Vasconcellos et al. 2001; Freitag and Tuxhorn 2005; Cormack et al. 2007; Vendrame et al. 2009; Berg et al. 2012). Importantly, in children with well-controlled epilepsy, there does not seem to be any association between age at onset and cognitive function (Berg et al. 2012). Children with more frequent seizures may experience greater cognitive impairment relative to those with less frequent, and this is independent of age (Vasconcellos et al. 2001).

The conceptualization of epileptic encephalopathy as a process also comes with important implications, chiefly that early diagnosis and effective intervention can bend the encephalopathy curve and lead to better, if not entirely normal, cognitive outcomes. Evidence from a few sources now links the delay to diagnosis and initiation of treatment with a decline in development (O'Callaghan et al. 2011; Auvin et al. 2012; Berg et al. 2014). The implications for ameliorating this source of negative impact on development are to identify and correct those reasons for delayed diagnosis and treatment (Auvin et al. 2012; Berg et al. 2014). Once a child is diagnosed, the decline in development continues in those whose seizures are treatment resistant (Berg et al. 2004; Humphrey et al. 2014). Following effective intervention for seizures, numerous studies demonstrate substantial cognitive improvement. Most of these studies are based upon surgical therapy (Jonas et al. 2004; Lee et al. 2010; Skirrow et al. 2011; Lee et al. 2014); however, survey data of parents and physicians suggest that this is also the case with nonsurgical interventions (Brunklaus et al. 2013).

While seizures are the obvious culprit in the concept of "epileptic encephalopathy," they are likely to be only part of the problem. The syndromes of continuous spike wave in sleep and Landau-Kleffner syndrome (LKS), which are addressed in Chapter 13, are a prime example of "epileptic encephalopathy." Few if any clinical seizures occur in these overlapping disorders, but the sleep EEG is dominated by a continuous spike wave pattern and is thought to be the source of the cognitive deficits that occur (Tassinari et al. 2009; Raha et al. 2012). By the same token, treatment goals for West syndrome include not only suppression of spasms but resolution of hypsarrhythmia, the chaotic EEG pattern that is practically pathognomic for this form of epilepsy (Pellock et al. 2010).

The natural response to seizures is to treat them and suppress them
The first-line approach is generally with pharmacologic agents that alter neuronal function and in doing so suppress seizures. Many antiseizure medications (ASMs) are excellent at doing this; however, the seizure suppression often comes at a cost: cognitive, and behavioral side effects. In healthy volunteer adults, these have been beautifully demonstrated in an elegant series of randomized experimental studies (Meador et al. 2001; 2003; 2005). Drugs such as phenytoin, phenobarbital, and sodium valproate are particularly associated with cognitive impacts. Levetiracetam and lamotrigine are much less likely to produce cognitive side effect; however, levetiracetam does have negative behavioral impacts in some individuals (Halma et al. 2014). In children with childhood absence epilepsy, a group already predisposed to attentional difficulties, valproate was found to be inferior to both lamotrigine and ethosuximide in terms of cognitive impact despite good efficacy for seizure control (Glauser et al. 2010).

Prenatal exposure to common ASMs has also been examined in two studies from the United States and the United Kingdom (Meador et al. 2013; Shallcross et al. 2014). These studies found that, in children exposed prenatally to sodium valproate, IQ was on average several points lower at age 6 than expected based upon maternal IQ (one of the strongest predictors of a child's IQ). Prenatal exposure to other ASMs was not found to be as strongly, if at all, associated with drops in IQ later in childhood. One study from Denmark did, however, report evidence of decreased IQ in young men prenatally exposed to phenobarbital compared to unexposed men (Reinisch et al. 1995).

Finally, a randomized trial of phenobarbital in young children with febrile seizures also demonstrated a several-point decline in developmental scores a few years after the medications had been stopped (Farwell et al. 1990; Sulzbacher et al. 1999). The evidence in humans thus supports reasons to be concerned about some of these medications.

In animal models, there is growing evidence that, at the right stage in development, exposure to many common ASMs can inappropriately increase programmed cell death (apoptosis) and that, in adulthood, exposed animals display selective cognitive and behavioral deficits (Bittigau et al. 2002; Bittigau et al. 2003; Forcelli et al. 2010). This finding was especially pronounced for phenobarbital. Lamotrigine by itself and levetiracetam appeared relatively safe with respect to apoptosis and later cognitive effects.

In all, when these drugs are effective in controlling seizures, there may be a price to pay in terms of some impacts on development. This means that, in the very young and rapidly developing brain, there is a balancing act between suppressing seizures and normalizing chaotic EEG activity to prevent interference with neurodevelopment versus potentially impairing those same neurodevelopmental processes with medications. There is currently no evidence to guide practice in this regard. It is likely, although again, there is no evidence, that most clinicians would emphasize seizure control initially.

Misdiagnosis

While there is undoubtedly an increased prevalence of intellectual disability among children with epilepsy and vice versa, not all diagnoses are equal. Several studies have examined the frequency of the misdiagnosis of epilepsy in children and young adults with intellectual disability and with autism, and the results are sobering. Children with intellectual disability or autism (and the two often co-occur together) have as part of their presentation a range of odd behaviors that can be interpreted as seizure-like (stereotypies, nonresponsiveness, motor tics, and other behavioral events). The standard EEG is often abnormal and results in an assumption that the behaviors must therefore be seizures. The criterion standard for diagnosis of epilepsy, however, is the recording of the "event" with simultaneous EEG and video. When this is done, a large proportion of children are found not to have epilepsy. This has been demonstrated from the perspective of a patient with intellectual disability (Chapman et al. 2011) as well as autism (Chez et al. 2006; Yasuhara 2010; Berg and Plioplys 2012).

Such an error can be serious and result in a child who is already intellectually and behaviorally challenged receiving treatments that pose their own array of cognitive and behavioral risks. Potentially, these may exacerbate cognitive and behavioral problems, and result in needless testing and use of multiple ASMs in an effort to control events that are not epileptic seizures.

The parents' role

A large literature on cognitive and behavioral problems in children with epilepsy is available. An important segment of this literature is based on parent-reported outcomes. The parent of a child with epilepsy, however, is often under considerable stress him or herself. Recent studies have highlighted the role that parents' stress and perceptions play in reporting children's outcomes (Ronen Gabriel et al. 2003; Verhey et al. 2009; Baca et al. 2010; Wu et al. 2014; Eom et al. 2016). While much of this may be avoided by direct testing of the children, this is not always possible in a research or even in a clinic setting. Consequently, parent reports must be taken for exactly that, parents' report. Even if some children do not themselves actually have the cognitive or behavioral problems reported by the parents, they are still living with the parent's perception that there is a problem. Thus, for the medical provider, just taking care of the child may not be enough. The parent is always part of the equation. The role of services directed to the parent may, in some cases, be extremely important and enable the parent to be a more effective member of the care team.

Conclusion

Cognitive disorders, whether they be frank and global intellectual disability, or more subtle disorders in otherwise normally developing children, are very common in children with epilepsy. The main types of reasons, reviewed above, have different implications for prevention, evaluation, and intervention. Perhaps most importantly is the need for developmental or cognitive screening to be a routine part of the initial evaluation of a child with epilepsy as well as part of routine follow-up care. The physician providing neurological care (a neurologist in the United States but typically a pediatrician in other settings) may assume that the primary care provider (the pediatrician in the United States but often the general practitioner elsewhere) has already performed recommended screening. A recent audit of a comorbidity screening program at a US tertiary epilepsy center found that one of five children with epilepsy (both new-onset and established patients) had developmental concerns that had not been previously recognized or addressed. This resulted in referrals for further evaluation for these children (Eom et al. 2014). Clearly early control of seizures is a goal of epilepsy care and may ameliorate some, although not necessarily all, of the cognitive impacts of the disorder. The implications that follow from this include the need for rapid and accurate diagnosis, and optimal treatment. Barriers obviously exist at each of these steps and need to be overcome. For children who might be surgical candidates, there is no reason to delay consideration of surgery, or at least a comprehensive evaluation, if there is any difficulty bringing seizure under complete control. Again, barriers exist in the form of physician and parent knowledge, availability of comprehensive epilepsy programs, and other parental concerns (Berg et al. 2013). While some drugs may induce a degree of cognitive dysfunction, few clinicians would use this as a reason to withhold therapy.

Involvement of parents as members of the care team and addressing their needs may help clarify the nature of some problems reportedly occurring in the child (Berg et al. 2013). Progress in this area hinges on filling in the evidence gaps that lead to uncertainty and training health care providers in the urgency to address cognitive concerns.

REFERENCES

Als LC, Nadel S, Cooper M et al. (2013) Neuropsychologic function three to six months following admission to the PICU with meningoencephalitis, sepsis, and other disorders: A prospective study of school-aged children. *Crit Care Med* 41: 1093–1103.

Auvin S, Hartman A, Desnous B et al. (2012) Diagnosis delay in West syndrome: Misdiagnosis and consequences. *Eur J Pediatr* 171: 1695–1701.

Baca CB, Vickrey BG, Hays RD et al. (2010) Differences in child versus parent reports of the child's health-related quality of life in children with epilepsy and healthy siblings. *Value Health* 13: 778–786.

Bai X, Guo J, Killory B et al. (2011) Resting functional connectivity between the hemispheres in childhood absence epilepsy. *Neurology* 76: 1960–1967.

Barkovich AJ, Guerrini R, Kuzniecky RI et al. (2012) A developmental and genetic classification for malformations of cortical development: Update 2012. *Brain* 135: 1348–1369.

Berg AT, Baca CB, Loddenkemper T et al. (2013) Priorities in pediatric epilepsy research: Improving children's futures today. *Neurology* 81: 1166–1175.

Berg AT, Berkovic SF, Brodie MJ et al. (2010) Revised terminology and concepts for organization of seizures and epilepsies: Report of the ILAE Commission on Classification and Terminology, 2005–2009. *Epilepsia* 51: 676–685.

Berg AT, Hesdorffer DC, Zelko FAJ (2011) Special education participation in children with epilepsy: What does it reflect? *Epilepsy Behav* 22: 336–341.

Berg AT, Langfitt JT, Testa FM et al. (2008) Global cognitive function in children with epilepsy: A community-based study. *Epilepsia* 49: 608–614.

Berg AT, Loddenkemper T and Baca CB (2014) Diagnostic delays in children with early onset epilepsy: Impact, reasons, and opportunities to improve care. *Epilepsia* 55: 123–132.

Berg AT, Mathern GW, Bronen RA et al. (2009) Frequency, prognosis and surgical treatment of structural abnormalities seen with magnetic resonance imaging in childhood epilepsy. *Brain* 132: 2785–2797.

Berg AT and Plioplys S (2012) Epilepsy and autism: Is there a special relationship? *Epilepsy Behav* 23: 193–198.

Berg AT, Shinnar S, Levy SR et al. (1999) Newly diagnosed epilepsy in children: Presentation at diagnosis. *Epilepsia* 40: 445–452.

Berg AT, Smith SN, Frobish D et al. (2004) Longitudinal assessment of adaptive behavior in infants and young children with newly diagnosed epilepsy: Influences of etiology, syndrome, and seizure control. *Pediatrics* 114: 645–650.

Berg AT, Zelko FA, Levy SR et al. (2012) Age at onset of epilepsy, pharmacoresistance, and cognitive outcomes: A prospective cohort study. *Neurology* 79: 1384–1391.

Bittigau P, Sifringer M, Genz K et al. (2002) Antiepileptic drugs and apoptotic neurodegeneration in the developing brain. *Proc Natl Acad Sci U S A* 99: 15089–15094.

Bittigau P, Sifringer M and Ikonomidou C (2003) Antiepileptic drugs and apoptosis in the developing brain. *Ann NY Acad Sci* 993: 103–114.

Brunklaus A, Dorris L, Ellis R et al. (2013) The clinical utility of an SCN1A genetic diagnosis in infantile-onset epilepsy. *Dev Med Child Neurol* 55: 154–161.

Callenbach PM, Geerts AT, Arts WF et al. (1998) Familial occurrence of epilepsy in children with newly diagnosed multiple seizures: Dutch Study of Epilepsy in Childhood. *Epilepsia* 39: 331–336.

Camfield C and Camfield P (2007) Preventable and unpreventable causes of childhood-onset epilepsy plus mental retardation. *Pediatrics* 120: e52–e55.

Carney PW and Jackson G. (2014) Insights into the mechanisms of absence seizure generation provided by EEG with Functional MRI. *Frontiers in Neurology* 5: 162.

Carney PW, Masterton RAJ, Flanagan D et al. (2012) The frontal lobe in absence epilepsy: EEG-fMRI findings. *Neurology* 78: 1157–1165.

Chan CH, Briellmann RS, Pell GS et al. (2006) Thalamic atrophy in childhood absence epilepsy. *Epilepsia* 47: 399–405.

Chapman M, Iddon P, Atkinson K et al. (2011) The misdiagnosis of epilepsy in people with intellectual disabilities: A systematic review. *Seizure* 20: 101–106.

Chez MG, Chang M, Krasne V et al. (2006) Frequency of epileptiform EEG abnormalities in a sequential screening of autistic patients with no known clinical epilepsy from 1996 to 2005. *Epilepsy Behav* 8: 267–271.

Chowdhury FA, Elwes RDC, Koutroumanidis M et al. (2014) Impaired cognitive function in idiopathic generalized epilepsy and unaffected family members: An epilepsy endophenotype. *Epilepsia* 55: 835–840.

Cormack F, Helen Cross J, Isaacs E et al. (2007) The development of intellectual abilities in pediatric temporal lobe epilepsy. *Epilepsia* 48: 201–204.

D'Agati E, Cerminara C, Casarelli L et al. (2012) Attention and executive functions profile in childhood absence epilepsy. *Brain Dev* 34: 812–817.

Danielsson J and Petermann F. (2009) Cognitive deficits in children with benign rolandic epilepsy of childhood or rolandic discharges: A study of children between 4 and 7 years of age with and without seizures compared with healthy controls. *Epilepsy Behav* 16: 646–651.

Dulac O (2001) Epileptic encephalopathy. *Epilepsia* 42: 23–26.

Ellenberg JH, Hirtz DG and Nelson KB (1984) Age at onset of seizures in young children. *Ann Neurol* 15: 127–134.

Eom S, Caplan R and Berg AT (2016) Behavioral problems and childhood epilepsy: Parent vs child perspectives. *J Pediatr* 179: 233–239.

Eom S, Fisher B, Dezort C et al. (2014) Routine developmental, autism, behavioral, and psychological screening in epilepsy care settings. *Dev Med Child Neurol* doi:0.1111/dmcn.12497

Farwell JR, Lee YJ, Hirtz DG et al. (1990) Phenobarbital for febrile seizures – Effects on intelligence and on seizure recurrence. *N Engl J Med* 322: 364–369.

Fastenau PS, Johnson CS, Perkins SM et al. (2009) Neuropsychological status at seizure onset in children: Risk factors for early cognitive deficits. *Neurology* 73: 526–534.

Forcelli PA, Janssen MJ, Stamps LA et al. (2010) Therapeutic strategies to avoid long-term adverse outcomes of neonatal antiepileptic drug exposure. *Epilepsia* 51: 18–23.

Freitag H and Tuxhorn I (2005) Cognitive function in preschool children after epilepsy surgery: Rationale for early intervention. *Epilepsia* 46: 561–567.

Geerts A, Brouwer O, van Donselaar C et al. (2011) Health perception and socioeconomic status following childhood-onset epilepsy: The Dutch study of epilepsy in childhood. *Epilepsia* 52: 2192–2202.

Glauser TA, Cnaan A, Shinnar S et al. (2010) Ethosuximide, valproic acid, and lamotrigine in childhood absence epilepsy. *N Engl J Med* 362: 790–799.

Gleeson JG, Minnerath S, Kuzniecky RI et al. (2000) Somatic and germline mosaic mutations in the doublecortin gene are associated with variable phenotypes. *Am J Hum Genet* 67: 574–581.

Guerrini R, Mei D, Sisodiya S et al. (2004) Germline and mosaic mutations of FLN1 in men with periventricular heterotopia. *Neurology* 63: 51–56.

Halma E, de Louw AJA, Klinkenberg S et al. (2014) Behavioral side-effects of levetiracetam in children with epilepsy: A systematic review. *Seizure* doi:10.1016/j.seizure.2014.06.004

Hermann B, Jones J, Sheth R et al. (2006) Children with new-onset epilepsy: Neuropsychological status and brain structure. *Brain* 129: 2609–2619.

Humphrey A, MacLean C, Ploubidis GB et al. (2014) Intellectual development before and after the onset of infantile spasms: A controlled prospective longitudinal study in tuberous sclerosis. *Epilepsia* 55: 108–116.

Jonas R, Nguyen S, Hu B et al. (2004) Cerebral hemispherectomy: Hospital course, seizure, developmental, language, and motor outcomes. *Neurology* 62: 1712–1721.

Kihara M, de Haan M, Were E et al. (2012) Cognitive deficits following exposure to pneumococcal meningitis: An event-related potential study. *BMC Infect Dis* 12: 79.

Lamprecht R and LeDoux J (2004) Structural plasticity and memory. *Nat Rev Neurosci* 5: 45–54.

Lee YJ, Kang H-C, Lee JS et al. (2010) Resective pediatric epilepsy surgery in Lennox-Gastaut syndrome. *Pediatrics* 125: e58–e66.

Lee YJ, Lee JS, Kang H-C et al. (2014) Outcomes of epilepsy surgery in childhood-onset epileptic encephalopathy. *Brain Dev* 36: 496–504.

Lemke JR, Riesch E, Scheurenbrand T et al. (2012) Targeted next generation sequencing as a diagnostic tool in epileptic disorders. *Epilepsia* 53: 1387–1398.

Lillywhite LM, Saling MM, Simon Harvey A et al. (2009) Neuropsychological and functional MRI studies provide converging evidence of anterior language dysfunction in BECTS. *Epilepsia* 50: 2276–2284.

Lucas MM, Lenck-Santini P-P, Holmes GL et al. (2011) Impaired cognition in rats with cortical dysplasia: Additional impact of early-life seizures. *Brain* 134: 1684–1693.

Lundberg S, Frylmark A and Eeg-Olofsson O. (2005) Children with rolandic epilepsy have abnormalities of oromotor and dichotic listening performance. *Dev Med Child Neurol* 47: 603–608.

Marini C, Scheffer IE, Crossland KM et al. (2004) Genetic architecture of idiopathic generalized epilepsy: Clinical genetic analysis of 55 multiplex families. *Epilepsia* 45: 467–478.

Mastrangelo M and Leuzzi V (2012) Genes of early-onset epileptic encephalopathies: From genotype to phenotype. *Pediatr Neurol* 46: 24–31.

Masur D, Shinnar S, Cnaan A et al. (2013) Pretreatment cognitive deficits and treatment effects on attention in childhood absence epilepsy. *Neurology* 81: 1572–1580.

Matsumoto N, Leventer RJ, Kuc JA et al. (2001) Mutation analysis of the DCX gene and genotype/phenotype correlation in subcortical band heterotopia. *Eur J Hum Genet* 9: 5–12.

Meador KJ, Baker GA, Browning N et al. (2013) Fetal antiepileptic drug exposure and cognitive outcomes at age 6 years (NEAD study): A prospective observational study. *Lancet Neurol* 12: 244–252.

Meador KJ, Loring DW, Hulihan JF et al. (2003) Differential cognitive and behavioral effects of topiramate and valproate. *Neurology* 60: 1483–1488.

Meador KJ, Loring DW, Ray PG et al. (2001) Differential cognitive and behavioral effects of carbamazepine and lamotrigine. *Neurology* 56: 1177–1182.

Meador KJ, Loring DW, Vahle VJ et al. (2005) Cognitive and behavioral effects of lamotrigine and topiramate in healthy volunteers. *Neurology* 64: 2108–2114.

Mefford HC, Batshaw ML and Hoffman EP (2012) Genomics, intellectual disability, and autism. *N Engl J Med* 366: 733–743.

Michelson DJ, Shevell MI, Sherr EH et al. (2011) Evidence report: Genetic and metabolic testing on children with global developmental delay: Report of the Quality Standards Subcommittee of the American Academy of Neurology and the Practice Committee of the Child Neurology Society. *Neurology* 77: 1629–1635.

Mirzaa GM, Riviere JB and Dobyns WB (2013) Megalencephaly syndromes and activating mutations in the PI3K-AKT pathway: MPPH and MCAP. *Am J Med Genet C Semin Med Genet* 163: 122–130.

Northcott E, Connolly AM, Berroya A et al. (2005) The neuropsychological and language profile of children with benign rolandic epilepsy. *Epilepsia* 46: 924–930.

Northcott E, Connolly AM, McIntyre J et al. (2006) Longitudinal assessment of neuropsychologic and language function in children with benign rolandic epilepsy. *J Child Neurol* 21: 518–522.

O'Callaghan FJK, Lux AL, Darke K et al. (2011) The effect of lead time to treatment and of age of onset on developmental outcome at 4 years in infantile spasms: Evidence from the United Kingdom Infantile Spasms Study. *Epilepsia* 52: 1359–1364.

Oostrom KJ, Smeets-Schouten A, Kruitwagen CLJJ et al. (2003) Not only a matter of epilepsy: Early problems of cognition and behavior in children with "epilepsy only"– A prospective, longitudinal, controlled study starting at diagnosis. *Pediatrics* 112: 1338–1344.

Oser N, Hubacher M, Specht K et al. (2014) Default mode network alterations during language task performance in children with benign epilepsy with centrotemporal spikes (BECTS). *Epilepsy Behav* 33: 12–17.

Paciorkowski AR, Thio LL and Dobyns WB (2011) Genetic and biologic classification of infantile spasms. *Pediatr Neurol* 45: 355–367.

Pardoe H, Pell GS, Abbott DF et al. (2008) Multi-site voxel-based morphometry: Methods and a feasibility demonstration with childhood absence epilepsy. *NeuroImage* 42: 611–616.

Pardoe HR, Berg AT, Archer JS et al. (2013) A neurodevelopmental basis for BECTS: Evidence from structural MRI. *Epilepsy Res* 105: 133–139.

Pellock JM, Hrachovy R, Shinnar S et al. (2010) Infantile spasms: A U.S. consensus report. *Epilepsia* 51: 2175–2189.

Qin W, Kozlowski P, Taillon BE et al. (2010) Ultra deep sequencing detects a low rate of mosaic mutations in tuberous sclerosis complex. *Hum Genet* 127: 573–582.

Raha S, Shah U and Udani V (2012) Neurocognitive and neurobehavioral disabilities in Epilepsy with Electrical Status Epilepticus in slow sleep (ESES) and related syndromes. *Epilepsy Behav* 25: 381–385.

Ramm-Pettersen A, Nakken KO, Skogseid IM et al. (2013) Good outcome in patients with early dietary treatment of GLUT-1 deficiency syndrome: Results from a retrospective Norwegian study. *Dev Med Child Neurol* 55: 440–447.

Reinisch J, Sanders SA, Mortensen E et al. (1995) IN utero exposure to phenobarbital and intelligence deficits in adult men. *JAMA* 274: 1518–1525.

Riviere J-B, Mirzaa GM, O'Roak BJ et al. (2012) De novo germline and postzygotic mutations in AKT3, PIK3R2 and PIK3CA cause a spectrum of related megalencephaly syndromes. *Nat Genet* 44: 934–940.

Ronen Gabriel M, Streiner David L, Rosenbaum P et al. (2003) Health-related quality of life in children with epilepsy: Development and validation of self-report and parent proxy measures. *Epilepsia* 44: 598–612.

Shallcross R, Bromley RL, Cheyne CP et al. (2014) In utero exposure to levetiracetam vs valproate: Development and language at 3 years of age. *Neurology* 82: 213–221.

Skirrow C, Cross JH, Cormack F et al. (2011) Long-term intellectual outcome after temporal lobe surgery in childhood. *Neurology* 76: 1330–1337.

Smith AB, Kavros PM, Clarke T et al. (2012) A neurocognitive endophenotype associated with rolandic epilepsy. *Epilepsia* 53: 705–711.

Sulzbacher S, Farwell JR, Temkin N et al. (1999) Late cognitive effects of early treatment with phenobarbital. *Clin Pediatr* 38: 387–394.

Tassinari CA, Cantalupo G, Rios-Pohl L et al. (2009) Encephalopathy with status epilepticus during slow sleep: "The Penelope syndrome". *Epilepsia* 50: 4–8.

Taylor J, Kolamunnage-Dona R, Marson AG et al. (2010) Patients with epilepsy: Cognitively compromised before the start of antiepileptic drug treatment? *Epilepsia* 51: 48–56.

Vadlamudi L, Andermann E, Lombroso CT et al. (2004a) Epilepsy in twins: Insights from unique historical data of William Lennox. *Neurology* 62: 1127–1133.

Vadlamudi L, Harvey AS, Connellan MM et al. (2004b) Is benign rolandic epilepsy genetically determined? *Ann Neurol* 56: 129–132.

Vasconcellos E, Wyllie E, Sullivan S et al. (2001) Mental retardation in pediatric candidates for epilepsy surgery: The role of early seizure onset. *Epilepsia* 42: 268–274.

Vendrame M, Alexopoulos AV, Boyer K et al. (2009) Longer duration of epilepsy and earlier age at epilepsy onset correlate with impaired cognitive development in infancy. *Epilepsy Behav* 16: 431–435.

Verhey LH, Kulik DM, Ronen GM et al. (2009) Quality of life in childhood epilepsy: What is the level of agreement between youth and their parents? *Epilepsy Behav* 14: 407–410.

Verrotti A, Matricardi S, Di Giacomo DL et al. (2013) Neuropsychological impairment in children with rolandic epilepsy and in their siblings. *Epilepsy Behav* 28: 108–112.

Washburn L, Dillard R, Goldstein D et al. (2007) Survival and major neurodevelopmental impairment in extremely low gestational age newborns born 1990–2000: A retrospective cohort study. *BMC Pediatr* 7: 20.

Wirrell EC, Grossardt BR, Wong-Kisiel LCL et al. (2011) Incidence and classification of new-onset epilepsy and epilepsy syndromes in children in Olmsted County, Minnesota from 1980 to 2004: A population-based study. *Epilepsy Res* 95: 110–118.

Wu YP, Follansbee-Junger K, Rausch J et al. (2014) Parent and family stress factors predict health-related quality in pediatric patients with new-onset epilepsy. *Epilepsia* 55: 866–877.

Yasuhara A (2010) Correlation between EEG abnormalities and symptoms of autism spectrum disorder (ASD). *Brain Dev* 32: 791–798.

Zelko FA, Pardoe HR, Blackstone SR et al. (2014) Regional brain volumes and cognition in childhood epilepsy: Does size really matter? *Epilepsy Res* 108: 692–700.

2
INTRODUCTORY REMARKS ON NEUROPSYCHOLOGICAL TESTING IN CHILDHOOD EPILEPSY

Agathe Laurent, Faustine Ilski-Lecoanet and Alexis Arzimanoglou

Neuropsychological evaluation of epilepsies considers everything that is essential or necessary for being able to identify specific abilities that are dysfunctional in children with a given type of epilepsy. Neuropsychological assessment seeks to evaluate adaptive behavioural deficits and abnormal developmental trajectories by considering key variables, including the type, number, combination and degree of any cognitive deficits, the presence or absence of associated or contributory impairments, the known or suspected aetiology, and the significance of any ability-related strengths. The aim is to be able, whenever possible, to suggest adequate measures for rehabilitation.

In children, dynamic epileptic processes interfere with typical maturational ones
The study of cognitive functions in children with epilepsy involves an examination of how the brain transforms environmental signals, processes and 'builds' information, and programs adaptive behaviour (including cognitive state). Consequently, it is necessary to take into account 'maturation' which refers to a dynamic process, of unknown duration, involving interactions between genetics and environment at every level, from molecules to the behaviour of the organism.

Schematically, cognitive development relies on the interaction between cerebral maturation and stimulation from the environment: typical developmental cognitive processes emerge from interactions between neural preorganization and environmental constraints, anticipated and selected by the neural organization.

The resulting new neural organization interacts, in turn, with new features of the environment. If no 'accident' occurs during this period of development, these snowball processes lead to cerebral functional specialization that will be more or less the same in all individuals. The time at which functional specialization becomes irreversible differs, according to the domains of cognitive development and to the kinds of networks involved.

Epilepsy also is a dynamic process that can start at any age and can result in morphological and functional localized/generalized cerebral network modifications. As a result, the pathological epileptic process interferes with normal cerebral development. It is known that structural damage to the brain associated with epilepsy differs, according to whether the first seizures occurred early in childhood or later in life. Onset during childhood has a more widespread structural effect on the brain than onset in adulthood. Brain connectivity reduction, as measured by volumetric reduction of white matter in the whole brain and the corpus callosum, seems to be greater in individuals with early rather than with late epilepsy onset. In individuals with early-onset epilepsy, the white matter volumetric reductions were found to be significantly associated with lower cognitive performances in some, but not all, cognitive domains. This pattern of results was not observed in patients with late-onset epilepsy (Hermann et al. 2002, 2003; Camfield and Camfield 2003; Ciumas et al. 2014).

Neuropsychological assessment should be performed as early as possible during the course of the disease

As in adults, many studies have shown the impact of epilepsy in children on various and specific aspects of somesthesic, olfactory, visual, auditory, spatial and temporal regulation and cognition, speech, and language, including arithmetic, social and emotional cognition, attention and memory, decision making, and reasoning. It is acknowledged that a variety of factors contribute to the development of those cognitive deficits. These factors include underlying neuropathology, age at onset, psychosocial problems, origin of seizures, treatment side effects, genetic factors, and sleep disturbances. For each child, the neuropsychological assessment should consider all the factors above, including the exact type of epilepsy.

More recent studies suggest that cognitive abnormalities may be present at baseline in children with new-onset epilepsies (Herman et al. 2006; Jackson et al. 2013; Kellermann et al. 2015). Some of those are remediable when appropriately treated early in the course of the disorder, reinforcing the need for an early neuropsychological assessment and regular follow-ups.

Neuropsychological assessment including cognitive and mood regulation evaluation

In addition to cognitive impairments, abnormalities in psychiatric status and social-adaptive behaviours are potential major sources of disability in children and adults with epilepsy disorders. In paediatrics, findings have unequivocally documented raised psychiatric comorbidities in children with epilepsy, particularly emotional regulation disorders such as depression, anxiety, and bipolar disorders, compared with both the general population and children with other medical disorders, neurological and non-neurological. A prevalence of 12–35% has been reported, compared to 3–8% in the general population (Reilly et al. 2011; Garcia et al. 2012; Salpekar et al. 2013; Andrade-Machado et al. 2015).

The link between an underlying brain disorder and psychiatric comorbidities has emerged in recent literature, with evidence, based on studies in adults, suggesting bidirectional relations between epilepsy and neurobehavioural comorbidities. Emotional regulation disorders can follow the onset of epilepsy, but they can also precede it, thus serving as a possible risk factor. The clinical implication of such a bidirectional association is that neurobehavioural comorbidities might be present at diagnosis and even before epilepsy onset. There is a need for greater understanding of the causes of these conditions in children.

Although assessment of syndrome-related comorbidities in epilepsy is logical, much remains unknown regarding the distribution of shared versus syndrome-specific mood/emotional regulation disorders. This is because of the scarcity of investigations incorporating standardized comprehensive assessments that could identify children at risk for neurobehavioural complications early in the course of epilepsy and standardize their access to optimal care.

Indeed, recent studies in children argue that mood regulation disorders are evident early in the course of the epilepsy and are not necessarily related to the chronicity of the disorder. Consequently, neuropsychological assessment should also explore for such deficits, known to have considerable impact in everyday life (Jones et al. 2015).

Neuropsychological assessment and intellectual impairment

In addition to the various difficulties in specific cognitive domains and in emotional regulation, childhood epilepsies are frequently associated with intellectual impairment (as assessed by low FSIQ [Full Scale Intellectual Quotient] – Wechsler scale). Although the vast majority of children with epilepsy present with normal intellectual abilities, 12–14% of them have a general intellectual deficit (Bulteau et al. 2000).

It has been shown that children with epilepsy when studied as a group have an IQ lower than controls (Nolan et al. 2003), regardless of the epilepsy type. However, prognosis at an individual level highly depends upon the type of epilepsy.

Given that intellectual abilities are crucial for building efficient compensatory strategies to cope with eventual impairments (cognitive, emotional, and behavioural), it is crucial that global intellectual level should be taken into account in neuropsychological assessment.

Screening in clinical practice

In everyday clinical practice, the high cost of neuropsychological screening prohibits a systematic and comprehensive evaluation of all children with newly diagnosed epilepsy. To overcome such difficulties, early detection is possible when using auto- and family questionnaires based on a broad approach. Such questionnaires do not necessarily imply prolonged involvement of staff competent in neuropsychology. Furthermore, not only professionals and controlled studies, but also parents report difficulties very early in the course of the disease, underscoring the repercussions in their children's life (Almane et al. 2014). We, therefore, strongly recommend the inclusion in preliminary assessments the points of view of usual caregivers (parents and school teachers).

On the basis of those preliminary results, but also considering the individual epilepsy profile and natural course, the clinician should then be able to prioritize the more focused neuropsychological investigations a child may or may not need.

A full review of current practices and future orientations is beyond the scope of this chapter. The reader is referred to a publication by Helmstaedter et al. (2011).

Conclusion

In contrast to rare epileptic encephalopathies, focal and generalized childhood epilepsies represent a frequent but heterogeneous group. Although most of them are controlled with antiepileptic drugs and/or surgical treatment, it is well known now that childhood-onset epilepsy is associated with an adverse neurodevelopmental impact on brain connectivity which has cognitive, emotional, and behavioural consequences.

Despite recent progresses in the field, the causal processes and the underlying mechanisms of dysfunction are poorly understood. Given that such information is a prerequisite for the future development of preventative measures, the ideal neuropsychological assessment of children with epilepsy should aim have a dual goal: at an individual level, the early detection of the deficits followed by optimization of rehabilitation and global care measures; at a group level, a better understanding of the specific repercussions of a given type of epilepsy on neurocognitive and emotional regulation development.

To achieve the goal of optimal individual care the scientific community, under the leadership of the International League Against Epilepsy, has to better promote the need for early access to specialized care for all newly diagnosed epilepsies. We need to better defend the value and impact of neuropsychological evaluation at the very first months from epilepsy onset.

Advancing the field will rely on continued research. Multiple reasons contribute to our limited knowledge. Examples are the heterogeneity of the epilepsies, both in terms of electroclinical expression and underlying aetiologies; the complexity of issues related to cognitive function and dysfunction; and the fact that neurodevelopment is a moving target, complicating long-term assessment. The community will need to agree upon a limited number of neuropsychological batteries, sensitive to the specific effects of cortical dysfunction in children, measuring 'overall intelligence', such as FSIQ measures, various aspects of language function, visuospatial and auditory processing, memory, attention, and executive function. Emotional regulation disorders also need to be detected and treated early. Prospective multicentre studies, tracking changes over time in large populations and using tests that can be applied in a large age range, are still needed.

Such an approach would increase our chances of having relatively homogeneous groups with comparable data for analysis leading to amelioration of clinical care and further improvement of assessment procedures.

REFERENCES

Almane D, Jones JE, Jackson DC, Seidenberg M, Hermann BP (2014) The social competence and behavioral problem substrate of new- and recent-onset childhood epilepsy. *Epilepsy Behav* 31: 91–96.

Andrade-Machado R, Ochoa-Urrea M, Garcia-Espinosa A, Benjumea-Cuartas V, Santos-Santos A (2015) Suicidal risk, affective dysphoric disorders, and quality-of-life perception in patients with focal refractory epilepsy. *Epilepsy Behav* 45: 254–260.

Bulteau C, Jambaqué I, Viguier D et al. (2000) Epileptic syndromes, cognitive assessment and school placement: A study of 251 children. *Dev Med Child Neurol* 42: 319–327.

Camfield P and Camfield C (2003) *Prognosis in epilepsies*. Montrouge, France: John Libbey Eurotext.

Ciumas C, Saignavongs M, Ilski F et al. (2014) White matter development in children with benign childhood epilepsy with centro-temporal spikes. *Brain* 137: 1095–1106.

Garcia CS (2012) Depression in temporal lobe epilepsy: A review of prevalence, clinical features, and management considerations. *Epilepsy Res Treat* 809–843.

Helmstaedter C, Hermann B, Lassonde M, Kahane P, Arzimanoglou A (2011). *Neuropsychology in the care of people with epilepsy*. Paris, France: John Libbey Eurotext.

Herman B, Jones J, Sheth R et al. (2006) Children with new-onset epilepsy: Neuropsychological status and brain structure. *Brain* 129: 2609–2619.

Hermann B, Hansen R, Seidenberg M et al. (2003) Neurodevelopmental vulnerability of the corpus callosum to childhood onset localization related epilepsy. *Neuroimage* 18: 284–292.

Hermann B, Seidenberg M, Bell B et al. (2002) The neurodevelopmental impact of childhood-onset temporal lobe epilepsy on brain structure and function. *Epilepsia* 43: 1062–1071.

Jackson DC, Dabbs K, Walker NM et al. (2013) The neuropsychological and academic substrate of new/recent-onset epilepsies. *J Pediatr* 162: 1047–1053.

Jones JE, Jackson DC, Chambers KL et al. (2015) Children with epilepsy and anxiety: Subcortical and cortical differences. *Epilepsia* 56: 283–290.

Kellermann TS, Bonilha L, Lin JJ, Hermann BP (2015) Mapping the landscape of cognitive development in children with epilepsy. *Cortex* 66: 1–8.

Nolan MA, Redoblado MA, Lah S et al. (2003) Intelligence in childhood epilepsy syndromes. *Epilepsy Res* 53: 139–150.

Reilly C, Agnew R, Neville BG (2011) Depression and anxiety in childhood epilepsy: A review. *Seizure* 20: 589–597.

Salpekar JA, Berl MM, Havens K et al. (2013) Psychiatric symptoms in children prior to epilepsy surgery differ according to suspected seizure focus. *Epilepsia* 54: 1074–1082.

3
BEHAVIOURAL PROBLEMS IN CHILDHOOD EPILEPSY

Melissa Filippini and Giuseppe Gobbi

Defining the problem: the 'what' and the 'how'

Epilepsy is the most common neurological disorder in childhood (Reilly et al. 2014). In addition to recurrent seizures, psychiatric, cognitive and social-adaptive behaviour disorders are major potential sources of disability, in many cases more challenging than epilepsy itself. These complications have been recently referred to collectively as the neurobehavioural comorbidities of the epilepsies (Lin et al. 2012).

In paediatrics, findings have unequivocally documented an increased rate of psychiatric comorbities in children with epilepsy compared with both the general population and children with other medical disorders, including non-neurological disorders (Jones et al. 2007; Hermann et al. 2008). Psychiatric problems occur typically in around 24–66% of children (Rodenburg et al. 2005; 2006; Austin et al. 2011). This risk is evident in children with uncomplicated epilepsies, for example, those with normal results on neurological examination and normal IQ, also attending mainstream schools (Sillanpää and Shinnar 2010), but is especially marked in those with complicated epilepsies, for example, epilepsy plus brain lesion and/or intellectual disability (e.g. IQ < 70) and in children with active epilepsy (Reilly et al. 2014), rating over 50%, as compared with 6.6% in the general child population (Choudhary et al. 2014). Similarly, uncomplicated epilepsies show, even with a normal IQ, an increased prevalence of impairment in some aspects of cognition, such as attention, memory and language (Høie et al. 2006; Fastenau et al. 2009). Prevalent academic achievement problems have also been characterised, with significantly higher rates of school-based interventions (e.g. repeating the same grade, summer schools, tutors) (Rantanen et al. 2010). In addition, the social and psychological effects of epilepsy can be profound. Epilepsy can exert a negative effect on the child and family quality of life (QOL), because of lower social competences, more physical and functional disabilities, more unmet medical and mental health needs than children without epilepsy, exposure to real and perceived stigma, financial stress, treatment-related adverse events and the general fear of seizures (Luoni et al. 2011; Russ et al. 2012).

Even if neurobehavioural comorbidities in children with epilepsy are frequent, few are assessed by mental health professionals, probably indicating either a lack of recognition of need for referral or a lack of appropriate services to meet this particular need (Reilly et al. 2014). In the former case, it is probable that children with epilepsy are subject to a form

17

of 'diagnostic overshadowing', with the neurological disorder overshadowing neurobehavioural problems (Fastenau et al. 2008). Similarly, when an intellectual disability is present, the assumption may be that the intervention is not needed because the abnormal or atypical behaviour is an inherent part of intellectual disability, leading to missed and untreated disorders (Reilly et al. 2014).

POSSIBLE BEHAVIOURAL DISORDERS

The phenomenology of psychiatric disorders associated with epilepsy is wide and variable (Choudhary et al. 2014). Adding to the diagnostic difficulty of neurobehavioural disorders in epilepsy is the fact that several psychiatric symptoms, recognised as diagnostic criteria, can occur secondary to seizure activity, EEG abnormalities or antiepileptic drugs (AEDs). Moreover, some authors have considered cognition and language as intrinsic components of behaviour since they play an important role in social functioning, as well as in the sense of competence and self-esteem (Austin and Caplan 2007). Consequently, in some articles it is difficult to discern between pure behavioural and cognitive problems.

The neurobehavioural comorbidities being various, the attempts of classification have been controversial. Some researchers contend that psychiatric syndromes in epilepsy can be characterised by atypical features that are poorly represented by conventional classification systems such as the fourth edition (text revised) of the Diagnostic and Statistical Manual of Mental Disorders (DSM IV-R) and the International Classification of disease (ICD) Version 10 (Krishnamoorthy et al. 2007). In 2007, the International League Against Epilepsy (ILAE) Commission on Psychobiology of Epilepsy developed a classification proposal of neuropsychiatric disorders in epilepsy with the aim to separate disorders comorbid with epilepsy and those that reflect ongoing epileptiform activity from epilepsy-specific disorders, and to attempt to subclassify the epilepsy-specific disorders alone (Krishnamoorthy et al. 2007). The classification was followed by international clinical practice consensus statements for the treatment of neuropsychiatric conditions associated with epilepsy, to provide guidance on the management of these conditions (Kerr et al. 2011a). These documents put together adult and childhood epilepsies.

Generally, there is a wide consensus regarding a greater association between epilepsy and the following behavioural disorders: attention-deficit–hyperactivity disorder (ADHD), autism spectrum disorders (ASD), anxiety, depression and psychosis.

ADHD is one of the most common comorbidities, being reported in about 30–40% of children with epilepsy compared to 3–6% of controls, especially in preschool and school-age children, without sex differences (Dunn and Kronenberger 2005; Hermann et al. 2007a; Parisi et al. 2010; Cohen et al. 2013; Socanski et al. 2013). Differently from children without epilepsy, children with epilepsy are most likely to present with an inattentive form (Reilly 2011). The symptoms of ADHD may not be the same as those of ADHD in other conditions, because of the comorbidity with psychiatric disorders, underlying brain abnormality, frequent epileptiform discharges, seizures and adverse effects of medication. A common pathogenic mechanism has been hypothesised: the animal models of ADHD suggest that synaptic abnormality in excitatory glutamergic transmission may contribute to vulnerability for epilepsy and ADHD (Jensen et al. 2009).

ASD have been reported in around 20% of children with epilepsy; estimates of epilepsy in autism range from 5–40%, compared to 1% of general population, depending on the samples chosen, on diagnostic criteria and on the age of participants (Berg et al. 2011c; Woolfenden et al. 2012). Indeed, there are two peaks of onset of epilepsy associated with autism: the first in infancy and the second in adolescent years. Moreover, the prevalence of autism in children with epilepsy also depends on the IQ level (the lower the IQ the higher the incidence of ASD) and on sex (being girls at higher risk) (Amiet et al. 2008; Tuchman et al. 2013). Despite the importance of this comorbidity, the rate of misdiagnosis of epilepsy is still high, typically around 20–25%, and despite the large number of studies performed, a full understanding of the possible links between epilepsy and ASD remains elusive (Uldall et al. 2006). So far, there is no evidence that typical autism can be attributed to an epileptic disorder, even in those children with a history of regression after normal early development (Deonna and Roulet 2006). The current evidence seems to point to a common underlying predisposition factor since a growing number of genetic defects leading to both conditions have been discovered (Betancur 2011; Brooks-Kayal 2011).

The increased prevalence of *anxiety and depression* has been found in epidemiological and clinical studies, and is frequently comorbid (Berg et al. 2011a; Russ et al. 2012). The reported prevalence of these internalising disorders from samples obtained in epilepsy clinics is higher than the prevalence reported in epidemiological surveys, namely 12–20% for depression and 10–20% for anxiety, compared to 1–7% of controls, going beyond 30% in patients with lower IQ, language delays, or neuropsychological deficits such as academic difficulties (Caplan et al. 2005b; Cushner-Weinstein et al. 2008; Ekinci et al. 2009; Austin et al. 2010b; Reilly 2011). The higher risk for anxiety includes specific phobias, panic disorder, and posttraumatic stress symptoms (Dunn et al. 2009). Age has been found to be a significant risk factor for both depression and anxiety, adolescents being more at risk than younger children, although findings are discordant (Ekinci et al. 2009). It also seems that adolescents report more symptoms than parents observe. For children and adolescents with primary depression, early age at onset and the severity of depressive symptoms are associated with non-adherence to treatment or lack of treatment and are predictive of both pharmaco-resistant epilepsy and recurrence of depressive symptoms during their adult age (Pereira and Valente 2013). The sex difference in the increased prevalence of anxiety and depression is inconsistent though the prevalence of depression is high in female adolescents (Pereira and Valente 2013). The symptoms are similar to those observed in peers without seizures (Vega et al. 2011). However, some symptoms may relate specifically to epilepsy: brief episodes of anxiety or fear can occur as an aura in children with focal epileptiform discharges frequently originating from the temporal lobe (Salpekar and Dunn 2007). For symptoms of depression and anxiety, some authors suggested distinguishing between epilepsy-related preictal, ictal, postictal and interictal symptoms and comorbid disorders unrelated to epilepsy. Specific epilepsy-related factors do not seem to be a major factor in the causation of anxiety or depression (Pereira and Valente 2013), and findings have shown that depression is more important than seizure frequency in determining perceived QOL (Hecimovic et al. 2012).

Psychosis or 'psychotic' features are significantly more frequent in patients with epilepsy than in the general population, with prevalence rates ranging between 2% and 8%, compared to less than 1% of controls (Helmstaedter et al. 2014). Nevertheless, in a large proportion of these reports no formal diagnosis has been made and the term is being used loosely to describe any behaviour that cannot be easily explained. No evidence of features such as hallucinations or thought disorder is provided; moreover, there is confusion surrounding the classification terms. Some authors suggested distinguishing at least four categories: psychosis related to seizures (e.g. ictal or postictal), psychosis related to seizure remission (alternative psychosis or forced normalization), interictal psychosis (i.e. psychosis between seizures without any clear time relationship to them) and iatrogenic psychosis related to AEDs or after temporal lobectomy. In adolescents, psychosis can be postictal, interictal, antiepileptic-drug induced or post-surgical; whether ictal psychosis occurs in teenagers remains open to debate.

In children occur also *psychogenic non-epileptic seizures* (*PNES*), even if no formal guidelines for diagnosing in children exist, and little is known about the clinical practice of diagnosing PNES in the paediatric setting (Wichaidit et al. 2014). PNES are paroxysmal events that resemble clinical signs and symptoms of epileptic seizures but are not associated with ictal epileptiform abnormalities in the EEG pattern. Some studies focused on the development or on the remission of PNES after cranial surgery for epilepsy, especially for right temporal dysplasia. The clinical semiology of PNES is very complex and belongs to the complicated phenomenon defined as 'dissociation', for example, 'a disruption of and/or discontinuity in the normal integration of consciousness, memory, identity, emotion, perception, body representation, motor control, and behavior' (Roberts and Reuber 2014).

Bipolar disorders are rarely diagnosed in the paediatric epilepsy population, rating around 1% (Berg 2011). Bipolar disorder symptoms have been more often reported as postictal phenomena and occasionally as ictal phenomena. The phenomenological understanding of childhood mania has changed over recent years to the extent that a bipolar disorder spectrum allows for better description of the patient presentations most commonly encountered in clinical practice. Symptoms such as explosive rage, extreme irritability, mood lability and agitation may not meet full criteria for traditional mania but may be consistent with a bipolar disorder spectrum especially in terms of treatment selection (Nishida et al. 2005; Schmitz 2005).

There does not appear to be a significant increase of *oppositional defiant disorder (ODD) or conduct disorder* in children with uncomplicated epilepsy, although results are not univocal (Jones et al. 2007).

Suicidal ideation has been reported in around 20% of children with epilepsy, compared to about 5% in general population (Caplan et al. 2005b; Wagner et al. 2009; Hesdorffer et al. 2012b). Adolescents with epilepsy are at higher risk, both as compared with general population and as compared with adults with older-onset epilepsy. The risk seems to be associated with the severity of epilepsy and with intellectual disability, but other factors are likely to be important and need to be discovered through further investigation and clinical practice advances (Rodenburg et al. 2011).

Compared to siblings and to children with other chronic conditions, *social difficulties* (e.g. difficulties in having a productive and mutually satisfying relationship with others) tend to be specific to children with epilepsy (Sillanpää and Cross 2009; Clary et al. 2010; Rantanen et al. 2009; 2012; Rodenburg et al. 2011). Measures of initiating behaviour, making conversation, responding to the actions of others, and assertiveness have proved significantly impaired (Tse et al. 2007). Poorer social competence may be related to a chronic condition or, as seen in typically developing children, peer problems may also be associated with neurocognitive functions (e.g. inattention and social cognition) (Drewel et al. 2009). Cognitive impairment or learning problems and verbal IQ are proposed to be moderators of development of social competence in children with epilepsy (Clary et al. 2010; Buelow et al. 2012; Byars et al. 2014). An individual with inadequately developed communication skills may not effectively express emotions, regulate behaviour, or develop and maintain interpersonal relationships (Clary et al. 2010). It is possible that early-onset epilepsy with comorbid cognitive impairment and a longer duration of seizures are associated with poorer social skills or delayed social skill acquisition (Cushner-Weinstein et al. 2008; Rantanen et al. 2009). Also, an abnormal family function has been shown to be strongly predictive of social skills impairment (Tse et al. 2007). Alternatively, psychosocial factors may play a role. Epilepsy remains a stigmatised condition and myths and misconceptions are still prevalent in society (Baxendale and O'Toole 2007). Because of this, children with epilepsy may feel less welcome in peer interactions and may avoid social situations for fear they may suffer a seizure or be restricted from participation by their parents and caregivers (Cheung and Wirrell 2006). Put together, findings regarding the importance of several epilepsy variables (e.g. aetiology, seizure frequency and seizure type) to be associated with problems in social competence are contradictory. The relationship between epilepsy-related variables and social competence is probably indirect rather than direct (Noeker et al. 2005). Nevertheless, problematic social skills during childhood and adolescence are related to subsequent psychopathology and may predispose to behavioural and adjustment problems in adulthood (Rantanen et al. 2012).

METHODOLOGICAL ISSUES

Consensus neurobehavioural diagnoses have been generally made using the DSM-IV criteria together with standardised scales. The ADHD Rating Scale-IV (ADHD-RS-IV; DuPaul et al. 1998) and Conners' Rating Scales (CRS-R, Conners 1997) have been used for ADHD diagnosis. The Childhood Depression Inventory (CDI, Kovacs 1985), the Short Mood and Feelings Questionnaire (SMFQ) (Angold et al. 1987), the Child or Adolescent Symptom Inventory (Sprafkin et al. 2002), the Beck Depression Inventory (BDI) (Beck et al. 1988) and the Children Depression Rating-Scale Revised (CDRS-R) (Poznanski and Mokros 1996) have been used to rate mood disorders. So far, the instruments most commonly used to assess anxiety disorders have been the Revised Children's Manifest Anxiety Scale (RCMAS) (Reynolds and Richmond 1985), the Multidimensional Anxiety Scale for Children (MASC, March et al. 1997), the Screen for Child Anxiety Related Emotional Disorders (SCARED, Birmaher et al. 1997).

Some studies used psychiatric diagnoses based on structured psychiatric interviews with the child or parent, such as the Child Global Assessment Scale (CGAS, Shaffer et al. 1983), the Kiddie Schedule for Affective Disorders and Schizophrenia (K-SADS)

(Kaufman et al. 1997), the Diagnostic Interview Schedule for Children (Shaffer et al. 2000), the Vineland Social Maturity Scale (VSMS, Doll 1965) and the Behaviour Assessment System for children, Second Edition (BASC-2) (Reynolds and Kamphaus 2004).

Among self-rating scales, the Child Behaviour Check List (CBCL) (Achenbach 1991) for children, parent and teacher has been highly used, confirming behavioural disorders associated with epilepsy, although with different results (Rantanen et al. 2012).

To rate parenting stress in relation to children with special needs and/or epilepsy, the Parenting Stress Index (PSI) has been developed (Abidin 1990).

To assess social skills, there are the CBCL, the CRS-R and the Social Skills Rating System (SSRS, Gresham and Elliott 1990). Together with the SSRS, the Strength and Difficulties Questionnaire (SDQ, Goodman 1997) is an example of possible and practical assessment tools for a broader perspective in the assessment of social competence, since they include all aspects (Dafoulis and Kalyva 2012). Studies have also provided evidence for a high sensitivity and specificity of SDQ among children with epilepsy (Hysing et al. 2007). Furthermore, since expectations of social competence increase as a function of child's age and developmental level, the division into subgroups according to their age has been suggested (Rantanen et al. 2012).

A novel approach using multiple instruments to assess ASD, developmental delay and behavioural/emotional difficulties has been proposed (Eom et al. 2014), including the Social Communication Questionnaire (SCQ) (Rutter et al. 2003), the Modified Checklist for Autism in Toddlers (mCHAT) (Robins et al. 2001), and the SDQ.

QOL scales specific for children with epilepsy have been developed to cover physical, psychological, social and academic functioning. Examples of tools include the Quality of Life in Epilepsy for Adolescents (QOLIE-AD-48) (Cramer et al. 1999), the Quality of Life in Childhood Epilepsy (QOLCE) (Sabaz et al. 2000), the Impact of Paediatric Epilepsy Scale (IPES) (Camfield et al. 2001) and the Impact of Childhood Illness Scale (Hoare and Russell 1995). The National Institute of Neurological Disorders and Stroke (NINDS) provided leadership to develop the Neuro-QOL, which provides psychometrically sound and clinically relevant QOL measures for children and adults with neurological disorders (Cella et al. 2012; Gershon et al. 2012).

The best way of obtaining accurate information on the prevalence of neurobehavioural comorbidities in children with epilepsy is to analyse data from well-designed, prospective epidemiological studies on large populations of children, including control groups. While interviewing patients, some strategies can be used that are both efficient and accurate (Salpekar and Dunn 2007). With younger children, a calm and reassuring stance will yield the most information, and a gradual process of general questions leading to more specific questions is often most effective. Especially for adolescents, to obtain a behavioural description every attempt should be made to interview the patient independently, since they may not reveal their symptoms in the presence of caregivers.

Nevertheless, findings may differ on the basis of the rate of the behaviour and type of measurement, which can lead to over- or underestimation of problems (Dafoulis and Kalyva 2012). Clinicians and researchers should be aware that using different rating scales may yield different results especially since they have not been designed specifically for children with epilepsy (Krishnamoorthy 2006). In addition, parents' psychiatric status might influence what information they provide and how they communicate it: depressed and/or anxious parents might be aware of the child's symptoms, but under- or overestimate their severity.

A lifespan perspective on behavioural disorders

Evidence has emerged suggesting bidirectional relations between epilepsy and various neurobehavioural comorbidities in paediatric epilepsy (Lin et al. 2012; Helmstaedter et al. 2014). Psychiatric disorders can either precede or follow the onset of epilepsy, which is the case for depression, anxiety, ADHD and psychosis (Jones et al. 2005; Hesdorffer et al. 2006; Wotton and Goldacre 2012). Seizure incidence has been shown to be higher in psychiatric patients, males and aged 6 to 12 years, even in those without seizure risk factors (McAfee et al. 2007).

THE ONSET

In a study, more than 40% of children with epilepsy met diagnostic criteria for a DSM-IV disorder before the diagnosis of epilepsy and the first recognised seizure (Jones et al. 2005), even without clinical evidence of brain structural abnormalities (Almane et al. 2014). The increased prevalence may be consistent with the presence of underlying neurobiological influences independent of seizures, epilepsy syndrome and AEDs (Jones et al. 2007).

ADHD is more prevalent in new-onset epilepsy than in healthy controls (31% vs 6%), even in idiopathic syndromes (Hermann et al. 2007a). More than 15% of the children with new-onset seizures fell in the clinical range of internalising and externalising problems (Dunn et al. 2009). About 25% of children with new-onset idiopathic epilepsies need special education services before clinical seizure onset (Berg et al. 2005). Behavioural complications do not necessarily respect traditional syndrome groupings in children with new- or recent-onset epilepsy, showing shared findings in localisation-related and generalised epilepsies, even if social difficulties and internalising behaviours are more frequent in the latter (Bhise et al. 2009; Almane et al. 2014). At the time of the first seizure episodes, the child must begin to adapt to an unpredictable and frightening disorder, causing him/her persisting worries about having another seizure (Choudhary et al. 2014). Anxiety, stress and emotions can trigger seizures and increase seizure frequency. This, in turn, can also trigger anticipatory anxiety and evoke stress, anger and frustration leading to a vicious circle of anxiety and seizures fuelling each other, further increasing the risk for behavioural problems (Lathers and Schraeder 2006).

THE OUTCOME

The effects of early disorders may be short-term on educational functioning and long-term on occupational, social and behavioural development. Though most studies of behaviour in children with epilepsy have been cross-sectional, several groups have assessed changes over time, finding in some cases a trend either of behavioural improvement with controlled seizures or of stability (Austin et al. 2012). However, longitudinal retesting of patients with epilepsy and controls has shown persistent neurobehavioural differences (such as lower levels of education and employment, less cognitive gaining in testing) even in adults with childhood-onset epilepsy who have been seizure free and off medication for many years and those with benign types of epilepsy. In particular, an earlier age at onset is associated with poorer cognitive function and, consequently, with an increasing risk for neurobehavioural comorbidities (Hermann et al. 2008). A 10-year follow-up population study of psychological and social outcome in well-functioning children and adolescents with childhood-onset epilepsy has shown some emotional, behavioural and social problems, especially in patients with active epilepsy (e.g. at least one seizure episode in the last 5y) and polytherapy, with a better outcome for idiopathic localization-related epilepsies (Jonsson et al. 2014). In a population-based study with a median follow-up duration of 28 years since the onset of epilepsy, compared to unaffected population, children with epilepsy with good cognitive development and without comorbidities have shown similar adult health, educational and employment outcomes but had difficulties with establishing and maintaining personal relationships (Chin et al. 2011). On the contrary, a combination of childhood epilepsy and poor cognitive development and/or comorbidities and/or difficulties in feeling accepted by peers at the age of 11 years is more likely to be associated with adverse outcomes compared to having poor cognitive development without childhood epilepsy. Consequently, a good childhood cognitive development can be considered as an important predictor of good adult outcomes. Higher IQ may relate to stronger strategies to handle with sickness, such as an active participation and compliance to pharmacological intake, reducing the specific impact of medical epilepsy-related variables, such as seizure severity (Pereira and Valente 2013). Moreover, the management of social/emotional problems around 11 years should have positive long-term impacts. It is generally recognised that the development of social competence is one of the best predictors of later social and academic success, and of present and future behavioural and emotional problems (Rantanen et al. 2012). Other studies have reported similar findings suggesting that negative societal attitudes towards epilepsy may cause isolation in later life (Camfield and Camfield 2007). With respect to factors predicting behavioural adaptation to epilepsy, early temperament (e.g. the early appearing, biologically based characteristic patterns of emotional reactivity and self-regulation) and neuropsychological functioning (especially executive functions also involved in behavioural control) in school-age children with new-onset seizures have shown to predict the outcome 3 years after seizure onset (Baum et al. 2010). In particular, novelty distress (perhaps an early marker of anxiety), unmanageability (perhaps an early marker of impulsivity and deviant behaviours) and cognitive self-regulatory difficulties may put children at risk for relatively long-term poor behaviour outcomes.

Authors have proposed that the concept of cerebral reserve might have important implications in understanding the life course of people with epilepsy who have an early brain insult, raising the question whether it confers an increased risk for disrupted cognitive development and accelerated ageing effects owing to reduced cerebral reserve (Deary et al. 2004). In the context of childhood-onset chronic epilepsy, this concept might help to conceptualise the lifespan course of cognition and brain structure in epilepsy (Hermann et al. 2008).

There are relatively few studies of the behavioural outcome of epilepsy surgery in children who have used standardised behavioural measures before and after the procedure. Moreover, homogeneous data are lacking because of groups with mixed pathology and retrospective studies. Characterising the long-term behavioural outcome for people with epilepsy previously admitted to surgery is complex, given the highly individual nature of patient response to illness and its treatment (Wilson et al. 2005). Increasing evidence supports the idea that epilepsy surgery early in life may be associated with a complex psychological process of postoperative adjustment, which persists for many years (McLellan et al. 2005).

Taken together, results show that the outcome in temporal and extra-temporal surgery is very variable, with few children improving and others deteriorating, and with a better outcome in younger children (Mclellan et al. 2005; Colonnelli et al. 2012). De novo depression is a common psychiatric sequela of temporal lobe epilepsy (TLE) surgery (McLellan et al. 2005; Wrench et al. 2009). The study of the psychological profile in childhood-onset TLE approximately 13 years after seizure onset showed that surgical non-seizure-free patients had the poorest outcome in terms of lowered mood and depression (Micallef et al. 2010), and are at higher risk for postictal psychosis (Cleary et al. 2013) . Lifetime psychiatric history predicts a worse seizure outcome following temporal lobectomy (Kanner et al. 2009). The outlook for hemispherectomy does not seem better, since psychopathology has been a common result either pre- or postoperatively, without post-surgical worsening or improvement, even in seizure-free patients (Danielsson et al. 2009; Colonnelli et al. 2012). Vagus nerve stimulation seems to increase QOL, even without a change of adaptive behaviour (Mikati et al. 2009; Zamponi et al. 2011).

Explicative models
Theoretical models propose that psychopathology in epilepsy can stem from a complex interplay of multiple aetiological variables (Choudhary et al. 2014). The prevalence of neurobehavioural comorbidities in epilepsy across the lifespan has triggered a concerted effort to uncover their potential mediators, including various epilepsy-related variables. Moreover, psychosocial models have been developed to depict the complexity of behavioural comorbidities in childhood epilepsy. Recent neuroimaging evidence contributes to the tracing of the neurobiological underpinnings of associated disorders, providing biological markers of increased risk.

Given that neurobehavioural comorbidities are especially recurrent in complicated epilepsies, it is important to distinguish the burden of the core clinical features of epilepsy. Among many possible factors, the most relevant to clinical practice include aetiology, syndrome, epileptiform discharges, seizure, age at epilepsy onset, years of epilepsy duration and prescribed drugs (Lin et al. 2012).

An assumption in the specialty is that epilepsy occurs in a fundamentally abnormal brain, which increases a person's risk not only for seizures, but also for neurobehavioural comorbidities (Salpekar and Dunn 2007). Hence, comorbid symptoms may be directly related to epilepsy and the underlying brain disorder. Despite their variability, structural-functional relations seem to be strong in *lesional* epilepsy such as malformation of cortical development, even before seizure onset (Freilinger et al. 2006; Chang et al. 2012). However, removing a lesion does not always improve symptoms, suggesting that this mechanism alone is not the entire explanation (Hamiwka and Wirrell 2009).

The *electro-clinical syndrome* is a factor which has received particular interest. For decades, the syndromic model has served as the basis for investigating the cognitive and psychiatric domains most at risk. The importance of the behavioural implications of syndrome classification could be considered in two broad categories: first, the behavioural effects of epilepsy syndromes and, second, the behavioural associations of childhood syndromes ('behavioural phenotypes') in which epilepsy occurs as a prominent feature. Even if different syndromes seem to have diverse comorbidities, the same disorders have been documented across a wide range of epilepsy syndromes: for example, psychiatric complications of TLE have been documented also in benign epilepsy with centrotemporal spikes (BECTS). Consequently, the decade-long controversy regarding the unique psychiatric vulnerability of some syndromes has been replaced by the opinion that psychiatric disorders occur across diverse epilepsy syndromes. This variability within and across syndromes suggests that phenotypic presentations might be driven by other factors.

In the following, we provide a description of behavioural disorders of some syndromes which will not be discussed in detail in the next chapters of the book. Generally speaking, there is a common consensus that localisation-related epilepsies have less behavioural problems than generalised epilepsies (Dafoulis and Kalyva 2012; Almane et al. 2014), even if in both AEDs, age at epilepsy onset and seizure frequency are shown to be related to the severity of behavioural and neuropsychological comorbidity (Freilinger et al. 2006; Caplan et al. 2008a). Core psychiatric deficits in TLE have been described as being depression and anxiety (Caplan et al. 2005b). Although behavioural disorders attributable to executive dysfunction are usually considered more indicative of frontal lobe pathology, patients with TLE may manifest at least a moderate degree of executive dysfunction, especially with earlier onset, longer duration of epilepsy and polytherapy (Rzezak et al. 2007). The impact of epilepsy-related variables such as severity of seizures on depression in TLE does not seem to be significant, especially in adolescents (Pereira and Valente 2013). Moreover, the executive dysfunction may reduce both academic achievements and daily life efficiency, leading to depression aggravation (Gois et al. 2011). Frontal lobe epilepsy (FLE) seems to be mostly associated with issues regarding impulse control, greater maladaptive behaviours, personality disorders, and ADHD linked to frontal dysfunction (Prévost et al. 2006; Ryvlin et al. 2006; Parisi et al. 2010; Braakman et al. 2011). High rates of ADHD have been reported in FLE associated with tuberous sclerosis; nevertheless, the majority (about 67%) of children affected by nonlesional FLE also exhibit symptoms of ADHD, and in these patients seizure control does not guarantee the concomitant improvement of the hyperactive/impulsive behaviour and of inattention (Prévost et al. 2006). Among generalised epilepsies, juvenile myoclonic epilepsy (JME) has also been characterised by a frontal lobe dysfunction. Although prior studies have reported patients with JME to have higher rates of immature, unstable and unreliable personalities leading to social maladjustment (Moschetta et al. 2011), these results have limited validity in that standardised scales were not used (Hamiwka and Wirrell 2009). Childhood absence epilepsy (CAE) is characterised by impaired behaviour, mostly ADHD with a prevalence of the inattentive type, in association with duration of illness, AEDs and seizure frequency (about 61% in Caplan et al. 2006; 2008b). Children with catastrophic epileptic encephalopathies such as Dravet syndrome and Lennox-Gastaut syndrome have more behavioural and cognitive problems (Wolff et al. 2006; Hamiwka and Wirrell 2009). There are several early epilepsies (infantile spasms, partial complex epilepsies, epilepsies with continuous spike-waves during slow sleep [CSWS], early forms of Landau-Kleffner syndrome) with different aetiologies (tuberous sclerosis is an important model of these situations) in which a direct relationship between epilepsy and some features of autism may be suspected (Deonna and Roulet 2006).

Interictal epileptiform discharges (IEDs) have been suggested to have important behavioural and cognitive consequences, determining 'subtle' effects not immediately obviously attributable to an epileptic seizure (Besag 2006). The most recent system of epilepsy classification (Berg et al. 2010) has defined the concept of 'epileptic encephalopathy' in which epileptiform discharges themselves can affect cognition and behaviour. The best-known example of major behavioural and cognitive disorder is the EEG pattern of CSWS (Tassinari et al. 2009). In transient cognitive impairment, discharges may cause inattention and slowing of motor speed, besides material-specific cognitive deficits, even if the application of these findings in the clinical setting is not straightforward (Nicolai et al. 2012). Findings are inconsistent in demonstrating that the lateralization and localization of IED in benign focal epilepsy are associated with behavioural problems (Northcott et al. 2005; Salpekar and Mishra 2014), even if rolandic, frontal or generalised spike-wave discharges have been associated with ADHD (Holtmann et al. 2006). Although a high percentage of children with ASD show IED (Baird et al. 2006), there appears to be no association with regression (Chez et al. 2006) and the role of EEG remains open to debate and has to be evaluated in longitudinal studies (Deonna and Roulet 2006).

Sleep disruption may be a comorbidity of epilepsy and can be the result of seizures and/or IEDs during sleep, AEDs, or behavioural problems (Rodenburg et al. 2011). Sleep activates both focal and generalised IED in about one third of all patients with epilepsy (Parisi et al. 2010). With or without nocturnal seizures, they reduce sleep efficiency. Prolonged focal epileptic activity such as CSWS interferes with slow wave activity, impairing the plastic changes associated with learning (Nickels and Wirrell 2008). Nocturnal seizures significantly increase in frequency during the first rapid eye movement period and during drowsiness (Foldvary-Schaefer and Grigg-Damberger 2006). Sleep fragmentation/disruption can cause hyperactivity, ADHD, learning and social problems (Tse et al. 2007; Parisi et al. 2010; Filippini et al. 2013).

Focusing on the role of seizures, the temporal relationship with psychiatric comorbidities is particularly relevant. Ictal and postictal depression has been described even if it seems less common in children rather than in adults, as well as interictal dysphoric disorder (Mula et al. 2008a; 2008b). A complicating factor in the temporal relationship between seizures and symptoms of anxiety and depression concerns whether or not seizures have been occurring before they are first reported, and whether they have been occurring during sleep or during wake but being interpreted as low mood or non-compliance. Moreover, EEG abnormalities without seizures may have occurred before a reported seizure (Reilly 2011).

Postictal psychoses account for approximately 25% of all psychoses of epilepsy. They usually occur after a cluster of secondary generalised tonic–clonic seizures in patients with TLE (Hersdorffer et al. 2006; Cleary et al. 2013). These psychotic episodes are usually brief, last from 1 to 6 days, and often remit spontaneously within days or weeks. However, they are characterised by mixed mood and paranoid ideas with religious content, with an increased risk of self-harm (McAfee et al. 2007). Peri-ictal psychoses are more frequently reported than interictal psychoses. Interictal psychoses are unrelated to seizures and typically develop after several years of active mesial TLE (Chang et al. 2012). Despite their chronic course, differences with schizophrenia are quite striking with low rates of long-term institutionalisation, a tendency of psychotic symptoms to attenuate over time, and the paucity of personality and cognitive deterioration (Adachi et al. 2011; 2012). Post- or interictal psychoses have been reported in two cases of FLE, presenting as delusional thinking, depression, paranoia, aggression and bizarre behaviour in conjunction with brief stereotypic events of sudden screaming, agitation and physical aggression, disappearing with adequate seizure control (Sinclair and Snyder 2008).

Age at onset is directly related to the severity of comorbid cognitive, linguistic and behavioural problems (Austin and Caplan 2007; Freilinger et al. 2006). In early onset, especially when difficult to control and accompanied by developmental delay, epilepsy impacts strongly on family functioning and on child behaviour. Onset prior to the age of 3–4 years is more likely to be associated with intellectual disability and with the linked comorbidities including behavioural problems (Clary et al. 2010). Indeed, population studies demonstrated a higher rate of psychopathology in children with epilepsy and intellectual disability (Hermann et al. 2008). In middle childhood, the child becomes aware of the ramifications of living with epilepsy in that he/she has to face school requests and develop peer relationships. On the one hand, this challenge may cause psychological difficulties; on the other, this process would be more difficult for the child with behaviour and/or cognitive problems. During adolescence, the onset of the illness and the need to be dependent on the parent hinder the normal process of increasing independence and evolving self-identity (De Souza and Salgado 2006). Opportunities may be rare for adolescents with epilepsy to be in social settings in which they feel normal and can interact without regard to their potentially isolating illness. Behavioural problems may further jeopardize the ability of the child to cope with epilepsy and may increase stress on the family (Salpekar and Dunn 2007).

Firm conclusions regarding the impact of early-life seizures on behaviour can be confounded by several methodological factors, such as the inclusion of a mixed spectrum of epilepsy syndromes, and possible confounding of earlier seizure onset with longer seizure duration: therefore, it is difficult to interpret these findings without controlling for variables such as IQ, seizure frequency and AEDs (Datta et al. 2005). Clinically, recognising that earlier seizure onset is an important, but not the only, contributor to neurobehavioural comorbidities in children is essential.

Whether patients' psychiatric status worsens with an increasing duration of epilepsy is a controversial topic. The progression of neurobehavioural problems has often been assessed in terms of cognitive decline, without focusing on specific behavioural problems (Jones et al. 2007).

A general consensus on the cognitive and psychiatric effects of AEDs has been reached, especially in polytherapy (Datta et al. 2005; Freilinger et al. 2006; Mula et al. 2009; Dafoulis and Kalyva 2012). See also Chapter 8 in this book for further details. Put together, results show that children differ in their vulnerability to the behavioural side effects of AEDs and several additional factors may contribute to this vulnerability (Freilinger et al. 2006; Choudhary et al. 2014). Indeed, patient-related factors such as age, epilepsy type and premorbid behavioural and/or cognitive problems may be implicated in the adverse behavioural effects of AEDs (Caplan et al. 2006). However, individual AEDs have been associated with specific behavioural side effects (Austin and Caplan 2007; Eddy et al. 2012, Halma et al. 2014), including depression in children on phenobarbital, primidone or valproic acid and mania in some children treated with felbamate; psychosis has been associated with topiramate, levetiracetam, zonisamide and vigabatrin. Irritability, aggression and hyperactivity have been reported with phenobarbital, benzodiazepines, gabapentin, levetiracetam, topiramate and vigabatrin. No behavioural adverse effects have been noted with lamotrigine. Beyond the specific side effects of each drug, rapid titration of the drug, polypharmacy, a history of psychiatric disorders and limbic system functional or structural abnormalities can increase the risk of developing drug-induced cognitive and psychiatric complications.

In conclusion, the variation across studies in terms of the association between epilepsy-related variables and behaviour might reflect methodological differences, including variations in the behavioural measures, informants, sample size, age range of participants, IQ, proportion of participants with early onset epilepsy, as well as the socioeconomic background. Unfortunately, being most studies cross-sectional, the possibility of reaching conclusions is limited. Nevertheless, there is increasing evidence indicating that the identification of the epilepsy syndrome can be of prognostic value also in terms of behavioural outcome. Moreover, epilepsy variables are associated with comorbidities (such as low IQ) which in turn contribute to behavioural difficulties, particularly in those children with earlier and difficult-to-control seizures.

THE NEUROBIOLOGICAL HYPOTHESIS
These distributed psychiatric and cognitive abnormalities have been linked to surprisingly widespread neuroanatomical derangements. Either structural or functional brain abnormalities that result in seizures or seizure-induced dysfunction in key areas such as the frontal lobe and the limbic system may lead to a behavioural change (Tse et al. 2007).

Such functional–structural relationships are best characterised in adult people with childhood- or adolescence-onset TLE (Lin et al. 2012). While the link between hippocampus and behavioural tasks is well documented (Berg et al. 2011b; Lugo et al. 2014), more data are needed on the structural abnormalities existing outside this region and subserving behaviour, including extratemporal lobes (i.e. frontal, parietal and occipital lobes) as well as subcortical (basal ganglia) and cerebellar regions and their direct and indirect connections (Riley et al. 2010). Likewise, the volume of the corpus callosum and the integrity of the frontostriatal connections are correlated with executive functions the control of behaviour. Temporal lobe abnormalities have also been implicated in the neurocircuitry of depression and TLE. For example, the degree of hippocampal atrophy is inversely correlated with the severity and/or duration of depression in TLE. Widespread functional and anatomical abnormalities are associated with mood disorders in TLE, including orbital frontal cortex, cingulate gyrus, subcortical regions and brainstem. Patients with TLE and psychosis had 16–18% larger amygdala volumes, when compared to TLE patients without psychosis. Abnormalities in advanced social cognition have been linked to mesial TLE (Schacher et al. 2006).

The high prevalence of similar psychiatric changes among patients with TLE and FLE has been related to the intimate white matter connection of the frontal and temporal limbic systems (Lin et al. 2012). In patients with FLE, psychoses or ictal fear has been related to the reciprocal connections between amygdala, orbitofrontal and anterior cingulated regions and between frontal and temporal lobes through the uncinate fasciculus and the superior longitudinal fasciculus. Aggressive behaviour has been related to the activation of limbic structures and loss of frontal suppression of limbic activity (Sumer et al. 2007). Dysfunction in frontal or temporal lobes may be involved in the aetiology of both epilepsy and depression (Kanner 2005).

In children with epilepsy and ADHD, magnetic resonance imaging volumetric analysis has shown increased frontal grey matter and decreased total brain stem volumes compared with those with epilepsy and no ADHD, likely to be linked to the subtype of ADHD which is predominantly inattentive (Hermann et al. 2007a). Recent advances in neuroimaging techniques have revealed white matter tracts linking specific brain regions such as caudate nucleus and prefrontal cortex, both of which seem to be constituents of ADHD pathophysiology (Seidman et al. 2005; Pavuluri et al. 2009).

Children with epilepsy exhibit abnormalities in brain structure at or near the time of seizure onset and an altered development trajectory early in the course of epilepsy (Tosun et al. 2011). At baseline, quantitative MRI studies have revealed enlarged ventricular and reduced thalamic volumes in new-onset idiopathic generalised epilepsy (Jackson et al. 2011). Over the prospective 2 years, children with epilepsy displayed a slowed white matter expansion and altered region-specific patterns of grey matter thinning, compared to age-matched controls. Cross-sectional studies supplement this literature, demonstrating the adverse impact of early-onset epilepsy on the brain structure. The posterior corpus callosum appears to be particularly vulnerable, with earlier age at seizure onset consistently linked to reduced white matter volume or microstructural integrity (Lin et al. 2012) In children with new-onset JME, baseline frontothalamic volume is correlated with deficits in higher-order executive function, and in children with new-onset BECTS, striatal enlargement predicts better executive function performances (Hermann et al. 2008).

Clearly, developmental trajectories in these children are divergent from those of their healthy peers, which becomes evident near the time of epilepsy onset, but the link between aberrant brain development and variable cognitive, psychiatric and social progress in children with epilepsy is uncertain.

Animal models are considered to be useful in understanding the basis of neurobehavioural disorders, as they afford reproducible systems in which either epilepsy or a neurobehavioural disorder represents an unequivocal and on-demand primary pathology. Furthermore, epilepsy comorbidities can be examined in their native states and/or in the absence of iatrogenic neurobehavioural abnormalities, the latter being for example attributed to AEDs (Pineda et al. 2014). There has been growing evidence that rodent models of acquired chronic epilepsy are not only characterised by spontaneous recurrent seizures but also produce a spectrum of neurobehavioural impairments, some of which have been validated as experimental equivalents of neurobehavioural comorbidities of epilepsy (Pineda et al. 2010; 2014).

Genetic studies have shown a sharing of genetic risk factors in psychiatric disorders (Cross-disorder Group of the Psychiatric Genomic Consortium 2013). There are a growing number of genetic defects recognised as being associated with epilepsy, intellectual disability and psychiatric problems (Battaglia et al. 2010; Brooks-Kayal 2011; Hesdorffer et al. 2012a) leading to the conclusion that neurobehavioural comorbidities may be a manifestation of the underlying pathophysiology involved in epilepsy. The assumption remains that a single genetic defect can be associated with more than one syndrome and more than one genetic defect can be associated with a single syndrome.

While various findings suggest that an intrinsic brain disorder, including a possible genetic predisposition, might underlie both epileptic and behavioural comorbidities, the effect of environmental factors remains to be clarified.

THE PSYCHOSOCIAL MODEL

Since the mid-1980s, psychological and social factors have started being reported to have potential influences on the behaviour of children with epilepsy (Rodenburg et al. 2011).

Focusing on an individual level, the patient's psychological response to illness may be a significant contributor to internalizing problems. Adolescents' attitude towards illness and external or unknown locus of control have proved to be predictors of depression; hopelessness is significantly associated with depression in children and adolescents (Wagner et al. 2009). Maternal depression is associated with depression in children and adolescents with epilepsy (Austin et al. 2010b).

In paediatrics, behavioural aspects are related to the family environment and have been studied mostly using ratings of symptoms by parents (e.g. CBCL). Family stress and coping models are considered as useful frameworks and focus on major concepts such as family demands caused by epilepsy as well as other events (stressors), family capabilities (adaptive) and coping behaviours (action strategies related to family relationships, parenting and supporting the child's successful adjustment), definition or meaning of epilepsy (perceptions), family adjustment (Austin 1996). The models propose that when a stressor occurs, the family's adaptive resources and perceptions related to the stressor interact to influence family coping behaviours. The latter, in turn, influence family adjustment related to the stressors. There is substantial evidence that epilepsy in a child is stressful for parents, especially at the onset: seizures are frightening to parents, their unpredictable and episodic nature adds stress, and parents may feel overwhelmed and fearful (Iseri et al. 2006). Intractable childhood epilepsy is associated with markedly increased maternal parenting stress (Wirrell et al. 2008). Parents also report stress as they worry about the child, about changes in family relationships because of epilepsy, problems obtaining support in the community and unsatisfactory interactions with their child's health care providers and school personnel (Buelow and Shore 2006). Additional impact may be represented by other stressors such as marital distress or divorce, and psychopathology in other family members (Oostrom et al. 2005). Low family communication has been widely associated with more behavioural problems in children with epilepsy. Stress in the family environment has the potential to disrupt parenting behaviours and erode parents' confidence in their ability to care for their child (Rodenburg et al. 2011). From a socioeconomic point of view, lower parental education level, poverty status and less extended family social support result in increasing stress (Austin et al. 2010a). Hence, greater family stress and abnormal family functioning coinciding with a heavier impact of epilepsy on family life are associated with more child behavioural and social problems (Tse et al. 2007). Family factors are major contributors to academic performance, which in turn determines child adaptive functioning (Dunn et al. 2010).

Family resources should be associated with fewer child problems and findings from most studies support this proposition, including in children with intractable epilepsy (Austin and Caplan 2007). Greater family mastery at seizure onset may be a predictor of less child behaviour problems 2 years later. Coping responses have shown to be the strongest predictors of child behavioural problems, with rejection being positively related and positive parent–child relationship being negatively related to psychopathology (Rodenburg et al. 2006). Families who are able to deal with the child's epilepsy, who feel confident that they can handle the problems associated with paediatric epilepsy, are the ones who are able to transfer this confidence to their children, resulting in a better QOL (Tse et al. 2007).

Stigma is commonly associated with epilepsy. More negative attitudes and greater perceived stigma on part of the family related to epilepsy are expected to be associated with greater child psychopathology. Moreover, in adolescents who had epilepsy during childhood, one factor strongly associated with behavioural problems in a long-term follow-up was represented by the adolescent's current negative feelings related to having had epilepsy (Chin et al. 2011). Perception of felt stigma had a stronger association with depression diagnoses in adolescents with epilepsy than did parent perceptions, family adaptive resources or family stress (Adewuya and Ola 2005).

Put together, findings have been very consistent in showing that family-related psychosocial variables are associated with child behaviour. In general, greater family stress, fewer family adaptive resources and more negative perceived stigma impact on family adjustment are associated with more child behaviour problems. A chronic condition such as childhood epilepsy with its unpredictable episodes and long-term prognosis, comorbid behavioural problems and possible cumulative effects on academic achievement is a continuing source of stress for families (Rodenburg et al. 2011).

Treatment of behavioural disorders
Systematic data on psychiatric treatment strategies for epilepsy remain limited, with clinical practice relying heavily on individual experience. If the need for mental health care at the acute stage is recognised, the importance of intervention at the chronic stage is underscored

(Austin and Caplan 2007). In a clinical based study, although 60% of children with epilepsy met criteria for one or more psychiatric diagnoses, nearly two-thirds of diagnosed children were not in receipt of treatment for the conditions (Reilly et al. 2011). International expert panels advocate that treatments for primary psychiatric disorders outside epilepsy are valuable if the underlying neurological disorder is taken into consideration (Barry et al. 2008; Kerr et al. 2011b).

The first-line treatment for children with *ADHD*, regardless of whether they have epilepsy or not, remains methylphenidate. Behavioural therapy in ADHD has proved less effective than medication, but it should be considered anyway (Dunn and Kronenberger 2005). Parent education about ADHD should include information about the usual behaviours of the child with ADHD and recommendations for interventions to modify inadequate behaviours. Increased structure, immediate feedback and frequent contacts with parents are an important component of intervention within the school system. Behavioural interventions are particularly needed when there are additional problems with depression, anxiety or with family relationships.

The management of the child with epilepsy and *ASD* basically consists of managing each of these conditions as they would be managed on their own. Even if most of the reports are single cases or open trials, it has been shown that emotional lability, aggression, impulsivity and self-injurious behaviour can be reduced with a number of AEDs including carbamazepine, valproic acid, divalproex sodium, lamotrigine and topiramate (Robinson 2012). Moreover, a comprehensive developmental behavioural intervention for toddlers with ASD can increase IQ, improve adaptive behaviour and ameliorate the diagnosis (Dawson 2010). The improvements in social behaviours are associated with normalised patterns of brain activity, and social-cognitive interventions in infants at risk for ASD positively alter the atypical development of the neural networks critical for social and communicative interactions (Dawson et al. 2010; 2012).

In the management of *depression and anxiety*, there are few controlled trials. A reasonable first step in treatment is the assessment for possible reversible causes of anxiety or depression, such as recent additions or changes in AEDs. Then, cognitive-behavioural therapy (CBT) has proved useful in children and adolescents, even to prevent depression (Martinovi et al. 2006) and to reduce parents' perceived anxiety (Blocher et al. 2013). At the 3-month post-treatment follow-up, parents reported to the CBCL an overall reduction in children's total problems, suggesting that the intervention may help to reduce problematic behaviours by targeting anxiety (Blocher et al. 2013). The combination of CBT and medication has been found to be superior to medication alone for the achievement of remission (Brent et al. 2008). Interventions may also involve psychotherapy (Martinovi et al. 2006) and family therapy (Barry et al. 2008). A recent consensus statement addressed the evaluation and treatment of affective disorders in people with epilepsy and recommended incorporation of psychoeducational, supportive and CBT, and family and school intervention, with medical therapies (Barry et al. 2008).

Generally speaking, besides pharmacological treatment, education should be a standard part of all treatment for patients with paediatric epilepsy, particularly those at risk of comorbid psychiatric and behavioural problems (Wagner et al. 2010; Rodenburg et al. 2011).

This includes informing parents about exactly what they may expect to happen in the course of the child's illness, teaching them how to manage epilepsy symptoms, explaining how to handle the medication and identifying symptoms they should watch for in their children. Moreover, interventions are needed to support parents in the accomplishment of further major tasks, such as facilitating the child's accomplishment of developmental tasks and helping the child to successfully cope with having a seizure condition. Training in coping techniques, decision making and communication enhances children's and parents' self-perceived social competency and behaviour, also in the long-term (May and Pfafflin 2005; Pfäfflin et al. 2012). Interventions have to be tailored to the needs of the child and of the family. For example, interventions might need to differ according to seizure variables (e.g. new onset, intractable epilepsy), child development (normal, delayed, neuropsychological difficulties) or the type of behavioural problems experienced by the child (attention problem, mood disorders, etc.) (Rodenburg et al. 2011).

Once the child has developed behavioural problems, group, individual and family therapies may be useful, through the teaching of relaxation techniques and coping skills. These techniques have resulted in improvement of self-concept as well as a significant reduction in seizure frequency. Specific issues to address may be the initial reactions to grief, anxiety, or anger related to the diagnosis of epilepsy, decreased competence and autonomy in the preschool child, attentional and learning problems in school-age child, and low self-esteem and social issues in the adolescent, coordinating treatment with neurological care (Rodenburg et al. 2011). Negative attitudes, overprotectivness and hostility in the family response to epilepsy may be amenable to family therapy. Group and individual therapies have been used to assess precipitants for emotionally-based seizures and then to teach self-relaxation or self-control techniques. Teaching the patient and the family the ability to cope with epilepsy may also reduce the perceived social stigma, providing a long-lasting reinforcement of self-esteem and social adjustment (McCagh et al. 2009).

Conclusion

Neurobehavioural comorbidities associated with childhood epilepsy are substantial and evident across the lifespan, and likely to be more common than in other medical disorders, significantly affecting QOL of children and families. Major advances have begun to uncover the potential mediators of neurobehavioural comorbidities in epilepsy, but gaps remain in the early detection, treatment and prevention of these disorders. The imperative is to screen all new-onset cases for comorbidities to facilitate early intervention. Brief and uniform aids are needed to identify individuals at risk for neurobehavioural comorbidities and standardise their access to care. Diagnostic and prognostic tools have to be evidence based and accurate to guide therapeutic decision. From a methodological point of view, investigators and clinicians will have to use the most rigorous approach, for example, prospective retesting of the same group of patients with epilepsy and controls over a fixed period. Longitudinal studies are needed to gain more insight into developmental trajectories and long-term outcomes of psychopathology, cognition, family factors and medical/neurological parameters. Moreover, it is essential to use more specialised scales to measure certain aspects of behavioural problems more accurately and use as many sources as possible. Once the biological basis and the psychosocial context of different epilepsies are better understood, large-scale, prospective and randomised trials are needed to develop epilepsy-specific and individualised treatment options, also including guidelines for pharmacological treatment of comorbidities. It will be important to identify which families need which type of intervention at what point in the epilepsy trajectory.

Management of neurobehavioural comorbidities is warranted as a patient's and his/her family QOL and the patient's outcome may improve, even more than by only reducing seizure frequency.

REFERENCES

Abidin RR (1990) *Parenting Stress Index.* Charlottesville, VA: Pediatric Psychology Press.

Achenbach T (1991) *Manual for the Child Behavior Checklist/4–18 and 1991 Profile.* Burlington, VT: University of Vermont Department of Psychiatry.

Adachi N, Akanuma N, Ito M et al. (2012) Interictal psychotic episodes in epilepsy: Duration and associated clinical factors. *Epilepsia* 53: 1088–1094. doi:10.1111/j.1528-1167.2012.03438.x.

Adachi N, Onuma T, Kato M et al. (2011) Analogy between psychosis antedating epilepsy and epilepsy antedating psychosis. *Epilepsia* 52: 1239–1244. doi:10.1111/j.1528-1167.2011.03039.x.

Adewuya AO and Ola BA (2005) Prevalence of and risk factors for anxiety and depressive disorders in Nigerian adolescents with epilepsy. *Epilepsy Behav* 6: 342–347.

Almane D, Jones JE, Jackson DC, Seidenberg M and Hermann BP (2014) The social competence and behavioral problem substrate of new- and recent-onset childhood epilepsy. *Epilepsy Behav* 31: 91–96. doi:10.1016/j.yebeh.2013.11.018.

Amiet C, Gourfinkel-An I, Bouzamondo A et al. (2008) Epilepsy in autism is associated with intellectual disability and sex: Evidence from a meta-analysis. *Biol Psychiatry* 64: 577–582. doi:10.1016/j.biopsych.2008.04.030.

Angold A, Costello EJ, Pickles A and Winder F (1987) *The Development of a Questionnaire for Use in Epidemiological Studies of Depression in Children and Adolescents.* London: The Medical Research Council, Child Psychiatry Unit.

Austin JK (1996) A model of family adaptation to new-onset childhood epilepsy. *J Neurosci Nurs* 28: 82–92.

Austin JK and Caplan R (2007) Behavioral and psychiatric comorbidities in pediatric epilepsy: Toward an integrative model. *Epilepsia* 48: 1639–1651.

Austin JK, Kakacek JR and Carr D (2010a) Impact of training program on school nurses' confidence levels in managing and supporting students with epilepsy and seizures. *J Sch Nurs* 26: 420–429. doi:10.1177/1059840510380206.

Austin JK, Perkins SM, Johnson CS et al. (2010b) Self-esteem and symptoms of depression in children with seizures: Relationships with neuropsychological functioning and family variables over time. *Epilepsia* 51: 2074–2083. doi:10.1111/j.1528-1167.2010.02575.x.

Austin JK, Perkins SM, Johnson CS et al. (2011) Behavior problems in children at time of first recognized seizure and changes over the following 3 years. *Epilepsy Behav* 21: 373–381. doi:10.1016/j.yebeh.2011.05.028.

Austin JK, Hesdorffer DC, Liverman CT and Schultz AM; Testimony Group (2012) Testimonies submitted for the Institute of Medicine report: Epilepsy across the spectrum: Promoting health and understanding. *Epilepsy Behav* 25: 634–661. doi:10.1016/j.yebeh.2012.10.003.

Baird G, Robinson RO, Boyd S and Charman T (2006) Sleep electroencephalograms in young children with autism with and without regression. *Dev Med Child Neurol* 48: 604–608.

Barry JJ, Ettinger AB, Friel P et al. (2008) Consensus statement: The evaluation and treatment of people with epilepsy and affective disorders. *Epilepsy Behav* 13: 1–29. doi:10.1016/j.yebeh.2008.04.005.

Battaglia A, Parrini B and Tancredi R (2010) The behavioral phenotype of the idic(15) syndrome. *Am J Med Genet C Semin Med Genet* 154C: 448–455. doi:10.1002/ajmg.c.30281.

Baum KT, Byars AW, deGrauw TJ et al. (2010) The effect of temperament and neuropsychological functioning on behavior problems in children with new-onset seizures. *Epilepsy Behav* 17: 467–473. doi:0.1016/j.yebeh.2010.01.010.

Baxendale S and O'Toole A (2007) Epilepsy myths: Alive and foaming in the 21st century. *Epilepsy Behav* 11: 192–196.

Beck AT, Steer RA and Carbin MG (1988) Psychometric properties of the Beck Depression Inventory: Twenty-five years of evaluation. *Clin Psychol Rev* 8: 77–100. doi:10.1016/0272-7358(88)90050-5.

Berg AT (2011) Epilepsy, cognition, and behavior: The clinical picture. *Epilepsia* 52: 7–12. doi:10.1111/j.1528-1167.2010.02905.

Berg AT, Berkovic SF, Brodie MJ et al. (2010) Revised terminology and concepts for organization of seizures and epilepsies: Report of the ILAE Commission on Classification and Terminology, 2005–2009. *Epilepsia* 51: 676–685. doi:10.1111/j.1528-1167.2010.02522.x.

Berg AT, Caplan R and Hesdorffer DC (2011a) Psychiatric and neurodevelopmental disorders in childhood-onset epilepsy. *Epilepsy Behav* 20: 550–555. doi:10.1016/j.yebeh.2010.12.038.

Berg AT, Pardoe HR, Fulbright RK, Schuele SU and Jackson GD (2011b) Hippocampal size anomalies in a community-based cohort with childhood-onset epilepsy. *Neurology* 76: 1415–1421. doi:10.1212/WNL.0b013e318216712b.

Berg AT, Plioplys S and Tuchman R (2011c) Risk and correlates of autism spectrum disorder in children with epilepsy: A community-based study. *J Child Neurol* 26: 540–547. doi:10.1177/0883073810384869.

Berg AT, Smith SN, Frobish D et al. (2005) Special education needs of children with newly diagnosed epilepsy. *Dev Med Child Neurol* 47: 749–753.

Besag FM (2006) Cognitive and behavioral outcomes of epileptic syndromes: Implications for education and clinical practice. *Epilepsia* 47: 119–125.

Betancur C (2011) Etiological heterogeneity in autism spectrum disorders: More than 100 genetic and genomic disorders and still counting. *Brain Res* 1380: 42–77. doi:10.1016/j.brainres.2010.11.078.

Bhise VV, Burack GD and Mandelbaum DE (2009) Baseline cognition, behavior, and motor skills in children with new-onset, idiopathic epilepsy. *Dev Med Child Neurol* 52: 22–26. doi:10.1111/j.1469-8749.2009.03404.x.

Birmaher B, Khetarpal S, Brent D et al. (1997) The Screen for Child Anxiety Related Emotional Disorders (SCARED): Scale construction and psychometric characteristics. *J Am Acad Child Adolesc Psychiatry* 36: 545–553.

Blocher JB, Fujikawa M, Sung C, Jackson DC, and Jones JE (2013) Computer-assisted cognitive behavioral therapy for children with epilepsy and anxiety: A pilot study. *Epilepsy Behav* 27: 70–76. doi:10.1016/j.yebeh.2012.12.014.

Braakman HM, Vaessen MJ, Hofman PA et al. (2011) Cognitive and behavioral complications of frontal lobe epilepsy in children: A review of the literature. *Epilepsia* 52: 849–856. doi:10.1111/j.1528-1167.2011.03057.x.

Brent D, Emslie G, Clarke G et al. (2008) Switching to another SSRI or to venlafaxine with or without cognitive behavioral therapy for adolescents with SSRI resistant depression: The TORDIA randomized controlled trial. *J Am Med Assoc* 299: 901–913.

Brooks-Kayal A (2011) Molecular mechanisms of cognitive and behavioral comorbidities of epilepsy in children. *Epilepsia* 52: 13–20. doi:10.1111/j.1528-1167.2010.02906.x.

Buelow JM, Perkins SM, Johnson CS et al. (2012) Adaptive functioning in children with epilepsy and learning problems. *J Child Neurol* 27: 1241–1249.

Buelow JM and Shore CP (2006) Childhood epilepsy: Failures along the path to diagnosis and treatment. *Epilepsy Behav* 9: 440–447.

Byars AW, deGrauw TJ, Johnson CS et al. (2014) Language and social functioning in children and adolescents with epilepsy. *Epilepsy Behav* 31: 167–171. doi:10.1016/j.yebeh.2013.11.007.

Camfield CS and Camfield PR (2007) Long-term social outcomes for children with epilepsy. *Epilepsia* 48: 3–5.

Camfield C, Breau L and Camfield P (2001) Impact of pediatric epilepsy on the family: A new scale for clinical and research use. *Epilepsia* 42: 104–112.

Caplan R, Sagun J, Siddarth P et al. (2005a) Social competence in pediatric epilepsy: Insights into underlying mechanisms. *Epilepsy Behav* 6: 218–228.

Caplan R, Siddarth P, Gurbani S et al. (2005b) Depression and anxiety disorders in pediatric epilepsy. *Epilepsia* 46: 720–730.

Caplan R, Siddarth P, Bailey CE et al. (2006) Thought disorder: A developmental disability in pediatric epilepsy. *Epilepsy Behav* 8: 726–735.

Caplan R, Levitt J, Siddarth P et al. (2008a) Thought disorder and frontotemporal volumes in pediatric epilepsy. *Epilepsy Behav* 13: 593–599. doi:10.1016/j.yebeh.2008.06.021.

Caplan R, Siddarth P, Stahl L et al. (2008b) Childhood absence epilepsy: Behavioral, cognitive, and linguistic comorbidities. *Epilepsia* 49: 1838–1846. doi:10.1111/j.1528-1167.2008.01680.x.

Cella D, Lai JS, Nowinski CJ et al. (2012) Neuro-QOL: Brief measures of health-related quality of life for clinical research in neurology. *Neurology* 78: 1860–1867. doi:10.1212/WNL.0b013e318258f744.

Chang CC, Lui CC, Lee CC et al. (2012) Clinical significance of serological biomarkers and neuropsychological performances in patients with temporal lobe epilepsy. *BMC Neurol* 14: 12–15. doi:10.1186/1471-2377-12-15.

Cheung C and Wirrell E (2006) Adolescents' perception of epilepsy compared with other chronic diseases: 'through a teenager's eyes'. *J Child Neurol* 21: 214–222.

Chez MG, Chang M, Krasne V et al. (2006) Frequency of epileptiform EEG abnormalities in a sequential screening of autistic patients with no known clinical epilepsy from 1996 to 2005. *Epilepsy Behav* 8: 267–271.

Chin RF, Cumberland PM, Pujar SS et al. (2011) Outcomes of childhood epilepsy at age 33 years: A population-based birth-cohort study. *Epilepsia* 52: 1513–1521. doi:10.1111/j.1528-1167.2011.03170.x.

Choudhary A, Gulati S, Sagar R, Kabra M and Sapra S (2014) Behavioral comorbidity in children and adolescents with epilepsy. *J Clin Neurosci* 21: 1337–1340. doi:10.1016/j.jocn.2013.11.023.

Clary LE, Vander Wal JS and Titus JB (2010) Examining health-related quality of life, adaptive skills, and psychological functioning in children and adolescents with epilepsy presenting for a neuropsychological evaluation. *Epilepsy Behav* 19: 487–493. doi:10.1016/j.yebeh.2010.08.002.

Cleary RA, Thompson PJ, Thom M and Foong J (2013) Postictal psychosis in temporal lobe epilepsy: Risk factors and postsurgical outcome? *Epilepsy Res* 106: 264–272. doi:10.1016/j.eplepsyres.2013.03.015.

Cohen R, Senecky Y, Shuper A et al. (2013) Prevalence of epilepsy and attention-deficit hyperactivity (ADHD) disorder: A population-based study. *J Child Neurol* 28: 120–123. doi:10.1177/0883073812440327.

Colonnelli MC, Cross JH, Davies S et al. (2012) Psychopathology in children before and after surgery for extratemporal lobe epilepsy. *Dev Med Child Neurol* 54: 521–526. doi:10.1111/j.1469-8749.2012.04293.x.

Conners P (1997) *Conners' Rating Scale-Revised (CRS-R)* A.D.D. WareHouse. www.addwarehouse.com

Cramer JA, Westbrook LE, Devinsky O et al. (1999) Development of the quality of life in epilepsy inventory for adolescents: The QOLIE-AD-48. *Epilepsia* 40: 1114–1121.

Cross-Disorder Group of the Psychiatric Genomics Consortium (2013) Identification of risk loci with shared effects on five major psychiatric disorders: A genome-wide analysis. *Lancet* 381: 1371–1379. doi:10.1016/S0140-6736(12)62129-1.

Cushner-Weinstein S, Dassoulas K, Salpekar JA et al. (2008) Parenting stress and childhood epilepsy: The impact of depression, learning, and seizure-related factors. *Epilepsy Behav* 13: 109–114. doi:10.1016/j.yebeh.2008.03.010.

Dafoulis V and Kalyva E (2012) Factors associated with behavioral problems in children with idiopathic epilepsy. *Epilepsy Res* 100: 104–112. doi:10.1016/j.eplepsyres.2012.01.014.

Danielsson S, Viggedal G, Steffenburg S et al. (2009) Psychopathology, psychosocial functioning, and IQ before and after epilepsy surgery in children with drug-resistant epilepsy. *Epilepsy Behav* 14: 330–337. doi:10.1016/j.yebeh.2008.10.023.

Datta SS, Premkumar TS, Chandy S et al. (2005) Behaviour problems in children and adolescents with seizure disorder: Associations and risk factors. *Seizure* 14: 190–197.

Dawson G (2010) Recent advances in research on early detection, causes, biology, and treatment of autism spectrum disorders. *Curr Opin Neurol* 23: 95–96. doi:10.1097/WCO.0b013e3283377644.

Dawson G, Jones EJ, Merkle K et al. (2012) Early behavioral intervention is associated with normalized brain activity in young children with autism. *J Am Acad Child Adolesc Psychiatry* 51: 1150–1159. doi:10.1016/j.jaac.2012.08.018.

Deary IJ, Bastin ME, Pattie A et al. (2006) White matter integrity and cognition in childhood and old age. *Neurology* 66: 505–512.

Deonna T and Roulet E (2006) Autistic spectrum disorder: Evaluating a possible contributing or causal role of epilepsy. *Epilepsia* 47: 79–82.

Doll EA (1965) *Vineland Social Maturity Scale*. American Guidance Service, Circle Pines, MN.

Drewel EH, Bell DJ and Austin JK (2009) Peer difficulties in children with epilepsy: Association with seizure, neuropsychological, academic, and behavioral variables. *Child Neuropsychol* 15: 305–320. doi:10.1080/09297040802537646.

Dunn DW and Kronenberger WG (2005) Childhood epilepsy, attention problems, and ADHD: Review and practical considerations. *Semin Pediatr Neurol* 12: 222–228.

Dunn DW, Austin JK and Perkins SM (2009) Prevalence of psychopathology in childhood epilepsy: Categorical and dimensional measures. *Dev Med Child Neurol* 51: 364–372. doi:10.1111/j.1469-8749.2008.03172.x.

Dunn DW, Johnson CS, Perkins SM et al. (2010) Academic problems in children with seizures: Relationships with neuropsychological functioning and family variables during the 3 years after onset. *Epilepsy Behav* 19: 455–461. doi:10.1016/j.yebeh.2010.08.023.

DuPaul GJ, Power TJ, Anastopoulos AD and Reid R (1998) *ADHD Rating Scale—IV: Checklists, norms, and clinical interpretation.* New York, NY: Guilford Press.

Eddy CM, Rickards HE and Cavanna AE (2012) Behavioral adverse effects of antiepileptic drugs in epilepsy. *J Clin Psychopharmacol* 32: 362–375. doi:10.1097/JCP.0b013e318253a186.

Ekinci O, Titus JB, Rodopman AA, Berkem M and Trevathan E (2009) Depression and anxiety in children and adolescents with epilepsy: Prevalence, risk factors, and treatment. *Epilepsy Behav* 14: 8–18. doi:10.1016/j.yebeh.2008.08.

Eom S, Fisher B, Dezort C and Berg AT (2014) Routine developmental, autism, behavioral, and psychological screening in epilepsy care settings. *Dev Med Child Neurol* 56: 1100–1105. doi:10.1111/dmcn.12497.

Fastenau PS, Jianzhao S, Dunn DW and Austin JK (2008) Academic underachievement among children with epilepsy: Proportion exceeding psychometric criteria for learning disability and associated risk factors. *J Learn Disabil* 41: 195–207. doi:10.1177/0022219408317548.

Fastenau PS, Johnson CS, Perkins SM et al. (2009) Neuropsychological status at seizure onset in children: Risk factors for early cognitive deficits. *Neurology* 73: 526–534. doi:10.1212/WNL.0b013e3181b23551.

Filippini M, Boni A, Giannotta M and Gobbi G (2013) Neuropsychological development in children belonging to BECTS spectrum: Long-term effect of epileptiform activity. *Epilepsy Behav* 28: 504–511. doi:10.1016/j.yebeh.2013.06.016.

Foldvary-Schaefer N and Grigg-Damberger M (2006) Sleep and epilepsy: What we know, don't know, and need to know. *J Clin Neurophysiol* 23: 4–20.

Freilinger M, Reisel B, Reiter E et al. (2006) Behavioral and emotional problems in children with epilepsy. *J Child Neurol* 21: 939–945.

Gershon RC, Lai JS, Bode R et al. (2012) Neuro-QOL: Quality of life item banks for adults with neurological disorders: Item development and calibrations based upon clinical and general population testing. *Qual Life Res* 21: 475–486. doi:10.1007/s11136-011-9958-8.

Georgia H, Cooper PJ and Creswell C (2015) Social communication deficits: Specific associations with Social Anxiety Disorder. *J Affect Disord* 172: 38–42. doi:10.1016/j.jad.2014.09.040.

Gois J, Valente K, Vicentiis S et al. (2011) Assessment of psychosocial adjustment in patients with temporal lobe epilepsy using a standard measure. *Epilepsy Behav* 20: 89–94. doi:10.1016/j.yebeh.2010.10.033.

Goodman R (1997) The strengths and difficulties questionnaire: A research note. *J Child Psychol Psychiatry* 38: 581–586.

Gresham FM and Elliott SN (1990) *Social Skills Rating System Manual.* Circle Pines, MN: AGS.

Halma E, de Louw AJ, Klinkenberg S, Aldenkamp AP and Majoie M (2014) Behavioral side-effects of levetiracetam in children with epilepsy: A systematic review. *Seizure* 23: 685–691. doi:10.1016/j.seizure.2014.06.004.

Hamiwka LD and Wirrell EC (2009) Comorbidities in pediatric epilepsy: Beyond 'just' treating the seizures. *J Child Neurol* 24: 734–742. doi:10.1177/0883073808329527.

Hecimovic H, Santos JM, Carter J et al. (2012) Depression but not seizure factors or quality of life predicts suicidality in epilepsy. *Epilepsy Behav* 24: 426–429. doi:10.1016/j.yebeh.2012.05.005.

Helmstaedter C, Aldenkamp AP, Baker GA et al. (2014) Disentangling the relationship between epilepsy and its behavioral comorbidities - The need for prospective studies in new-onset epilepsies. *Epilepsy Behav* 31: 43–47. doi:10.1016/j.yebeh.2013.11.010.

Hermann B, Jones J, Dabbs K et al. (2007a) The frequency, complications and aetiology of ADHD in new onset paediatric epilepsy. *Brain* 130: 3135–3148.

Hermann B, Seidenberg M, Lee EJ, Chan F and Rutecki P (2007b) Cognitive phenotypes in temporal lobe epilepsy. *J IntNeuropsychol Soc* 13: 12–20.

Hermann B, Seidenberg M, Sager M et al. (2008) Growing old with epilepsy: The neglected issue of cognitive and brain health in aging and elder persons with chronic epilepsy. *Epilepsia* 49: 731–740.

Hermann BP, Jones J, Sheth R and Seidenberg M (2007c) Cognitive and magnetic resonance volumetric abnormalities in new-onset pediatric epilepsy. *Semin Pediatr Neurol* 14: 173–180.

Hesdorffer DC, Caplan R and Berg AT (2012a) Familial clustering of epilepsy and behavioral disorders: Evidence for a shared genetic basis. *Epilepsia* 53: 301–307. doi:10.1111/j.1528-1167.2011.03351.x.

Hesdorffer DC, Hauser WA, Olafsson E, Ludvigsson P and Kjartansson O (2006) Depression and suicide attempt as risk factors for incident unprovoked seizures. *Ann Neurol* 59: 35–41.

Hesdorffer DC, Ishihara L, Mynepalli L et al. (2012b) Epilepsy, suicidality, and psychiatric disorders: A bidirectional association. *Ann Neurol* 72: 184–191. doi:10.1002/ana.23601.

Hoare P and Russell M (1995) The quality of life of children with chronic epilepsy and their families: Preliminary findings with a new assessment measure. *Dev Med Child Neurol* 37: 689–696.

Høie B, Sommerfelt K, Waaler PE et al. (2006) Psychosocial problems and seizure-related factors in children with epilepsy. *Dev Med Child Neurol* 48: 213–219.

Holtmann M, Matei A, Hellmann U et al. (2006) Rolandic spikes increase impulsivity in ADHD - A neuro-psychological pilot study. *Brain Dev* 28: 633–640.

Hysing M, Elgen I, Gillberg C, Lie SA and Lundervold AJ (2007) Chronic physical illness and mental health in children. Results from a large-scale population study. *J Child Psychol Psychiatry* 48: 785–792.

Iseri PK, Ozten E and Aker AT (2006) Posttraumatic stress disorder and major depressive disorder is common in parents of children with epilepsy. *Epilepsy Behav* 8: 250–255.

Jackson DC, Irwin W and Dabbs K (2011) Ventricular enlargement in new-onset pediatric epilepsies. *Epilepsia* 52: 2225–2232.

Jensen V, Rinholm JE, Johansen TJ et al. (2009) N-methyl-D-aspartate receptor subunit dysfunction at hip-pocampal glutamatergic synapses in an animal model of attention-deficit/hyperactivity disorder. *Neuroscience* 158: 353–364. doi:10.1016/j.neuroscience.2008.05.016.

Jones JE, Hermann BP, Barry JJ et al. (2005) Clinical assessment of Axis I psychiatric morbidity in chronic epilepsy: A multicenter investigation. *J Neuropsychiatry Clin Neurosci* 17: 172–179.

Jones JE, Bell B, Fine J et al. (2007) A controlled prospective investigation of psychiatric comorbidity in temporal lobe epilepsy. *Epilepsia* 48: 2357–2360.

Jonsson P, Jonsson B and Eeg-Olofsson O (2014) Psychological and social outcome of epilepsy in well-functioning children and adolescents. A 10-year follow-up study. *Eur J Paediatr Neurol* 18: 381–390. doi:10.1016/j.ejpn.2014.01.010.

Kanner AM, Byrne R, Chicharro A, Wuu J and Frey M (2009) A lifetime psychiatric history predicts a worse seizure outcome following temporal lobectomy. *Neurology* 72: 793–799. doi:10.1212/01.wnl.0000343850.85763.9c.

Kanner AM (2005) Depression in epilepsy: A neurobiologic perspective. *Epilepsy Curr* 5: 21–27.

Kaufman J, Birmaher B, Brent D et al. (1997) Schedule for affective disorders and schizophrenia for school-age children-present and lifetime version (K-SADS-PL): Initial reliability and validity data. *J Am Acad Child Adolesc Psychiatry* 36: 980–988. doi:10.1097/00004583-199707000-00021.

Kerr C, Nixon A and Angalakuditi M (2011a) The impact of epilepsy on children and adult patients' lives: Development of a conceptual model from qualitative literature. *Seizure* 20: 764–774. doi:10.1016/j.seizure.2011.07.007.

Kerr MP, Mensah S, Besag F et al. (2011b) International consensus clinical practice statements for the treatment of neuropsychiatric conditions associated with epilepsy. *Epilepsia* 52: 2133–2138. doi:10.1111/j.1528-1167.2011.03276.x.

Kovacs M (1985) The children's depression, inventory (CDI). *Psychopharmacol Bull* 21: 995–998.

Krishnamoorthy ES (2006) The evaluation of behavioral disturbances in epilepsy. *Epilepsia* 47: 3–8.

Krishnamoorthy ES, Trimble MR and Blumer D (2007) The classification of neuropsychiatric disorders in epilepsy: A proposal by the ILAE Commission on Psychobiology of Epilepsy. *Epilepsy Behav* 10: 349–353.

Lathers CM and Schraeder PL (2006) Stress and sudden death. *Epilepsy Behav* 9: 236–242.

Lin JJ, Mula M and Hermann BP (2012) Uncovering the neurobehavioural comorbidities of epilepsy over the lifespan. *Lancet* 380: 1180–1192. doi:10.1016/S0140-6736(12)61455-X.

Lugo JN, Swann JW and Anderson AE (2014) Early-life seizures result in deficits in social behavior and learning. *Exp Neurol* 256: 74–80. doi:10.1016/j.expneurol.2014.03.014.

Luoni C, Bisulli F, Canevini MP et al. (2011) Determinants of health-related quality of life in pharmacoresistant epilepsy: Results from a large multicenter study of consecutively enrolled patients using validated quantitative assessments. *Epilepsia* 52: 2181–2191. doi:10.1111/j.1528-1167.2011.03325.x.

March JS, Parker JD, Sullivan K, Stallings P and Conners CK (1997) The Multidimensional Anxiety Scale for Children (MASC): Factor structure, reliability, and validity. *J Am Acad Child Adolesc Psychiatry* 36: 554–565.

Martinović Z, Simonović P and Djokić R (2006) Preventing depression in adolescents with epilepsy. *Epilepsy Behav* 9: 619–624.

May TW and Pfäfflin M (2002) The efficacy of an educational treatment program for patients with epilepsy (MOSES): Results of a controlled, randomized study. *Epilepsia* 43: 539–549.

McAfee AT, Chilcott KE, Johannes CB et al. (2007) The incidence of first provoked and unprovoked seizure in pediatric patients with and without psychiatric diagnoses. *Epilepsia* 48: 1075–1082.

McCagh J, Fisk JE and Baker GA (2009) Epilepsy, psychosocial and cognitive functioning. *Epilepsy Res* 86: 1–14. doi:10.1016/j.eplepsyres.2009.04.007.

McLellan A, Davies S, Heyman I et al. (2005) Psychopathology in children with epilepsy before and after temporal lobe resection. *Dev Med Child Neurol* 47: 666–672.

Micallef S, Spooner CG, Harvey AS, Wrennall JA and Wilson SJ (2010) Psychological outcome profiles in childhood-onset temporal lobe epilepsy. *Epilepsia* 51: 2066–2073. doi:10.1111/j.1528-1167.2010.02664.x.

Mikati MA, Ataya NF, El-Ferezli JC et al. (2009) Quality of life after vagal nerve stimulator insertion. *Epileptic Disord* 11: 67–74. doi:10.1684/epd.2009.0244.

Moschetta S, Fiore LA, Fuentes D, Gois J and Valente KD (2011) Personality traits in patients with juvenile myoclonic epilepsy. *Epilepsy Behav* 21: 473–477. doi:10.1016/j.yebeh.2011.03.036.

Mula M, Hesdorffer DC, Trimble M and Sander JW (2009) The role of titration schedule of topiramate for the development of depression in patients with epilepsy. *Epilepsia* 50: 1072–1076. doi:10.1111/j.1528-1167.2008.01799.x.

Mula M, Jauch R, Cavanna A et al. (2008a) Clinical and psychopathological definition of the interictal dysphoric disorder of epilepsy. *Epilepsia* 49: 650–666.

Mula M, Schmitz B, Jauch R et al. (2008b) On the prevalence of bipolar disorder in epilepsy. *Epilepsy Behav* 13: 658–661. doi:10.1016/j.yebeh.2008.08.002.

Nickels K and Wirrell E (2008) Electrical status epilepticus in sleep. *Semin Pediatr Neurol* 15: 50–60. doi:10.1016/j.spen.2008.03.002.

Nicolai J, Ebus S, Biemans DP et al. (2012) The cognitive effects of interictal epileptiform EEG discharges and short nonconvulsive epileptic seizures. *Epilepsia* 53: 1051–1059. doi:10.1111/j.1528-1167.2012.03491.x.

Nishida T, Kudo T, Nakamura F et al. (2005) Postictal mania associated with frontal lobe epilepsy. *Epilepsy Behav* 6: 102–110.

Noeker M, Haverkamp-Krois A and Haverkamp F (2005) Development of mental health dysfunction in childhood epilepsy. *Brain Dev* 27: 5–16.

Northcott E, Connolly AM, Berroya A et al. (2005) The neuropsychological and language profile of children with benign rolandic epilepsy. *Epilepsia* 46: 924–930.

Oostrom KJ, van Teeseling H, Smeets-Schouten A et al. (2005) Three to four years after diagnosis: Cognition and behaviour in children with 'epilepsy only'. A prospective, controlled study. *Brain* 128: 1546–1555.

Parisi P, Moavero R, Verrotti A and Curatolo P (2010) Attention deficit hyperactivity disorder in children with epilepsy. *Brain Dev* 32: 10–16. doi:10.1016/j.braindev.2009.03.005.

Pavuluri MN, Yang S, Kamineni K et al. (2009) Diffusion tensor imaging study of white matter fiber tracts in pediatric bipolar disorder and attention-deficit/hyperactivity disorder. *Biol Psychiatry* 65: 586–593. doi:10.1016/j.biopsych.2008.10.015.

Pereira A and Valente KD (2013) Severity of depressive symptomatology and functional impairment in children and adolescents with temporal lobe epilepsy. *Seizure* 22: 708–712. doi:10.1016/j.seizure.2013.05.008.

Pfäfflin M, Petermann F, Rau J and May TW (2012) The psychoeducational program for children with epilepsy and their parents (FAMOSES): Results of a controlled pilot study and a survey of parent satisfaction over a five-year period. *Epilepsy Behav* 25: 11–16. doi:10.1016/j.yebeh.2012.06.012.

Pineda E, Jentsch JD, Shin D et al. (2014) Behavioral impairments in rats with chronic epilepsy suggest comorbidity between epilepsy and attention deficit/hyperactivity disorder. *Epilepsy Behav* 31: 267–275. doi:10.1016/j.yebeh.2013.10.004.

Pineda E, Shin D, Sankar R and Mazarati AM (2010) Comorbidity between epilepsy and depression: Experimental evidence for the involvement of serotonergic, glucocorticoid, and neuroinflammatory mechanisms. *Epilepsia* 51: 110–114. doi:10.1111/j.1528-1167.2010.02623.x.

Poznanski E and Mokros H (1996) *Children's Depression Rating Scale–Revised (CDRS-R)*. Los Angeles: WPS.

Prévost J, Lortie A, Nguyen D, Lassonde M and Carmant L (2006) Nonlesional frontal lobe epilepsy (FLE) of childhood: Clinical presentation, response to treatment and comorbidity. *Epilepsia* 47: 2198–2201.

Rantanen K, Timonen S, Hagström K et al. (2009) Social competence of preschool children with epilepsy. *Epilepsy Behav* 14: 338–343. doi:10.1016/j.yebeh.2008.10.022.

Rantanen K, Nieminen P and Eriksson K (2010) Neurocognitive functioning of preschool children with uncomplicated epilepsy. *J Neuropsychol* 4: 71–87. doi:10.1348/174866409X451465.

Rantanen K, Eriksson K and Nieminen P (2012) Social competence in children with epilepsy – A review. *Epilepsy Behav* 24: 295–303. doi:10.1016/j.yebeh.2012.04.117.

Reilly CJ (2011) Attention deficit hyperactivity disorder (ADHD) in childhood epilepsy. *Res Dev Disabil* 32: 883–893. doi:10.1016/j.ridd.2011.01.019.

Reilly C, Atkinson P, Das KB et al. (2014) Neurobehavioral comorbidities in children with active epilepsy: A population-based study. *Pediatrics* 133: 1586–1593. doi:10.1542/peds.2013-3787.

Reynolds CR and Kamphaus RW (2004) *Behavior Assessment System for Children—Second edition (BASC-2)*. Circle Pines, MN: AGS.

Reynolds CR and Richmond BO (1985) *Revised Children's Manifest Anxiety Scale. RCMAS Manual.* Los Angeles: Western Psychological Services.

Riley JD, Franklin DL, Choi V et al. (2010) Altered white matter integrity in temporal lobe epilepsy: Association with cognitive and clinical profiles. *Epilepsia* 51: 536–545. doi:10.1111/j.1528-1167.2009.02508.x.

Roberts NA and Reuber M (2014) Alterations of consciousness in psychogenic nonepileptic seizures: Emotion, emotion regulation and dissociation. *Epilepsy Behav* 30: 43–49. doi:0.1016/j.yebeh.2013.09.035.

Robins DL, Fein D and Barton ML (1999) *The Modified Checklist for Autism in Toddlers (M-CHAT)*. Storrs, CT: Self-published.

Robinson SJ (2012) Childhood epilepsy and autism spectrum disorders: Psychiatric problems, phenotypic expression, and anticonvulsants. *Neuropsychol Rev* 22: 271–279. doi:10.1007/s11065-012-9212-3.

Rodenburg R, Stams GJ, Meijer AM, Aldenkamp AP and Deković M (2005) Psychopathology in children with epilepsy: A meta-analysis. *J PediatrPsychol* 30: 453–468.

Rodenburg R, Marie A, Deković M and Aldenkamp AP (2006) Family predictors of psychopathology in children with epilepsy. *Epilepsia* 47: 601–614.

Rodenburg R, Wagner JL, Austin JK, Kerr M and Dunn DW (2011) Psychosocial issues for children with epilepsy. *Epilepsy Behav* 22: 47–54. doi:10.1016/j.yebeh.2011.04.063.

Russ SA, Larson K and Halfon N (2012) A national profile of childhood epilepsy and seizure disorder. *Pediatrics* 129: 256–264. doi:10.1542/peds.2010-1371.

Ryvlin P, Rheims S and Risse G (2006) Nocturnal frontal lobe epilepsy. *Epilepsia* 47: 83–86. Review.

Rzezak P, Fuentes D, Guimarães CA et al. (2007) Frontal lobe dysfunction in children with temporal lobe epilepsy. *Pediatr Neurol* 37: 176–185.

Sabaz M, Cairns DR, Lawson JA et al. (2000) Validation of a new quality of life measure for children with epilepsy. *Epilepsia* 41: 765–774.

Salpekar JA and Dunn DW (2007) Psychiatric and psychosocial consequences of pediatric epilepsy. *Semin Pediatr Neurol* 14: 181–188.

Salpekar JA and Mishra G (2014) Key issues in addressing the comorbidity of attention deficit hyperactivity disorder and pediatric epilepsy. *Epilepsy Behav* 37: 310–315. doi:10.1016/j.yebeh.2014.04.021.

Schacher M, Winkler R, Grunwald T et al. (2006) Mesial temporal lobe epilepsy impairs advanced social cognition. *Epilepsia* 47: 2141–2146.

Schmitz B (2005) Depression and mania in patients with epilepsy. *Epilepsia* 46: 45–49.

Shaffer D, Fisher P, Lucas C, Dulcan M and Schwab-Stone M (2000) NIMH Diagnostic Interview Schedule for Children, Version IV (NIMH DISC-IV): Description, differences from previous versions, and reliability of some common diagnoses. *J Am Acad Child Adolesc Psychiatry* 39: 28–38.

Shaffer D, Gould MS and Brasic J (1983) A children's global assessment scale (CGAS). *Arch Gen Psychiatry* 40: 1228–1231.

Sillanpää M and Cross JH (2009) The psychosocial impact of epilepsy in childhood. *Epilepsy Behav* 15: 5–10. doi:10.1016/j.yebeh.2009.03.007.

Sillanpää M and Shinnar S (2010) Long-term mortality in childhood-onset epilepsy. *N Engl J Med* 363: 2522–2529. doi:10.1056/NEJMoa0911610.

Sinclair DB and Snyder T (2008) Psychosis with frontal lobe epilepsy responds to carbamazepine. *J Child Neurol* 23: 431–434. doi:10.1177/0883073807307107.

Socanski D, Aurlien D, Herigstad A, Thomsen PH and Larsen TK (2013) Epilepsy in a large cohort of children diagnosed with attention deficit/hyperactivity disorders (ADHD). *Seizure* 22: 651–655. doi:10.1016/j.seizure.2013.04.021.

Sprafkin J, Gadow K, Salisbury H, Schneider J and Loney J (2002) Further evidence of reliability and validity of the child symptom inventory-4: Parent checklist in clinically referred boys. *J Clin Child Adolesc Psychol* 31: 513–524. doi:10.1207/S15374424JCCP3104_10.

Sumer MM, Atik L, Unal A, Emre U and Atasoy HT (2007) Frontal lobe epilepsy presented as ictal aggression. *Neurol Sci* 28: 48–51.

Tassinari CA, Cantalupo G, Rios-Pohl L, Giustina ED and Rubboli G (2009) Encephalopathy with status epilepticus during slow sleep: 'the Penelope syndrome'. *Epilepsia* 50: 4–8. doi:10.1111/j.1528-1167. 2009.02209.x.

Tosun D, Dabbs K, Caplan R et al. (2011) Deformation-based morphometry of prospective neurodevelopmental changes in new onset paediatric epilepsy. *Brain* 134: 1003–1014. doi:10.1093/brain/awr027.

Tse E, Hamiwka L, Sherman EM and Wirrell E (2007) Social skills problems in children with epilepsy: Prevalence, nature and predictors. *Epilepsy Behav* 11: 499–505.

Tuchman R, Hirtz D, Mamounas LA (2013) NINDS epilepsy and autism spectrum disorders workshop report. *Neurology* 81: 1630–1636. doi:10.1212/WNL.0b013e3182a9f482. Review.

Uldall P, Alving J, Hansen LK, Kibaek M and Buchholt J (2006) The misdiagnosis of epilepsy in children admitted to a tertiary epilepsy centre with paroxysmal events. *Arch Dis Child* 91: 219–221.

Vega C, Guo J, Killory B et al. (2011) Symptoms of anxiety and depression in childhood absence epilepsy. *Epilepsia* 52: 70–74. doi:10.1111/j.1528-1167.2011.03119.x.

Wagner JL, Smith GM, Ferguson PL and Wannamaker BB (2009) Caregiver perceptions of seizure severity in pediatric epilepsy. *Epilepsia* 50: 2102–2109. doi:10.1111/j.1528-1167.2009.02146.x.

Wichaidit BT, Ostergaard JR and Rask CU (2014) Diagnostic practice of psychogenic nonepileptic seizures (PNES) in the pediatric setting. *Epilepsia*. doi:10.1111/epi.12881.

Wilson SJ, Bladin PF, Saling MM and Pattison PE (2005) Characterizing psychosocial outcome trajectories following seizure surgery. *Epilepsy Behav* 6: 570–580.

Wirrell EC, Wood L, Hamiwka LD and Sherman EM (2008) Parenting stress in mothers of children with intractable epilepsy. *Epilepsy Behav* 13: 169–173. doi:10.1016/j.yebeh.2008.02.011.

Wolff M, Cassé-Perrot C and Dravet C (2008) Severe myoclonic epilepsy of infants (Dravet syndrome): Natural history and neuropsychological findings. *Epilepsia* 47: 45–48.

Woolfenden S, Sarkozy V, Ridley G, Coory M and Williams K (2012) A systematic review of two outcomes in autism spectrum disorder - Epilepsy and mortality. *Dev Med Child Neurol* 54: 306–312. doi:10.1111/j.1469-8749.2012.04223.x.

Wotton CJ and Goldacre MJ (2012) Coexistence of schizophrenia and epilepsy: Record-linkage studies. *Epilepsia* 53: 71–74. doi:190.1111/j.1528-1167.2011.03390.x.

Wrench JM, Wilson SJ, O'Shea MF and Reutens DC (2009) Characterising de novo depression after epilepsy surgery. *Epilepsy Res* 83: 81–88. doi:10.1016/j.eplepsyres.2008.09.007.

Zamponi N, Passamonti C, Cesaroni E, Trignani R and Rychlicki F (2011) Effectiveness of vagal nerve stimulation (VNS) in patients with drop-attacks and different epileptic syndromes. *Seizure* 20: 468–474. doi:10.1016/j.seizure.2011.02.011.

4
THE INTERACTION BETWEEN CHILDHOOD-ONSET EPILEPSY AND COGNITION: LONG-TERM FOLLOW UP

Peter Camfield and Carol Camfield

Introduction

The long-term outcome of childhood epilepsy has two main themes: seizure remission and social success. Seizure outcome is generally straightforward and is typically defined at the end of follow-up as a terminal remission from seizures for several years, persistent infrequent seizures despite treatment, and intractable epilepsy. Social outcome is more complex and depends on many factors including the culture where the person lives and cognitive ability. Few studies have specifically addressed the issue of long-term cognitive outcome for children with epilepsy. There is no standard definition for long-term – publications have used this honorific concept with definitions ranging from 1 year all the way to 50 years. For this chapter we have only included studies with a follow-up of greater than 3 years.

Cognitive outcome and seizure outcome may have a bidirectional effect. Cognitive problems at the onset of epilepsy influence the likelihood of seizure remission. Presumably an unsatisfactory evolution of seizures is not caused by cognitive difficulties; rather cognitive difficulties are associated with more severe brain difficulties that somehow render seizure remission less likely. Seizures or the accompanying EEG discharges may influence brain development leading to long-term cognitive difficulties or actual damage to the brain causing deteriorating cognitive function.

Cognitive difficulties lie along a spectrum from mild specific learning problems with preserved overall intelligence to profound intellectual disability. The term "learning disorder" is problematic because in some parts of the world it implies intellectual disability (mental impairment) and in others, normal overall intelligence with a specific learning problem. In this chapter, we will use intellectual disability to mean "mental impairment" or an IQ < 70. Very little literature has explored specific learning problems as a long-term cognitive outcome for childhood epilepsy.

Population-based studies that establish that long-term cognitive deterioration is uncommon

The US National Collaborative Perinatal Project followed approximately 55 000 children from the prenatal period to age 7 years. There were 83 children who had standardized psychometric assessments before 4 years of age followed by one or more seizures between age 4 and 7 years and then repeat psychometric testing at age 7 (Ellenberg et al. 1986). Half of this group had three or more seizures although the exact number of seizures was not always clear. There was no decline or gain in IQ between the two assessments indicating that a modest number of seizures had no effect on cognitive outcome. This conclusion was unchanged even for children who had an episode of status epilepticus.

By contrast, the Connecticut study explored adaptive behavior in a more selected group of children who had epilepsy with onset before 3 years of age (Berg et al. 2004). Of 613 patients in the cohort, 172 (28%) fulfilled this age criterion and had at least 3 years of follow-up. Because of their age and coexistent neurological problems, standard psychometric assessment was deemed infeasible. The authors used the Vineland Scales of Adaptive Behavior (VABS) as a proxy for intellectual assessment and repeated this assessment on an annual basis. Fifty of the children with epilepsy onset before 3 years were considered to have an epileptic encephalopathy. Overall, there was a decline in VABS scores over the 3-year follow-up. The decline was almost exclusively in children with remote symptomatic etiology or epileptic encephalopathy or intractable epilepsy. At baseline these special patients already had below average VABS scores and over time their scores fell further away from normal. Those with all three of these factors were of special concern and showed an average decline in VABS scores of 12 points/year. It is not clear if the decline represents actual developmental deterioration or failure to progress because VABS scores are based on age. A child who makes no developmental gains between 1 and 3 years of age would have a significant decline in VABS scores. Approximately 75% of the 172 patients did not have remote symptomatic etiology, epileptic encephalopathy, or intractable epilepsy, and as a group they showed no decline. Although the follow-up in this study is not very long, it does suggest that very severe epilepsy starting before age 3 years may have a serious effect on cognition.

Clinic-based studies of children with mixed epilepsy syndromes that establish that cognitive deterioration is uncommon

Only a few studies have used standardized measures of cognition at the time of diagnosis of epilepsy in children and then compared the results with standardized testing after follow-up. Approximately 25% of children with epilepsy have seizure onset in the first 2 years of life when standard testing is either not possible or only loosely associated with later cognitive skills (Camfield et al. 1996). Therefore, outcome studies with pre- and postcognitive testing only apply to older children.

One of the first of these studies was carried out in the United States. Seventy-two children with epilepsy were tested within 2 weeks of diagnosis and then annually for 4 years (Bourgeois et al. 1983). IQ decreased by 10 points or more in 11%, increased in 17%, fluctuated 40%, and did not change in 32%. The number of seizures did not predict a decrease in IQ. The strongest predictors were antiepileptic drug (AED) intoxication and younger age at onset.

A Dutch study enrolled 42 children with "epilepsy only" shortly after diagnosis and before AED treatment (Oostrom et al. 2005). They were compared with 30 classmate controls matched for sex. Baseline neuropsychology testing showed poorer function in the children with epilepsy, but there was no group deterioration when they were retested 3.5 years later. Poor academic and social success was related to parental dysfunction and not to epilepsy variables such as seizure type and frequency or AED burden.

A further US study documented academic achievement in 98 school children with recent onset of epilepsy compared with 96 children with asthma (McNelis et al. 2007). Not unexpectedly, at baseline and 4 years later, those with epilepsy had poorer academic performance in all five areas assessed – Composite, Reading, Mathematics, Language, and Vocabulary. Children with high severity epilepsy had the lowest levels of academic achievement; however, there was no evidence of deterioration over time in any of the groups of children with epilepsy.

Based on these studies, it is safe to conclude that cognitive abilities do not deteriorate over 4 to 5 years in the vast majority of children with epilepsy. Cognitive deficits persist if they are present at epilepsy onset. The cognitive profile at onset is the cognitive profile at follow-up.

Case series of specific epilepsy syndromes reporting cognitive outcome but without baseline assessment

Individual epilepsy syndromes are dealt with in greater detail in other chapters in this book. Here, we provide a brief review of publications about long-term cognitive outcome for individual epilepsy syndromes but only if the study included standard psychometric testing of at least 20 patients with $\geq$ 3 years of follow-up. To identify relevant publications we searched in PubMed with the name of each syndrome from the International League Against Epilepsy 2010 epilepsy syndrome list coupled with "cognitive outcome." We reviewed the abstracts and then the papers if they seemed relevant. We also reviewed the reference lists for each selected paper to search for other relevant papers. We did not undertake a formal systematic review, and we hope that we have not overlooked important studies.

BENIGN MYOCLONIC EPILEPSY OF INFANCY

A retrospective Argentinean study described 38 patients with benign myoclonic epilepsy of infancy (brief generalized myoclonic seizures associated with generalized spike-wave EEG paroxysms without other seizure types occurring in the first 3 years of life in developmentally normal children) (Caraballo et al. 2013). After a mean follow-up of 13.5 years, 32 had normal neuropsychological evaluations. Two children had cognitive impairment (IQ 60 and 63) and four had significant learning impairment coupled with attention deficit hyperactivity disorder.

A multicentered study from France included 20 children with the onset of myoclonic epilepsy of infancy at a median age of 12 months with follow-up at a median age of 9 years (Auvin et al. 2006). At follow-up one of the following neuropsychological studies was carried out: Brunet–Lezine scale, Wechsler Intelligence Scale for Preschool and Primary Children (WIPPSI-R), Wechsler Intelligence Scale for Children, 3rd edition (WISC-III), Wechsler Intelligence Scale for Adults (WAIS), and VABS. In 85% the assessment was normal, but one had mild intellectual disability and two had severe.

MYOCLONIC ASTATIC EPILEPSY

An Italian clinic reported their longitudinal experience with 18 patients with myoclonic astatic epilepsy (Trivisano et al. 2011). Age at onset averaged 3.6±0.7 years and follow-up was 6.5±2.9 years later. At the end of follow-up, there was a wide range in intellectual ability: 67% had a normal IQ, 17% borderline, 22% mild intellectual disability, and 5% moderate intellectual disability. Details of the clinical course did not predict the intellectual outcome, although the small sample size precluded statistical modeling.

WEST SYNDROME

Although a number of studies have addressed the intellectual outcome of children with West syndrome (infantile spasms plus hypsarrhythmia), the largest study with the longest follow-up is from Finland (Riikonen 1996). Of 214 children with a diagnosis of West syndrome who were born between 1960 and 1976 and followed at the Children's Hospital, University of Helsinki, 147 survivors were assessed at a mean age of 25.6 years. The intelligence quotient at the end of follow-up was greater than 80 in 17%, 60–80 in 6.5%, 40–60 in 25%, and less than 40 in 51%.

Childhood absence epilepsy with onset less than 3 years of age

A retrospective Italian study from 8 academic centers identified 40 unusual children with the onset of absence seizures before the age of 3 years (Verrotti et al. 2011). Age at follow-up ranged from 5.1 to 15.8 years. Thirty-four were said to be of normal intelligence although it is not clear if all of these children had formal psychometric testing. Of the remaining 6, IQ ranged from 60 to 71.

DRAVET SYNDROME

An Italian multicentered study followed 26 patients with Dravet syndrome from diagnosis to ages 5 to 19 years (Ragona et al. 2011). Testing with either Griffiths Scale or Wechsler Preschool Primary Scale of Intelligence (according to the child's age and level of cooperation) was completed within 12 months of diagnosis and again before they reached 5 years of age. All children had a decrease in global developmental quotient from baseline to second testing. The decrease varied widely with a mean of 33 points (range 6–77 points). No correlation was found between the severity of epilepsy and cognitive outcome and prolonged convulsive seizures or status epilepticus. Of course, virtually all patients with Dravet syndrome have these severe seizures.

Thirty-one patients with Dravet syndrome (14 with typical Dravet syndrome, and 17 with borderline Dravet syndrome) were followed up at a mean age of 24 years (range 18–43 years) in Japan (Akiyama et al. 2010).

One had borderline IQ and could live independently, four were testable, and each had an IQ < 40. The remaining 26 were untestable with severe intellectual disability. Less severe intellectual disability was correlated with the presence of occipital alpha rhythms in the background activity of the follow-up EEGs, whereas the lack of occipital alpha rhythms correlated with severe intellectual disability. The authors suggested that slow EEG background represents underlying brain dysfunction.

A second Japanese study of 44 patients with typical Dravet syndrome and 20 with atypical Dravet syndrome was followed for more than 10 years (Takayama et al. 2014). Individuals included were older than 19 years (median 34 years) with a median follow-up age of 24 years. Intellectual disability was observed in all patients with Dravet syndrome: severe in 49 patients (76.5%), moderate in 12 patients (18.8%), and mild in three patients (4.7%), with most patients having severe intellectual disability. Among the 44 patients with typical Dravet syndrome, intellectual disability was moderate in 8 patients and severe in 36 patients. No patient had mild intellectual disability. On the other hand, among 20 patients with atypical Dravet syndrome, there were 3 with mild, 4 with moderate, and 13 with severe intellectual disability. Overall, those with atypical Dravet syndrome tended to have milder intellectual disability compared to those with typical Dravet syndrome ($p = 0.03$). Interestingly, those with more severe cognitive delay had a higher frequency of generalized tonic clonic seizures ($p = 0.002$). As in the study summarized above, occipital alpha rhythms were associated with milder intellectual disability than those with none ($p = 0.009$).

LENNOX-GASTAUT SYNDROME

A retrospective study from France and Denmark examined the adult outcome (age 40–59 years) of 27 "consecutive" adult patients with Lennox-Gastaut syndrome who had received this diagnosis between 5 and 10 years of age and had medical records available at the respective hospitals (Ferlazzo et al. 2010). It is unclear what "consecutive" meant and how many patients did not have early diagnosis. The authors noted: "Neuropsychological evaluation was based on assessment of verbal and performance intelligence by means of Wechsler Intelligence Scale for Children or Wechsler Adult Intelligence Scale, although in most patients intellectual disability was too severe to allow formal testing." Of the 27, 26 were found to have moderate-to-severe intellectual disability "at last observation." One woman had mild cognitive impairment although her case description might allow some doubt about the diagnosis.

CONTINUOUS SPIKE WAVE IN SLOW SLEEP AND ENCEPHALOPATHY WITH STATUS EPILEPTICUS IN SLEEP

There are many small case series of continuous spike wave in slow sleep (CSWS) or encephalopathy with status epilepticus in sleep (ESES) with short follow-up. The most comprehensive study that we encountered is from Helsinki, Finland (Liukkonen et al. 2010). Thirty-two cases with various etiologies were identified from a single video EEG center and followed for at least 3 years. The mean age at onset was 3.1 years (range 0.4–7.6 years) and 13 had standard psychological assessments before the onset of ESES. Twenty-eight had several neuropsychological assessments after diagnosis with the last one at 4.5–18 years of age. Cognitive outcome was good in 10 (pre-ESES cognitive level was regained), moderate in 7 (mild decrement in IQ), and poor in 14 (deterioration in IQ). Overall 22 had an "unfavorable outcome." Favorable outcome was associated with a prompt EEG response to AED treatment.

ROLANDIC EPILEPSY

A variety of studies have established that approximately 20–40% of children with rolandic epilepsy have measurable neuropsychological problems detectable within a few years of diagnosis. These problems vary from study to study but tend to be correlated with EEG spike frequency, especially during sleep. Few studies have examined the long-term outcome. An Italian study of 33 children with rolandic epilepsy found some persistence of verbal deficits during a 2- to 8-year follow-up (Filippini et al. 2013). Others have suggested that these cognitive problems may improve over time (Kavros et al. 2008). We have argued that if there are transient or even persistent cognitive deficits, they have little functional importance in adult life (Camfield and Camfield 2014).

TEMPORAL LOBE EPILEPSY

An Australian community-based study from the State of Victoria identified 54 patients with the onset of temporal lobe epilepsy with a mean age at onset of 6±4 years (Wilson et al. 2012). Patients were followed up when they had a mean age of 20±4.1 years with a minimum of 11 years. At the end of follow-up, they underwent an Austin Comprehensive Epilepsy Program Interview that assesses (1) academic achievement, (2) peer social competence, and (3) independence. For patients in late adolescence (16–18 years) and young adulthood (19–30 years), two additional domains were assessed: (4) occupational achievement and (5) relationship status. In addition, at follow-up 36 patients had a neuropsychological evaluation. Overall 28 (52%) had a normal developmental trajectory, 20 (37%) had an "altered" developmental trajectory, and 6 (11%) were considered "delayed." The normal group had epilepsy for fewer years and was more likely to be seizure free at follow-up. Overall there was a high correlation between the developmental trajectory and the neuropsychological function, especially full-scale IQ.

JUVENILE MYOCLONIC EPILEPSY

Fifty patients with juvenile myoclonic epilepsy (JME) from São Paulo, Brazil, underwent neuropsychological testing and were compared with controls matched for age, sex, and educational achievement (Pascalicchio et al. 2007). The duration of epilepsy prior to testing was less than 10 years in 21, 11–19 years in 19, and greater than 20 years in 10. The age at onset was not specified but all were at least 17 years of age when tested. As a group those with JME scored significantly below controls on "measures of attention, immediate verbal memory, cognitive flexibility, control of inhibition, working memory, processing speed, verbal delayed memory, visual delayed memory, naming, and verbal fluency."

Another study from Turkey compared 35 patients with JME with 35 controls who did not have epilepsy and were matched for age and educational achievement (Sonmez et al. 2004). The duration of seizures in the JME group averaged 7 years. Neuropsychological testing found that patients with JME had preserved overall intelligence but had impaired verbal and visual memory, were less capable on visuospatial tests, and showed several problems on frontal lobe tests.

Epilepsy syndromes without studies addressing long-term cognitive outcome (based on our selection criteria and search strategy)

Childhood absence epilepsy
Juvenile absence epilepsy
Panayiotopoulos syndrome
Autosomal dominant nocturnal frontal epilepsy
Epilepsy with myoclonic absences
Late onset childhood occipital epilepsy (Gastaut type)
Epilepsy with myoclonic absences
Epilepsy with generalized tonic–clonic seizures alone
Autosomal dominant epilepsy with auditory features
Familial focal epilepsy with variable foci (childhood to adult)
Reflex epilepsies

Population-based studies of incidence cases that have investigated cognitive function as a predictor/correlate of epilepsy outcome

Several population-based studies have studied the influence of cognitive function on long-term seizure remission. On the basis of the literature reviewed above, we have assumed that most children with epilepsy do not have cognitive decline during follow-up. We have restricted this review to studies of incidence cases. Prevalence cases always have an over-representation of severe epilepsies.

The Connecticut study is close to population-based and recruited 613 patients from pediatric neurologists from a regional area (Berg et al. 2008). All patients had newly diagnosed epilepsy and the cohort included the full spectrum of epileptic syndromes, causes, and severities. Approximately 8–9 years after seizure onset, 66% had a psychometric assessment (55% for the study protocol and 11% in another setting). The distribution of IQ scores was as follows: normal 73.6%, mild intellectual disability 3.4%, moderate–severe 7.3%, neurologically devastated 4.7%, untestable but impaired 5.9%. Overall 26.4% were said to have "subnormal intelligence." The level of intellectual function was associated with remission. Terminal remission of 5 years or more was noted with normal intelligence in 59%, mild intellectual disability 33%, moderate–severe 22%, neurologically devastated 3%, and untestable but impaired 28%.

The Nova Scotia population-based study of children with new onset epilepsy (incidence cases) included 504 with epilepsies characterized by convulsive and focal seizures. In this group of patients over the next 7 years, 55% entered remission (seizure-free and no longer receiving AED medications) (Camfield et al. 1993a). Multivariate predictive modeling found that intellectual disability was an independent predictor of lack of remission along with age at onset greater than 12 years, neonatal seizures, and greater than 21 seizures before treatment.

The overall Nova Scotia Cohort including all types of epilepsies was composed of 692 patients. Twenty-one percent had intellectual disability (Camfield and Camfield 2007). During an average follow-up of greater than 21 years, 29 (20%) of those with intellectual disability died, all from causes related to their comorbid neurological disorder rather than the seizures. Overall only 36% of survivors with intellectual disability were in remission at the end of follow-up and 39% were considered to have intractable epilepsy (Camfield unpublished data). Approximately 56% of those with intellectual disability had epilepsy syndromes grouped under the umbrella term of "symptomatic generalized epilepsy (SGE)," whereas 40% had focal epilepsies. At the end of follow-up for survivors, the remission rate for those with SGE was 25% and for those with focal epilepsy 44%. Children with focal epilepsy and mild intellectual disability (IQ 50–69) had a remission rate of 52%, which was statistically the same as the remission rate for children with normal intelligence and focal epilepsy (68%).

A population-based cohort of children with epilepsy from Turku, Finland, has been followed for 30–40 years. The cohort contains a mixture of incidence and prevalence cases. Of 242 cases in the cohort, 92 (38%) had intellectual disability of whom 54% had at least 5 years' remission (with or without medication) compared with approximately 80% of those with normal intelligence (Sillanpää et al. 1998; Sillanpää 2004).

The Dutch study of childhood epilepsy identified 413 children with newly diagnosed epilepsy. The study is not quite population-based but case evaluation was very comprehensive. In that study, intellectual disability was sufficient in itself for a diagnosis of "remote symptomatic etiology" (Arts et al. 2004). With a 5- and 15-year follow-up, intellectual disability was not an independent predictor of outcome; however, remote symptomatic etiology was strongly predictive (Arts et al. 2004; Geerts et al. 2010). When the Dutch study was combined with the Nova Scotia study, intellectual disability was considered separately from remote symptomatic etiology and was found to be a strong predictor of seizure outcome in multivariate analysis (Geelhoed et al. 2005).

A retrospective population-based study was reported from the catchment area of Uwajima City Hospital in Japan (Wakamoto et al. 2000). All patients had new onset epilepsy and follow-up was up to 20 years. Of 148 survivors, 62.5% were in remission at the end of follow-up. Remission for those with normal intelligence was 75.8% but only 36.7% for those with intellectual disability.

Based on these population-based studies, it is very clear that children with epilepsy and intellectual disability are one third to one half less likely to have seizure remission over 5–30 years of follow-up compared with children with normal intelligence. This explains why prevalence studies of childhood epilepsy show a higher rate of intellectual disability than incidence studies.

Social outcome and cognition

Very few studies have addressed the relationship between cognitive abilities and social outcome. The UK study followed 17 414 children born in 1 week in the United Kingdom in 1958 (Chin et al. 2011). One hundred and one developed epilepsy and 66 were still followed in the study at age 33 years. Those with cognitive scores in the lowest quintile had more social difficulties. Of special interest, those in the cohort with cognitive scores in the lowest quintile but without epilepsy had better social outcomes than those with epilepsy.

The Finnish study of Dr. Sillanpaa described above investigated social outcome for 242 patients followed for 45 years (Sillanpaa 2004). Psychometric testing divided patients into five categories – normal (IQ > 85), normal with learning disorder, near normal (IQ 70–85), near normal with learning disorder, and intellectual disability (IQ < 70). There was a strong relationship between these categories and academic achievement and eventual social success.

The Nova Scotia population-based study investigated psychosocial outcome in 337 patients with IQ in the normal range and epilepsy characterized by focal or convulsive seizures at the end of an average follow-up of 7.5 years (Camfield et al. 1993b). Overall 42% had an adverse social outcome. School failure occurred in 34%, use of special education resources 34%, a mental health consultation 22%, psychotropic medication 5%, unemployment 20%, social isolation 27%, inadvertent pregnancy 12%, and a criminal conviction 2%. In multivariate analysis, most epilepsy-related variables did not predict these outcomes; however, the presence of a specific learning disorder was strongly associated ($p < 0.0001$).

The social outcome of children with epilepsy and intellectual disability has not been extensively reported. In the Nova Scotia study, 80 of the 692 (12%) symptomatic generalized epilepsy and nearly all were intellectually disabled (Camfield and Camfield 2008). Nineteen died during follow-up and 52 were followed until they were at least 18 years of age. There were seven (13%) with good social outcome (capable of independent living), and six of these seven had normal intelligence. Fifteen (29%) had moderate social outcome (independent for most basic activities of daily living but not judged able to live independently), and all had intellectual disability, mostly mild-moderate. Thirty (58%) had poor social outcome (dependent on others for nearly all activities of daily living).

Conclusion

Serious cognitive difficulties are present at the time of diagnosis in many children with childhood onset epilepsy but are typically not exacerbated by seizures. In a few with very severe epilepsy, especially with early onset (the "epileptic encephalopathies"), there may be a cognitive decline or at least stagnation. This group of patients is challenging to study because the early age at onset makes standardized psychometric testing difficult and because many have major neurological deficits that precede the onset of their epilepsy. The cognitive outcome of many epilepsy syndromes is not well described and population-based incidence studies have typically not addressed the cognition of children with these individual syndromes. Many syndromes are sufficiently uncommon that population-based studies will include few or no affected children. For example, in the Nova Scotia cohort ($n = 692$), there are no patients with Landau Kleffner syndrome or Ohtahara syndrome.

The presence of intellectual disability undoubtedly has a major effect on adult social success. Specific learning disorders despite normal overall intelligence are less well studied but also appear to have an important relationship with adverse adult social outcome, although interventions to improve this outcome are not well studied.

The long-term cognitive outcome for children with epilepsy is of major importance because it is likely to be the major determinant of adult social success. We hope that future research will include further follow-up studies with psychometric assessment shortly after diagnosis and many years later to better define the complicated relationship between childhood epilepsy and cognitive outcome.

REFERENCES

Akiyama M, Kobayashi K, Yoshinaga H and Ohtsuka Y (2010) A long-term follow-up study of Dravet syndrome up to adulthood. *Epilepsia* 51: 1043–1052. doi:10.1111/j.1528-1167.2009.02466.x.

Arts WF, Brouwer OF, Peters AC et al. (2004) Course and prognosis of childhood epilepsy: 5-year follow-up of the Dutch study of epilepsy in childhood. *Brain* 127: 1774–1784.

Auvin S, Pandit F, De Bellecize J et al. (2006) Benign myoclonic epilepsy in infants: Electroclinical features and long-term follow-up of 34 patients. *Epilepsia* 47: 387–393.

Berg AT, Smith SN, Frobish D et al. (2004) Control with newly diagnosed epilepsy: Influences of etiology, syndrome, and seizure longitudinal assessment of adaptive behavior in infants and young children. *Pediatrics* 114: 645. doi:10.1542/peds.2003-1151-L.

Berg AT, Langfitt JT, Testa FM et al. (2008) Global cognitive function in children with epilepsy: A community-based study. *Epilepsia* 49: 608–614.

Bourgeois BF, Prensky AL, Palkes HS, Talent BK and Busch SG (1983) Intelligence in epilepsy: A prospective study in children. *Ann Neurol* 14: 438–444.

Camfield C, Camfield P, Gordon K, Smith B and Dooley J (1993a) Outcome of childhood epilepsy: A population-based study with a simple predictive scoring system for those treated with medication. *J Pediatr* 122: 861–868.

Camfield C, Camfield P, Smith B, Gordon K and Dooley J (1993b) Biologic factors as predictors of social outcome of epilepsy in intellectually normal children: A population-based study. *J Pediatr* 122: 869–873.

Camfield C and Camfield P (2007) Preventable and unpreventable causes of childhood-onset epilepsy plus mental retardation. *Pediatrics* 120: e52–e55.

Camfield C and Camfield P (2008) Twenty years after childhood-onset symptomatic generalized epilepsy the social outcome is usually dependency or death: A population-based study. *Dev Med Child Neurol* 50: 859–863. doi:10.1111/j.1469-8749.2008.03165.x.

Camfield CS, Camfield PR, Wirrell E, Gordon KG and Dooley JM (1996) Incidence of epilepsy in childhood and adolescents: A population based study in Nova Scotia from 1977 to 1985. *Epilepsia* 37: 19–23.

Camfield CS and Camfield PR (2014) Rolandic epilepsy has little effect on adult life 30 years later: A population-based study. *Neurology* 82: 1162–1166. doi:10.1212/WNL.0000000000000267.

Caraballo RH, Flesler S, Pasteris MC et al., (2013) Myoclonic epilepsy in infancy: An electroclinical study and long-term follow-up of 38 patients. *Epilepsia* 54: 1605–1612. doi:10.1111/epi.12321.

Chin RF, Cumberland PM, Pujar SS et al. (2011) Outcomes of childhood epilepsy at age 33 years: A population-based birth-cohort study. *Epilepsia* 52: 1513–1521. doi:10.1111/j.1528-1167.2011.03170.

Ellenberg JH, Hirtz DG and Nelson KB (1986) Do seizures in children cause intellectual deterioration? *N Engl J Med* 314: 1085–1088.

Ferlazzo E, Nikanorova M, Italiano D et al. (2010) Lennox-Gastaut syndrome in adulthood: Clinical and EEG features. *Epilepsy Res* 89: 271–277. doi:10.1016/j.eplepsyres.2010.01.012.

Filippini M, Boni A, Giannotta M and Gobbi G (2013) Neuropsychological development in children belonging to BECTS spectrum: Long-term effect of epileptiform activity. *Epilepsy Behav* 28: 504–511. doi:10.1016/j.yebeh.2013.06.016.

Geelhoed M, Boerrigter A, Camfield PR et al. (2005) The accuracy of outcome prediction models for childhood-onset epilepsy. *Epilepsia* 46: 526–532.

Geerts A, Arts WF, Stroink H et al. (2010) Course and outcome of childhood epilepsy: A 15-year follow-up of the Dutch Study of Epilepsy in Childhood. *Epilepsia* 51: 1189–1197. doi:10.1111/j.1528-1167.2010.02546.x.

Liukkonen E, Kantola-Sorsa E, Paetau R et al. (2010) Long-term outcome of 32 children with encephalopathy with status epilepticus during sleep, or ESES syndrome. *Epilepsia* 51: 2023–2032. doi: 10.1111/j.1528-1167.2010.02578.x.

McNelis AM, Dunn DW, Johnson CS, Austin JK and Perkins SM (2007) Academic performance in children with new-onset seizures and asthma: A prospective study. *Epilepsy Behav* 10: 311–318.

Oostrom KJ, van Teeseling H, Smeets-Schouten A et al. (2005) Dutch Study of Epilepsy in Childhood (DuSECh). Three to four years after diagnosis: Cognition and behaviour in children with "epilepsy only." A prospective, controlled study. *Brain* 128: 1546–1555. doi:10.1093/brain/awh494.

Pascalicchio TF, de Araujo Filho GM, da Silva Noffs MH et al. (2007) Neuropsychological profile of patients with juvenile myoclonic epilepsy: A controlled study of 50 patients. *Epilepsy Behav* 10: 263–267.

Ragona F, Granata T, Dalla Bernardina B et al. (2011) Cognitive development in Dravet syndrome: A retrospective, multicenter study of 26 patients. *Epilepsia* 52: 386–392. doi:10.1111/j.1528-1167.2010.02925.x.

Riikonen R (1996) Long-term outcome of West syndrome: A study of adults with a history of infantile spasms. *Epilepsia* 37: 367–372.

Sillanpää M, Jalava M, Kaleva O and Shinnar S (1998) Long-term prognosis of seizures with onset in childhood. *N Engl J Med* 338: 1715–1722.

Sillanpää M (2004) Learning disability: Occurrence and long-term consequences in childhood-onset epilepsy. *Epilepsy Behav* 5: 937–944.

Sonmez F, Atakli D, Sari H, Atay T and Arpaci B (2004) Cognitive function in juvenile myoclonic epilepsy. *Epilepsy Behav* 5: 329–336.

Takayama R, Fujiwara T, Shigematsu H et al. (2014) Long-term course of Dravet syndrome: A study from an epilepsy center in Japan. *Epilepsia* 55: 528–538. doi:10.1111/epi.12532.

Trivisano M, Specchio N, Cappelletti S et al. (2011) Myoclonic astatic epilepsy: An age-dependent epileptic syndrome with favorable seizure outcome but variable cognitive evolution. *Epilepsy Res* 97: 133–141. doi:10.1016/j.eplepsyres.2011.07.021.

Verrotti A, Olivieri C, Agostinelli S et al. (2011) Long term outcome in children affected by absence epilepsy with onset before the age of three years. *Epilepsy Behav* 20: 366–369. doi:10.1016/j.yebeh.2010.12.015.

Wakamoto H, Nagao H, Hayashi M and Morimoto T (2000) Long-term medical, educational, and social prognoses of childhood-onset epilepsy: A population-based study in a rural district of Japan. *Brain Dev* 22: 246–255.

Wilson SJ, Micallef S, Henderson A et al. (2012) Developmental outcomes of childhood-onset temporal lobe epilepsy: A community-based study. *Epilepsia* 53: 1587–1596. doi:10.1111/j.1528-1167.2012.03632.x.

5
USE OF FUNCTIONAL IMAGING TO STUDY COGNITIVE FUNCTIONS

Madison M Berl and Leigh N Sepeta

Introduction

The use of neuroimaging tools to study the neural correlates of cognitive functioning has become a staple in clinical neuroscience endeavors (Cabeza and Nyberg 2000; Smith et al. 2009). Epilepsy populations are uniquely poised to be a model for comparing how neurological disruption due to a disease disrupts normal development because patients with epilepsy often undergo neuroimaging studies as part of their direct clinical care. Specifically, functional magnetic resonance imaging (fMRI) is a noninvasive method for mapping eloquent cortex and is often an integral step for planning epilepsy surgery (Loring et al. 2014). While the goals of fMRI for presurgical mapping are to map cognitive functions individually in patients with focal epilepsy to identify areas to spare during surgery, this same tool is also valuable in a research context for group comparisons. Moreover, because it is noninvasive, a typically developing control group can be included as a comparison group.

This chapter will address several topics related to functional imaging of cognition in children with epilepsy, including: (1) review of methodological approaches using functional imaging; (2) review by domain of extant literature with summarization of how results have informed us about the functioning of patients with childhood epilepsy; and (3) practical information about strategies for successfully imaging children with epilepsy for clinical studies.

Functional magnetic resonance imaging approaches

Functional neuroimaging has expanded exponentially from the early 1990s, and several design and analysis options exist but, fundamentally, the techniques discussed here rely on the detection of magnetic resonance signal as a result of blood flow over a period of time. The blood-oxygen-level-dependent technique (BOLD) is presumed to be an indirect measure of neural activity.

TASK-BASED ACTIVATION

Seminal fMRI paradigm designs are task based and require active engagement to garner robust activation at the individual level. In epilepsy, language and sensorimotor tasks have been studied the most and are accepted as standard clinical tools for mapping individuals (Woermann et al. 2003; Gaillard 2004; Binder 2011; Bauer et al. 2014). Motor mapping tasks include simple (tongue wiggling, finger tapping, or toe/foot tapping) or more complex

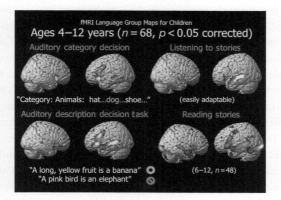

Fig. 5.1. Group activation (*p* < 0.05) from children across four language tasks. A colour version of this figure can be seen in the plate section at the end of the book.

tasks (sequence of moves) to activate the motor strip. Simple or complex motor movements can also activate the supplementary motor area. Even imagined movements (e.g. finger tapping) in hemiparetic patients can activate motor cortex (Bartsch et al. 2006). Sensory tasks include sensory stimulation (e.g. brushing of cheek). Also visual tasks, such as a flashing checkerboard, reliably activate primary occipital cortex (Kwong et al. 1992). The range of language paradigms used and the areas they activate have been described extensively elsewhere (Gaillard 2004; Klein et al. 2015). In brief, tasks may be presented in visual or auditory formats and include passive listening to sentences or stories, reading sentences or stories, word generation to semantic or phonemic prompts, sentence judgment, rhyming, and others. Other tasks including object naming, single-word reading, and repetition have not been effective for individual language mapping due to low task burden and/ or poor lateralizing effects (Gaillard 2004). Memory tasks have also not been established because of poor activation on an individual basis (Gabrieli et al. 1997; McAndrews 2014). Memory paradigms include word/object recognition, paired associate, scene encoding, and autobiographical (hometown walk) (McAndrews 2014).

Depending on the area of interest (i.e. temporal/Wernicke's; frontal/Broca's; sensorimotor, hippocampus), task selection is based on burdening the area of interest (Fig 5.1). For example, frontal language activation is often an area of interest for presurgical planning; however, choosing a passive listening task may not achieve the goal as a task such as listening to a story does not consistently activate frontal language areas on an individual basis (Berl et al. 2010). As fMRI analysis consists of the comparison of two conditions (e.g. task versus control), another factor in paradigm design is the choice of the control (baseline) condition (Gaillard 2004). For example, language tasks that involve listening to stimuli often have some type of auditory stimuli (e.g. tones, reverse speech) during the baseline condition to remove primary auditory cortex activation, which is bilaterally represented. In doing so, the subtraction yields a lateralized language map, assuming that the patient is lateralized. The drawback is that the subtraction may also remove activation in critical language areas. The clinician/ investigator will want to optimize his or her task selection based on the goal for the study.

In addition to paradigm design, data analysis techniques impact findings and conclusions. The issue of which threshold has been discussed in the literature (Seghier 2008) and tools to account for different thresholds are useful (Wilke and Lidzba 2007). Nevertheless, for clinical interpretation, efforts to eliminate spurious activation via rigorous thresholds may then underrepresent neural areas involved in the task. Related to threshold is the decision to conduct whole brain versus region of interest (ROI) analyses. An ROI analysis restricts the number of voxels under consideration, which then lowers the number of comparisons that need to be corrected for to reach significance. While there is strong a priori rationale for particular regions associated with language, motor, and memory, ROI selection is not entirely straightforward. Using a smaller language ROI based on Brodmann's area 44 or 45 versus a larger ROI based on the entire inferior frontal gyrus is one example. Our group often uses a larger ROI because we want to account for the possibility that a patient has shifted language within the hemisphere and may extend beyond the boundaries of a smaller ROI (Berl et al. 2014). Another aspect of the fMRI data processing pipeline that can impact on activation results is motion correction, which can be particularly challenging in pediatric populations. Postprocessing methods exist to help salvage data (Power et al. 2012; Wilke 2014; NITRC n.d.); however, the best method for ensuring that data do not get lost because of motion is to familiarize the child with the fMRI procedures and practice staying still (Byars et al. 2002; Yerys et al. 2009; Rothman et al. 2016). Activation in terms of extent and magnitude remain core parameters for clinical interpretation of task-based fMRI, but new parameters based on functional connectivity are being explored within active task paradigms (Fig 5.2) (Sepeta et al. 2015). Please see below for more details.

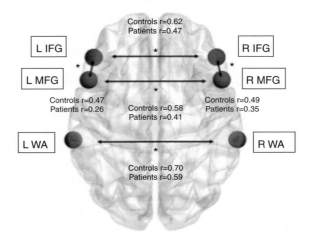

Fig. 5.2. Functional connectivity between specific language regions for children with epilepsy compared to typically developing controls. (*) indicates language connections with a significant difference between groups. IFG, inferior frontal gyrus; MFG, middle frontal gyrus, WA, Wernicke area.

Similar to task-based fMRI, resting-state (or task-free) fMRI (rs-fMRI) is based on the BOLD signal, but the participant does not explicitly engage in a task. Functional connectivity is the parameter used to quantify the signal changes across brain regions over time (Friston et al. 1993). Functional connectivity is presumed to represent functional organization of different regions because it consists of simple correlations between regions (Fox and Raichle 2007; Smith et al. 2009). Other methods include effective connectivity, which purports to represent a model of neuronal interaction where one neural system exerts an influence over another (Friston et al. 1997). Different analyses are used with functional and effective connectivity, and include model-independent (e.g. graph analysis, independent components analysis) or model-dependent approaches (e.g. Granger causality, structural equation modeling). Discussion of these methods is not within the scope of this chapter; however, the important point is that different conclusions about how epilepsy affects neuronal networks can be made with different analysis methods.

A potential advantage of rs-fMRI is that several functional networks (e.g. motor, language) may be identified simultaneously (Damoiseaux et al. 2006; Biswal et al. 2010) and the lack of a performance demand might be used in young or low functioning patients who are often precluded from task-based fMRI. In addition, rs-fMRI not only maps functional networks but is promising as a tool to localize seizure focus (Lang et al. 2014). A primary disadvantage of rs-fMRI is that the physiological basis of the resting-state signal is not completely understood and the state is unmonitored; therefore, information about the cognitive processes during the resting state (inner speech, etc.) is not available (for review, see Goodyear et al. 2014). This is important because certain cognitive states may potentially interfere with detecting resting-state networks.

Functional magnetic resonance imaging: Contributions to our understanding of childhood epilepsy

fMRI has enhanced our understanding of how function, particularly language, is represented in epilepsy populations. Language mapping with the same — or developmentally adapted paradigms — yields fundamentally similar activation maps in children as in adults such that typical language is a left-lateralized frontotemporal network (Berl et al. 2014). Nonetheless, fMRI studies also demonstrate how language differs from typically developing controls as well as adults with epilepsy. fMRI studies of language confirm findings from prior studies using invasive mapping techniques that show that atypical language representation occurs in 25–30% of individuals with epilepsy and is associated with clinical factors such as early age at onset (<5 years old), atypical handedness, and developmental pathology (Pujol et al. 1999; Springer et al. 1999; Berl et al. 2005). fMRI studies expanded upon these findings to demonstrate the range of atypical language patterns (Berl et al. 2014). fMRI studies confirmed that atypical activation commonly occurs in homologous regions in the right hemisphere and revealed that cross-dominance is a rare, but existing pattern such that frontal and temporal language dominance are in separate hemispheres (Staudt et al. 2001; Berl et al. 2014b). Moreover, reorganization of only frontal language is associated with specific factors including degree of frontal lobe periventricular white matter injury

(Staudt et al. 2001) and atypical handedness (Berl et al. 2014b). fMRI studies with typically developing children inform our understanding of the timing of lateralization such that language becomes more lateralized with age and that temporal regions lateralize earlier than frontal regions (Holland et al. 2007; Berl et al. 2014a), which has implications for the developmental timing of epilepsy surgery and its impact on language functioning. Despite these associations, patients with similar clinical factors do not uniformly shift their language and recent study explores other factors that potentially influence language reorganization such as features of the structures in the contralateral hemisphere (Pahs et al. 2013).

fMRI studies in epilepsy populations have contributed to our ability to predict outcomes. Motor fMRI accurately predicts the location of the motor cortex compared to electrical stimulation (Mehta and Klein 2010) with high sensitivity and specificity and contributes to clinical decision making (De Tiège et al. 2009). Similarly, language fMRI has been found to modify surgical planning and predict postoperative language deficits (Sabsevitz et al. 2003). In adults with temporal lobe epilepsy (TLE), activation in mesial structures predicts memory outcome after temporal lobe resection. Specifically, patients with greater ipsilateral compared to contralateral mesial temporal lobe (MTL) activation on pre-operative fMRI memory testing demonstrate greater memory decline following temporal lobe resection (Jokeit et al. 2001; Rabin 2004; Richardson 2004; Janszky et al. 2005; Richardson et al. 2006; Powell et al. 2007; Bonelli et al. 2010; Negishi et al. 2011). These outcome studies with adults inform models of hippocampal functioning that posit that postoperative memory outcome is predicted by activation in the hippocampus to be resected (*hippocampal adequacy*) rather than activation in the nonresected hippocampus (*hippocampal reserve*) (Chelune 1995). Resting-state connectivity is also emerging as a predictor of outcomes in epilepsy populations (Lang et al. 2014). rs-fMRI studies have found that patients who continued to have seizures following surgery had less lateralized functional connectivity than those who were seizure free (Negishi et al. 2011) and the strength of left hippocampus and posterior cingulate functional connectivity was associated with greater decline following left temporal resection (McCormick et al. 2013). Similar to activation studies, these functional connectivity results support the *hippocampal adequacy* theory, such that the connectivity in the to-be-resected tissue predicts cognitive outcome.

fMRI studies inform another theory of hippocampal functioning, *material specificity*, which posits that each hippocampus is specialized to process-specific types of information, namely the left hippocampus processes verbal information and the right hippocampus processes visual information. Group results of fMRI studies in typical adults support that verbal encoding is left lateralized and visual encoding is right lateralized (Kelley et al. 1998; Golby et al. 2002). Material-specific memory deficits ipsilateral to seizure foci are found in adults with TLE; some patients with left TLE perform worse on verbal memory and some with right TLE perform worse on visual memory measures (Helmstaedter et al. 1997; Bell and Davies 1998; Kim et al. 2003). In addition, postoperative decline in memory skills correlates with the side of focus/surgical intervention (Hermann et al. 1995; Gleissner et al. 2002; Henke et al. 2003; Janszky et al. 2005; Powell et al. 2008; Bonelli et al. 2010). While there is evidence for material specificity, there is also the lateralizing effect of which memory process (encoding vs retrieval) is being contrasted such that the left hemisphere is engaged preferentially during encoding while the right side preferentially retrieves regardless of stimulus type (Raslau et al. 2015).

As with language functions, but perhaps over a more protracted developmental window, memory functions in children may specialize and lateralize over time. Support for this hypothesis includes the finding that there are no consistent presurgical lateralizing memory impairments in children (Smith et al. 2002; Gonzalez et al. 2007), but adolescents with TLE show laterality differences in memory performance (Helmstaedter and Elger 2009). A review of 13 pediatric studies reported that postoperative memory decline occurred in four studies compared to six with no change, and three with improvement in memory functioning (Lah 2004). A recent study found that verbal memory is at risk in children with specific temporal lobe pathology (hippocampal sclerosis) more than frank temporal involvement and regardless of side of focus (Cormack et al. 2012). To date, no task-based fMRI studies of memory functioning in children with TLE have been published that would further inform our understanding of the impact of epilepsy on memory functions in children.

fMRI studies support the idea that epilepsy is a network disorder that not only impacts on normal development of neural networks but that even focal epilepsy does not lead to focal disruption (Hermann 2006; Kramer and Cash 2012). Within language fMRI studies, there is evidence that regions beyond traditional language areas are impacted (Berl et al. 2005; Ibrahim et al. 2015). One study demonstrated that language fMRI was more predictive of postoperative memory outcome than direct memory performance during Wada testing (Binder et al. 2008), which illustrates the relatedness between different cognitive networks and how epilepsy affects both. Several resting-state and task-based connectivity studies in adults with epilepsy reveal a reduction in functional connectivity among regions including the hippocampus (Waites et al. 2006; Frings et al. 2008; Liao et al. 2010; Pereira et al. 2010; Zhang et al. 2010; Pravatà et al. 2011; Vlooswijk et al. 2011; Stretton et al. 2012; James et al. 2013) and functional connectivity is associated with cognitive performance (Pravatà et al. 2011; Holmes et al. 2014). Research using rs-fMRI in children with focal epilepsy is limited but promising as it has been shown that resting-state networks similar to adults are identified in children (Fair et al. 2007; 2008; Thomason et al. 2008; Kelly et al. 2009) even as young as 26 weeks' gestation (Smyser et al. 2010). Similar to adults with epilepsy, studies of functional connectivity in children with focal epilepsy also found reduced connectivity (Fig 5.2), and higher functional connectivity among certain regions was positively associated with better performance (Braakman et al. 2012; Besseling et al. 2013; Vaessen et al. 2013; Croft et al. 2014; Sepeta et al. 2015).

Considerations for clinical functional magnetic resonance imaging in pediatric epilepsy

Several important factors to consider exist when conducting fMRI studies with pediatric populations. First, presurgical fMRI requires participant cooperation, which can be difficult with pediatric patients, particularly if they have cognitive impairments or if they are anxious and/or claustrophobic. fMRI is sensitive to motion, and thus it is important that the participant remain as still as possible. Extensive preparation provides the best way to increase participation and reduce motion. Preparation should include as much familiarization with

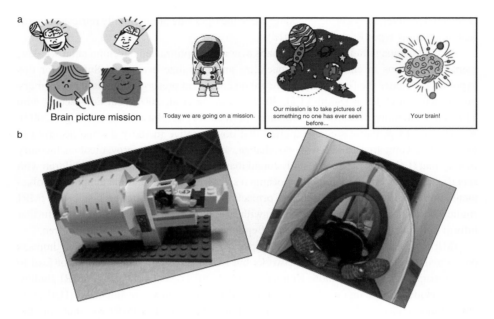

Fig. 5.3. fMRI preparation with children: (a) Social story for scanning session (courtesy of Center for Autism Spectrum Disorders at Children's National and Developmental Cognitive Neuroscience Lab at Georgetown University); (b) Lego set of fMRI environment; and (c) play tunnel to practice staying still in the bore of the MR scanner.

the procedures as possible. Effective techniques include the use of a mock scanner, social stories, and/or talking through the procedure in a manner tailored to children (Fig 5.3). The importance of being still can be explicitly addressed in a fun way through metaphors that appeal to a child such as "being still as a statue" or "going into a rocket ship like an astronaut." It can also be effective to use small incentives (e.g. a prize box, picture of the brain for show and tell) to encourage participation.

For task-based fMRI, participants need to perform and actively engage in the task. As previously stated, this can be difficult in a pediatric epilepsy population where cognitive impairments may be common. The paradigm design needs to be appropriate for age and ability level. It is important to consider adapting the paradigm to have several variations to use with individuals of different ages and ability levels rather than using the same stimuli for all. For higher level skills, such as reading, the participant needs to be able to read in order to complete the task, and the specific reading level should be known. Recent work also suggests using a self-paced paradigm (Máté et al. 2016). A final concern is that of covert versus monitored tasks. It is ideal to have the patients speak their answers in the scanner but the movement artifact is extensive; however, some groups are creating methods of turning the scanner on and off and modeling movement to solve the problem (Croft et al. 2013). A way to circumvent this problem is to use push button responses in order to assess performance and confirm that the patient is actively engaged in the task. However, this changes cognitive aspects of the paradigm (i.e. does not allow for the generation of responses) and may involve additional cognitive networks.

Conclusion

fMRI is an invaluable tool for clinical and experimental aspects of caring for and making discoveries with children with epilepsy. While historical trends tend to initiate new research in adult populations, it is also important to appreciate that epilepsy is a childhood disorder and that discovery, particularly related to prevention, requires working with pediatric populations. In addition, clinical trends toward earlier age of surgery also put fMRI studies with children at the forefront. The extant literature of fMRI studies demonstrates the contributions already made to the field; however, there remain many more areas of investigation that should be pursued especially as clinical fMRI is more in demand.

REFERENCES

Bartsch AJ, Homola G, Biller A, Solymosi L and Bendszus M (2006) Diagnostic functional MRI: Illustrated clinical applications and decision-making. *J Magn Reson Imaging* 23: 921–932. doi:10.1002/jmri.20579.

Bauer PR, Reitsma JB, Houweling BM, Ferrier CH and Ramsey NF (2014) Can fMRI safely replace the Wada test for preoperative assessment of language lateralisation? A meta-analysis and systematic review. *J Neurol Neurosurg Psychiatry* 85: 581–588. doi:10.1136/jnnp-2013-305659.

Bell BD and Davies KG (1998) Anterior temporal lobectomy, hippocampal sclerosis, and memory: Recent neuropsychological findings. *Neuropsychol Rev* 8: 25–41.

Berl MM, Balsamo LM, Xu B et al. (2005) Seizure focus affects regional language networks assessed by fMRI. *Neurology* 65: 1604–1611.

Berl MM, Duke ES, Mayo J et al. (2010) Functional anatomy of listening and reading comprehension during development. *Brain Lang* 114: 115–125. doi:10.1016/j.bandl.2010.06.002.

Berl MM, Mayo J, Parks EN et al. (2014a) Regional differences in the developmental trajectory of lateralization of the language network: Developmental trajectories of lateralization of language. *Hum Brain Mapp* 35: 270–284. doi:10.1002/hbm.22179.

Berl MM, Zimmaro LA, Khan OI et al. (2014b) Characterization of atypical language activation patterns in focal epilepsy. *Ann Neurol* 75: 33–42. doi:10.1002/ana.24015.

Besseling RMH, Jansen JFA, Overvliet GM et al. (2013) Reduced functional integration of the sensorimotor and language network in Rolandic epilepsy. *NeuroImage Clin* 2: 239–246. doi:10.1016/j.nicl.2013.01.004.

Binder JR (2011) FMRI is a valid noninvasive alternative to Wada testing. *Epilepsy Behav* 20: 214–222. doi:10.1016/j.yebeh.2010.08.004.

Binder JR, Sabsevitz DS, Swanson SJ et al. (2008) Use of preoperative functional MRI to predict verbal memory decline after temporal lobe epilepsy surgery. *Epilepsia* 49: 1377–1394. doi:10.1111/j.1528-1167.2008.01625.x.

Biswal BB, Mennes M, Zuo X-N et al. (2010) Toward discovery science of human brain function. *Proc Natl Acad Sci U S A* 107: 4734–4739. doi:10.1073/pnas.0911855107.

Bonelli SB, Powell RHW, Yogarajah M et al. (2010) Imaging memory in temporal lobe epilepsy: Predicting the effects of temporal lobe resection. *Brain* 133: 1186–1199. doi:10.1093/brain/awq006.

Braakman HMH, Vaessen MJ, Jansen JFA et al. (2012) Frontal lobe connectivity and cognitive impairment in pediatric frontal lobe epilepsy. *Epilepsia*. doi: 10.1111/epi.12044.

Byars AW, Holland SK, Strawsburg RH et al. (2002) Practical aspects of conducting large-scale functional magnetic resonance imaging studies in children. *J Child Neurol* 17: 885–890.

Cabeza R and Nyberg L (2000) Imaging cognition II: An empirical review of 275 PET and fMRI studies. *J Cogn Neurosci* 12: 1–47.

Chelune GJ (1995) Hippocampal adequacy versus functional reserve: Predicting memory functions following temporal lobectomy. *Arch Clin Neuropsychol* 10: 413–432.

Cormack F, Vargha-Khadem F, Wood SJ, Cross JH and Baldeweg T (2012) Memory in paediatric temporal lobe epilepsy: Effects of lesion type and side. *Epilepsy Res* 98: 255–259. doi:10.1016/j.eplepsyres.2011.09.004.

Croft LJ, Baldeweg T, Sepeta L et al. (2014) Vulnerability of the ventral language network in children with focal epilepsy. *Brain* 137: 2245–2257. doi:10.1093/brain/awu154.

Croft LJ, Rankin PM, Liégeois F et al. (2013) To speak, or not to speak? The feasibility of imaging overt speech in children with epilepsy. *Epilepsy Res* 107: 195–199. doi:10.1016/j.eplepsyres.2013.08.008.

Damoiseaux JS, Rombouts SARB, Barkhof F et al. (2006) Consistent resting-state networks across healthy subjects. *Proc Natl Acad Sci U S A* 103: 13848–13853. doi:10.1073/pnas.0601417103.

De Tiège X, Connelly A, Liégeois F et al. (2009) Influence of motor functional magnetic resonance imaging on the surgical management of children and adolescents with symptomatic focal epilepsy. *Neurosurgery* 64: 856–864; discussion 864. doi:10.1227/01.NEU.0000343741.54200.58.

Fair DA, Cohen AL, Dosenbach NUF et al. (2008) The maturing architecture of the brain's default network. *Proc Natl Acad Sci U S A* 105: 4028–4032. doi:10.1073/pnas.0800376105.

Fair DA, Dosenbach NUF, Church JA et al. (2007) Development of distinct control networks through segregation and integration. *Proc Natl Acad Sci U S A* 104: 13507–13512. doi:10.1073/pnas.0705843104.

Fox MD and Raichle ME (2007) Spontaneous fluctuations in brain activity observed with functional magnetic resonance imaging. *Nat Rev Neurosci* 8: 700–711. doi:10.1038/nrn2201.

Frings L, Wagner K, Halsband U et al. (2008) Lateralization of hippocampal activation differs between left and right temporal lobe epilepsy patients and correlates with postsurgical verbal learning decrement. *Epilepsy Res* 78: 161–170.

Friston KJ, Buechel C, Fink GR et al. (1997) Psychophysiological and modulatory interactions in neuroimaging. *Neuroimage* 6: 218–229.

Friston KJ, Frith CD, Liddle PF and Frackowiak RS (1993) Functional connectivity: The principal-component analysis of large (PET) data sets. *J Cereb Blood Flow Metab Off J Int Soc Cereb Blood Flow Metab* 13: 5–14.

Gabrieli JDE, Brewer JB, Desmond JE and Glover GH (1997) Separate neural bases of two fundamental memory processes in the human medial temporal lobe. *Science* 276: 264–266.

Gaillard W (2004) Functional MR imaging of language, memory, and sensorimotor cortex. *Neuroimaging Clin N Am* 14: 471–485. doi:10.1016/j.nic.2004.04.005.

Gleissner U, Sassen R, Lendt M, Clusmann H, Elger CE and Helmstaedter C (2002) Pre- and postoperative verbal memory in pediatric patients with temporal lobe epilepsy. *Epilepsy Res* 51: 287–296.

Golby AJ, Poldrack RA, Illes J et al. (2002) Memory lateralization in medial temporal lobe epilepsy assessed by functional MRI. *Epilepsia* 43: 855–863. doi:10.1046/j.1528-1157.2002.20501.x.

Gonzalez LM, Anderson VA, Wood SJ, Mitchell LA and Harvey AS (2007) The localization and lateralization of memory deficits in children with temporal lobe epilepsy. *Epilepsia* 48: 124–132. doi:10.1111/j.1528-1167.2006.00907.x.

Goodyear B, Liebenthal E and Mosher V (2014) Active and passive fMRI for presurgical mapping of motor and language cortex. In: Papageorgiou TD, Christopoulos GI and Smirnakis SM, editors. *Advanced Brain Neuroimaging Topics in Health and Disease—Methods and Applications*. InTech.

Helmstaedter C and Elger CE (2009) Chronic temporal lobe epilepsy: A neurodevelopmental or progressively dementing disease? *Brain* 132: 2822–2830.

Helmstaedter C, Grunwald T, Lehnertz K, Gleißner U and Elger CE (1997) Differential involvement of left temporolateral and temporomesial structures in verbal declarative learning and memory: Evidence from temporal lobe epilepsy. *Brain Cogn* 35: 110–131. doi:10.1006/brcg.1997.0930.

Henke K, Treyer V, Weber B et al. (2003) Functional neuroimaging predicts individual memory outcome after amygdalohippocampectomy. *Neuroreport* 14: 1197–1202.

Hermann B (2006) The effects of localization-related epilepsy on language lateralization and networks. *Epilepsy Curr* 6: 114–116.

Hermann BP, Seidenberg M, Haltiner A and Wyler AR (1995) Relationship of age at onset, chronologic age, and adequacy of preoperative performance to verbal memory change after anterior temporal lobectomy. *Epilepsia* 36: 137–145.

Holland SK, Vannest J, Mecoli M et al. (2007) Functional MRI of language lateralization during development in children. *Int J Audiol* 46: 533–551.

Holmes M, Folley BS, Sonmezturk HH et al. (2014) Resting state functional connectivity of the hippocampus associated with neurocognitive function in left temporal lobe epilepsy. *Hum Brain Mapp* 35: 735–744. doi:10.1002/hbm.22210.

Ibrahim GM, Morgan BR, Doesburg SM et al. (2015) Atypical language laterality is associated with large-scale disruption of network integration in children with intractable focal epilepsy. *Cortex J Devoted Study Nerv Syst Behav* 65: 83–88. doi:10.1016/j.cortex.2014.12.016.

James GA, Tripathi SP, Ojemann JG, Gross RE and Drane DL (2013) Diminished default mode network recruitment of the hippocampus and parahippocampus in temporal lobe epilepsy: Clinical article. *J Neurosurg* 119: 288–300. doi:10.3171/2013.3.JNS121041.

Janszky J, Jokeit H, Kontopoulou K et al. (2005) Functional MRI predicts memory performance after right mesiotemporal epilepsy surgery. *Epilepsia* 46: 244–250. doi:10.1111/j.0013-9580.2005.10804.x.

Jokeit H, Okujava M and Woermann FG (2001) Memory fMRI lateralizes temporal lobe epilepsy. *Neurology* 57: 1786–1793. doi:10.1212/WNL.57.10.1786.

Kelley WM, Miezin FM, McDermott KB et al. (1998) Hemispheric specialization in human dorsal frontal cortex and medial temporal lobe for verbal and nonverbal memory encoding. *Neuron* 20: 927–936.

Kelly AMC, Di Martino A, Uddin LQ et al. (2009) Development of anterior cingulate functional connectivity from late childhood to early adulthood. *Cereb Cortex N Y N 1991* 19: 640–657. doi:10.1093/cercor/bhn117.

Kim H, Yi S, Son EI and Kim J (2003) Material-specific memory in temporal lobe epilepsy: Effects of seizure laterality and language dominance. *Neuropsychology* 17: 59

Klein AP, Sabsevitz DS, Ulmer JL and Mark LP (2015) Imaging of cortical and white matter language processing. *Semin Ultrasound CT MRI* 36: 249–259. doi:10.1053/j.sult.2015.05.011.

Kramer MA and Cash SS (2012) Epilepsy as a disorder of cortical network organization. *Neuroscientist* 18: 360–372. doi:10.1177/1073858411422754.

Kwong KK, Belliveau JW, Chesler DA et al. (1992) Dynamic magnetic resonance imaging of human brain activity during primary sensory stimulation. *Proc Natl Acad Sci U S A* 89: 5675–5679.

Lah S (2004) Neuropsychological outcome following focal cortical removal for intractable epilepsy in children. *Epilepsy Behav* 5: 804–817. doi:10.1016/j.yebeh.2004.08.005.

Lang S, Duncan N and Northoff G (2014) Resting-state functional magnetic resonance imaging: Review of neurosurgical applications. *Neurosurgery* 74: 453–465. doi:10.1227/NEU.0000000000000307.

Liao W, Zhang Z, Pan Z et al. (2010) Altered functional connectivity and small-world in Mesial temporal lobe epilepsy. *PLoS ONE* 5: e8525. doi:10.1371/journal.pone.0008525.

Loring DW, Gaillard WD, Bookheimer SY, Meador KJ, Ojemann JG (2014) Cortical cartography reveals political and physical maps. *Epilepsia* 55: 633–637. doi:10.1111/epi.12553.

Máté A, Lidzba K, Hauser T-K, Staudt M, Wilke M (2016) A "one size fits all" approach to language fMRI: increasing specificity and applicability by adding a self-paced component. *Exp Brain Res* 234: 673–684. doi:10.1007/s00221-015-4473-8.

McAndrews MP (2014) Memory assessment in the clinical context using functional magnetic resonance imaging. *Neuroimaging Clin N Am* 24: 585–597. doi:10.1016/j.nic.2014.07.008.

McCormick C, Quraan M, Cohn M, Valiante TA and McAndrews MP (2013) Default mode network connectivity indicates episodic memory capacity in mesial temporal lobe epilepsy. *Epilepsia* 54: 809–818. doi:10.1111/epi.12098.

Mehta AD and Klein G (2010) Clinical utility of functional magnetic resonance imaging for brain mapping in epilepsy surgery. *Epilepsy Res* 89: 126–132. http://dx.doi.org/10.1016/j.eplepsyres.2009.12.001.

Negishi M, Martuzzi R, Novotny EJ, Spencer DD and Constable RT (2011) Functional MRI connectivity as a predictor of the surgical outcome of epilepsy. *Epilepsia* 52: 1733–1740. doi:10.1111/j.1528-1167.2011.03191.x.

NITRC (n.d.) Artifact Detection Tools (ART): Tool/Resource Info. http://www.nitrc.org/projects/artifact_detect/ (Accessed 20 June 2016).

Pahs G, Rankin P, Helen Cross J et al. (2013) Asymmetry of planum temporale constrains interhemispheric language plasticity in children with focal epilepsy. *Brain* 136: 3163–3175. doi:10.1093/brain/awt225.

Pereira FR, Alessio A, Sercheli MS et al. (2010) Research article Asymmetrical hippocampal connectivity in mesial temporal lobe epilepsy: Evidence from resting state fMRI. *BMC Neurosci* 11: 1

Powell HWR, Richardson MP, Symms MR et al. (2007) Preoperative fMRI predicts memory decline following anterior temporal lobe resection. *J Neurol Neurosurg Psychiatry* 79: 686–693. doi:10.1136/jnnp.2007.115139.

Powell HWR, Parker GJ, Alexander DC et al. (2008) Imaging language pathways predicts postoperative naming deficits. *J Neurol Neurosurg Psychiatry* 79: 327–330.

Power JD, Barnes KA, Snyder AZ, Schlaggar BL and Petersen SE (2012) Spurious but systematic correlations in functional connectivity MRI networks arise from subject motion. *NeuroImage* 59: 2142–2154. doi:10.1016/j.neuroimage.2011.10.018.

Pravatà E, Sestieri C, Mantini D et al. (2011) Functional connectivity MR imaging of the language network in patients with drug-resistant epilepsy. *Am J Neuroradiol* 32: 532–540. doi:10.3174/ajnr.A2311.

Pujol J, Deus J, Losilla JM and Capdevila A (1999) Cerebral lateralization of language in normal left-handed people studies by functional fMRI. *Neurology* 52: 1038–1043.

Rabin ML (2004) Functional MRI predicts post-surgical memory following temporal lobectomy. *Brain* 127: 2286–2298. doi:10.1093/brain/awh281.

Raslau FD, Mark LP, Sabsevitz DS and Ulmer JL (2015) Imaging of functional and dysfunctional episodic memory. *Semin Ultrasound CT MRI* 36: 260–274. doi:10.1053/j.sult.2015.05.010.

Richardson MP (2004) Pre-operative verbal memory fMRI predicts post-operative memory decline after left temporal lobe resection. *Brain* 127: 2419–2426. doi:10.1093/brain/awh293.

Richardson MP, Strange BA, Duncan JS and Dolan RJ (2006) Memory fMRI in left hippocampal sclerosis: Optimizing the approach to predicting postsurgical memory. *Neurology* 66: 699–705. doi:10.1212/01. wnl.0000201186.07716.98.

Rothman S, Gonen A, Vodonos A, Novack V and Shelef I (2016) Does preparation of children before MRI reduce the need for anesthesia? Prospective randomized control trial. *Pediatr Radiol.* doi: 10.1007/ s00247-016-3651-6.

Sabsevitz DS, Swanson SJ, Hammeke TA et al. (2003) Use of preoperative functional neuroimaging to predict language deficits from epilepsy surgery. *Neurology* 60: 1788–1792.

Seghier ML (2008) Laterality index in functional MRI: Methodological issues. *Magn Reson Imaging* 26: 594–601. doi:10.1016/j.mri.2007.10.010.

Sepeta LN, Croft LJ, Zimmaro LA et al. (2015) Reduced language connectivity in pediatric epilepsy. *Epilepsia* 56: 273–282. doi:10.1111/epi.12859.

Smith ML, Elliott IM and Lach L (2002) Cognitive skills in children with intractable epilepsy: comparison of surgical and nonsurgical candidates. *Epilepsia* 43: 631–637.

Smith SM, Fox PT, Miller KL et al. (2009) Correspondence of the brain's functional architecture during activation and rest. *Proc Natl Acad Sci U S A* 106: 13040–13045.

Smyser CD, Inder TE, Shimony JS et al. (2010) Longitudinal analysis of neural network development in preterm infants. *Cereb Cortex N Y N 1991* 20: 2852–2862. doi:10.1093/cercor/bhq035.

Springer JA, Binder JR, Hammeke TA et al. (1999) Language dominance in neurologically normal and epilepsy subjects: A functional MRI study. *Brain* 122: 2033–2046.

Staudt M, Grodd W, Niemann G et al. (2001) Early left periventricular brain lesions induce right hemispheric organization of speech. *Neurology* 57: 122–125.

Stretton J, Winston G, Sidhu M et al. (2012) Neural correlates of working memory in temporal lobe epilepsy — An fMRI study. *NeuroImage* 60: 1696–1703. doi:10.1016/j.neuroimage.2012.01.126.

Thomason ME, Chang CE, Glover GH et al. (2008) Default-mode function and task-induced deactivation have overlapping brain substrates in children. *NeuroImage* 41: 1493–1503. doi:10.1016/j. neuroimage.2008.03.029.

Vaessen MJ, Braakman HMH, Heerink JS et al. (2013) Abnormal modular organization of functional networks in cognitively impaired children with frontal lobe epilepsy. *Cereb Cortex N Y N 1991* 23: 1997–2006. doi:10.1093/cercor/bhs186.

Vlooswijk MCG, Vaessen MJ, Jansen JFA et al. (2011) Loss of network efficiency associated with cognitive decline in chronic epilepsy. *Neurology* 77: 938–944. doi:10.1212/WNL.0b013e31822cfc2f.

Waites AB, Briellmann RS, Saling MM, Abbott DF and Jackson GD (2006) Functional connectivity networks are disrupted in left temporal lobe epilepsy. *Ann Neurol* 59: 335–343. doi:10.1002/ana.20733.

Wilke M (2014) Isolated assessment of translation or rotation severely underestimates the effects of subject motion in fMRI data. *PLoS ONE* 9: e106498. http://dx.doi.org/10.1371/journal.pone.0106498.

Wilke M and Lidzba K (2007) LI-tool: A new toolbox to assess lateralization in functional MR-data. *J Neurosci Methods* 163: 128–136.

Woermann FG, Jokeit H, Luerding R et al. (2003) Language lateralization by Wada test and fMRI in 100 patients with epilepsy. *Neurology* 61: 699–701.

Yerys BE, Jankowski KF, Shook D et al. (2009) The fMRI success rate of children and adolescents: Typical development, epilepsy, attention deficit/hyperactivity disorder, and autism spectrum disorders. *Hum Brain Mapp* 30: 3426–3435. doi:10.1002/hbm.20767.

Zhang Z, Lu G, Zhong Y et al. (2010) Altered spontaneous neuronal activity of the default-mode network in mesial temporal lobe epilepsy. *Brain Res* 1323: 152–160. doi:10.1016/j.brainres.2010.01.042.

6
DISENTANGLING THE ROLE OF SEIZURES AND EEG ABNORMALITIES IN THE PATHOPHYSIOLOGY OF COGNITIVE DYSFUNCTION

Jonathan K Kleen and Gregory L Holmes

Introduction

Although seizures are the most striking clinical manifestation of the epilepsies, children with epilepsy are at risk not only for seizures but also for a number of comorbid health problems defined as conditions that occur in children with epilepsy at a higher rate than would be expected by chance (Committee on the Public Health Dimensions of the Epilepsies et al. 2012). Common comorbidities that occur in children with epilepsy include cognitive dysfunction, such as memory, attention, or processing difficulties; mental health conditions, including depression, anxiety, and oppositional-defiant disorder; and somatic comorbidities, such as sleep disorders and migraines. Epilepsy comorbidities are common and often severe. Many parents of children with epilepsy consider the comorbidities to outweigh the burden of the seizures themselves.

Cognitive abnormalities and behavioral disorders are among the most common and troublesome comorbidities associated with epilepsy in children. In children with epilepsy, there is an associated high rate of cognitive difficulties that compromise educational progress and achievement throughout their life (Berg et al. 2008). In addition to a higher incidence of low IQ scores (Farwell et al. 1985), approximately half of the children with epilepsy have a discrepancy between IQ and achievement (Fastenau et al. 2008). Lower IQ scores are particularly common in children with poorly controlled (pharmacoresistant) seizures (Berg et al. 2012). Likewise, children with epilepsy are at very high risk of attention-deficit–hyperactivity, anxiety, and conduct disorders (Cavazzuti and Nalin 1990; Dunn et al. 1997; Austin and Dunn 2002; Austin et al. 2004; Pellock 2004).

The major determinant of outcome in children with epilepsy is the etiology of their illness. However, there is increasing evidence that seizures, antiepileptic drugs, and interictal EEG abnormalities can contribute to adverse outcomes. In children, it is often difficult to differentiate the adverse cognitive effects of seizures and their treatment from transient EEG abnormalities because they all tend to converge. In animal studies, one can induce seizures, interictal spikes (IISs), or both in the normal brain without antiepileptic drug treatment. This allows investigation into the biological mechanisms underpinning independent influences of IISs or seizures on cognitive impairment. In this chapter, pertinent data from immature animals will be discussed in relationship to human studies.

Recurrent seizures

ANIMAL STUDIES

Substantial literature shows that recurrent seizures in the developing brain can result in long-term adverse consequences. Rat pups that are subjected to multiple recurrent seizures in the first weeks of life have considerable cognitive and behavioral abnormalities later on. This includes deficits of spatial cognition in the Morris water maze (Holmes et al. 1998; Huang et al. 1999; Liu et al. 1999; Karnam et al. 2009a; 2009b) and delayed non-match-to-sample task (Kleen et al. 2011b), auditory discrimination impairments (Neill et al. 1996), abnormal activity level (Karnam et al. 2009a), increased emotionality (Holmes et al. 1993), and reduced behavioral flexibility (Kleen et al. 2011a). Recurrent early-life seizures also produce physiological changes including a persistent decrease in GABA currents in the hippocampus (Isaeva et al. 2006) and neocortex (Isaeva et al. 2009), enhanced excitation in the neocortex (Isaeva et al. 2010), impairment in spike frequency adaptation (Villeneuve et al. 2000), and marked reductions in after-hyperpolarizing potentials following spike trains (Villeneuve et al. 2000). They are also associated with impaired long-term potentiation (Karnam et al. 2009a), enhanced short-term plasticity (Hernan et al. 2013), alterations in theta oscillation power (Karnam et al. 2009b), and impaired place cell coherence and stability (Karnam et al. 2009b).

Although early-life seizures have detrimental effects on cognitive function, recurrent seizures during the first 2 weeks of life do not produce cell loss (Holmes et al. 1998; Liu et al. 1999; Riviello et al. 2002). However, seizures in immature rats can produce synaptic reorganization as evidenced by CA3 sprouting (Holmes et al. 1998; Huang et al. 1999; Sogawa et al. 2001; Huang et al. 2002) and decreased neurogenesis (McCabe et al. 2001).

In the majority of studies, recurrent seizures have been induced in rats with "normal" brains. Using normal developing rats, investigators have been able to differentiate the effects of seizures from the etiological cause of epilepsy. However, in children, seizures do not occur in the "normal brain." As such, results from studies with animal models of epilepsy must be taken with a degree of reserve before applying to patients. Few investigators have studied the consequences of seizures in animals with structural abnormalities of the brain. In one of the few studies of this type, Lucas et al. (2011) found that seizures induced in rat pups with malformations of cortical development but without seizures had severe spatial cognitive deficits in the water maze. When the rat pups were subjected to recurrent flurothyl-induced seizures and tested at 25 days of age (immediate postweaning), their cognitive performance was worse. In contrast, in animals tested during adolescence, seizures had no additional adverse effect. The authors also investigated whether the severity of the structural abnormality and seizures affected brain weight, cortical thickness, hippocampal area, and cell dispersion area. Early-life seizures did not have a significant impact on any of these parameters, although the size of the dysplasia did have a significant effect.

STUDIES IN CHILDREN

Childhood epilepsy carries a significant risk for a variety of problems involving cognition. IQ scores in children with epilepsy have a skewed distribution toward lower values (Farwell et al. 1985; Neyens et al. 1999). The number of children with epilepsy and learning disabilities in school or behavioral problems is greater than that of the normal population (Sillanpaa et al. 1998; Williams et al. 1998; Bailet and Turk 2000; Wakamoto et al. 2000). Predictors of poor cognitive outcome include higher seizure frequencies (Hermann et al. 2008) and longer duration of the epilepsy (Farwell et al. 1985; Seidenberg et al. 1986).

Most children with epilepsy do not have a decline in intelligence or behavior, however. It could also be fairly argued that children with a high seizure frequency and a long duration of epilepsy have a more severe underlying brain abnormality than those with less severe epilepsy. Many children that develop epilepsy appear to have cognitive deficits that precede the onset of the seizures. This might suggest again that the etiology of the seizures, not the seizures themselves, is responsible for the impaired cognition (Fastenau et al. 2009). Nevertheless, some children with epilepsy slow in their cognitive development (Neyens et al. 1999) or even have progressive declines of IQ on serial intelligence tests over time (Bourgeois et al. 1983). Similarly, increasing duration of epilepsy in temporal lobe epilepsy is associated with declining performance across both intellectual and memory measures (Hermann et al. 2002). It is difficult to ascertain whether this is related to the underlying etiology causing progressive dysfunction or more so to the cumulative effects of seizures over time.

Animal data suggest that seizures in early childhood are more detrimental than those occurring at an older age. Risk factors for cognitive impairment in children with epilepsy include an early age at onset of seizures (Huttenlocher and Hapke 1990; Glosser et al. 1997; Bulteau et al. 2000; Bjornaes et al. 2001; Hermann et al. 2002; Cormack et al. 2007), particularly during the neonatal period (Glass et al. 2009). Epileptic syndromes in which psychomotor deterioration occurs have an early age at onset. These include early infantile epileptic encephalopathy with suppression burst (Ohtahara syndrome), early myoclonic encephalopathy, migrating partial epilepsy in infancy, infantile spasms (West syndrome), severe myoclonic epilepsy of infancy (Dravet syndrome), Lennox–Gastaut syndrome, myoclonic-astatic epilepsy, continuous spike–wave discharges during sleep (CSWS), and Landau–Kleffner syndrome (LKS) (Genton and Dravet 1997; Panayiotopoulos 2002; Nabbout and Dulac 2003). It is likely that pediatric seizures affect the activity-dependent processes among developing networks. They may thus be more detrimental than seizures in older individuals, in whom neural circuitry is relatively more fixed and less malleable. For example, infants with infantile spasms and hypsarrhythmia have EEGs that have high coherences, a measure of connectivity, predominately at long interelectrode distances. At short interelectrode distances, coherences are decreased in the theta and beta range, particularly in the frontal region (Burroughs et al. 2014). This suggests impaired local cortical integration in frontal regions (which are important for executive function development), yet abnormal congruence between areas that would normally have functional differentiation. Altered connectivity may thus underlie cognitive impairment among children with infantile spasms, and this may extend to other children with both seizures and developmental delay.

Although the etiology of the seizures clearly plays the major role in cognitive and behavioral development, childhood seizures themselves (i.e. independent of etiology) can lead to cognitive impairment (Glass et al. 2009; Korman et al. 2013; Payne et al. 2014). Among children with focal cortical dysplasia, Korman et al. (2013) found that the age at onset of epilepsy and the extent of the dysplasia each contributed independently to cognitive dysfunction. They suggested that the early onset of epilepsy led to poor cognitive outcomes potentially through disrupting critical periods of development. Furthermore, it was suggested that even a localized lesion could engender developmental deficits if the age at onset of epilepsy was early. In a pediatric intensive care unit, it was found that seizures, even without a behavioral correlate, were strongly associated with neurological decline that could not be accounted for by the etiology (Payne et al. 2014).

Interictal spikes

Although seizures themselves are significantly related to worse cognitive outcomes as described previously, there is an extensive literature on the topic of whether the IIS activity also contributes independently to cognitive impairment. Despite being quite transient and usually without overt clinical manifestations, these brief bursts of activity are hypothesized to affect cognition both dynamically and cumulatively over time.

RODENT STUDIES

Both the acute (transient) and chronic (cumulative) effects of IISs have been studied in rats. Animal models fortunately allow intracranial recordings (increasing sensitivity and specificity of IISs on EEG) and more controlled testing on large numbers of trials in cognitive tasks. The latter is often difficult to attain in patients with epilepsy given attentional, motivational, and situational (e.g. EEG lead discomfort) issues. The majority of studies dealing with the acute effects of IISs have been conducted in adult rats because it has been difficult to induce sustained IISs in immature rats. For example, following status epilepticus induced by kainic acid, pilocarpine, or electrical stimulation, IISs occur within days of the status epilepticus in adult rats, whereas in immature rats, status epilepticus rarely results in IISs. Although the acute effects of IISs in adult rats are remarkably similar to those found in adult patients with epilepsy, caution is required in extrapolating results from adult rats to children.

IISs have been shown to result in a task-specific cognitive impairment in adult rats. Using a within-subject analysis to analyze how IISs might independently affect memory processing in the hippocampus, Kleen et al. (2010) studied rats that developed chronic IIS following intrahippocampal pilocarpine in a hippocampal-dependent operant behavior task (delayed match-to-sample test). Although IISs that occurred during memory encoding or memory maintenance did not affect performance, hippocampal IISs that occurred during memory retrieval strongly impaired performance. Memory retrieval is especially reliant on hippocampal activation (Montgomery and Buzsaki 2007). Thus, IISs were most disruptive when the active engagement of neurons involved in performing this stage of the task was critical (Fig 6.1).

The physiological effects of IIS have been investigated. There is a sustained reduction of action potentials in the hippocampus for up to 2 seconds following a local IIS

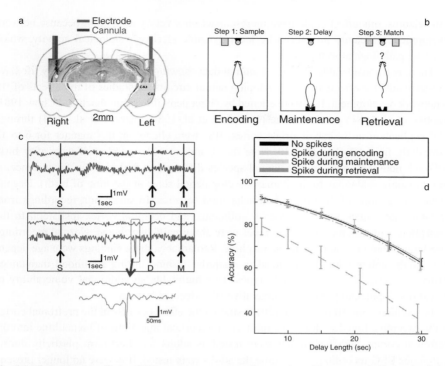

Fig. 6.1. To assess the effects of IISs on memory rats underwent intra-hippocampal pilocarpine injections to induced status epilepticus. (a) Bilateral electrodes are placed in the ventral hippocampus. (b) In the delayed match-to-sample test during the sample step, one of the two levers is randomly presented (right or left) and is pressed by the rat. Then, in the delay step, the rat has to poke its nose into a hole in the opposite wall for a random length of time (6–30s). After this time period has elapsed, the first nose poked into the hole turns off the stimulus light above and extends both the levers. Then, in the match step, the rat has to remember which lever it pressed during the sample phase and press the same lever again to procure a food reward. During the sampling stage, memory is encoded; during the delay phase memory is maintained; and during the match phase, memory is retrieved. Performance is recorded for trials without spikes (c, top trace) and trials with spikes (c, bottom). (d) Among trials in which an IIS occurs during the encoding or maintenance epoch of short-term memory, accuracy does not differ from trials without IIS. However, IISs during the retrieval phase produce a marked decrease in accuracy. Increasing delays produce decreases in accuracy, regardless of IIS epoch timing. (Modified from Kleen JK et al., *Ann Neurol*, 67, 250–257, 2010.) A colour version of this figure can be seen in the plate section at the end of the book.

(Zhou et al. 2007a) and up to 6 seconds following flurries of spikes (Zhou et al. 2007b). The extensive inhibitory wave immediately after IIS can also reduce the power of gamma oscillations and other important oscillatory signals in the hippocampus (Urrestarazu et al. 2006). Because oscillations are closely linked with ongoing learning and memory function (Halasz et al. 2005), this type of transient disruption likely contributes to cognitive deficits. As noted previously, whether IIS in immature rats also causes a transient impairment in cognition is known. However, in view of the physiological effects IISs have in the mature brain, the same phenomenon would likely occur in the immature brain. Furthermore, as with seizures, this effect could have more impact on a very young brain because network development is heavily influenced by local dynamic electrophysiological activity, which would be pathological in this case.

There is a considerable amount of animal data showing that IISs during early life have long-term adverse effects on the developing neural circuits. In studies of the effects of IIS on network development, IISs were elicited by either penicillin (Baumbach and Chow 1981; Crabtree et al. 1981) or bicuculline (Campbell et al. 1984; Ostrach et al. 1984) through focal application in the rabbit striate cortex. IISs were elicited in this manner for 6 to 12 hours daily from P8–9 to P24–30. Note that P indicates the number of days after birth (although note that there are substantial species differences; P10 in a rat, for instance, is approximately analogous to the human developmental stage at the time of birth). Despite frequent IISs, none of the rabbits had behavioral seizures. In single-unit recordings from the lateral geniculate nucleus, superior colliculus, and occipital cortex ipsilateral to the hemisphere with IIS, receptive field types were abnormally distributed. Normal recordings were found from the contralateral hemisphere. Remarkably, these findings were age dependent. Adult rabbits with IISs induced in a similar fashion during adulthood maintained normal disruption of receptive field types. This highlights an additional vulnerability of critical developmental periods to cumulative IIS effects over time.

In a similar vein, Hernan et al. (2013) studied the effects of IISs in the prefrontal cortex on the executive function. Rat pups received intracortical injections of bicuculline into the prefrontal cortex, and the animals were tested as adults for short-term plasticity during continuous EEG recording. At the time the adults were tested, IISs were no longer present. However, the IISs in early life resulted in a significant increase in short-term plasticity bilaterally in the prefrontal cortex. These rats also showed marked inattentiveness in a delayed non-match-to-sample task, despite no clear deficits in working memory. Rats also demonstrated deficits in sociability, showing an autism-like behavior. Similarly, generalized and multifocal IISs have also been elicited in young rats with flurothyl (Khan et al. 2010). When these rats with IISs were tested as adults, they had impairments in reference memory in the water maze and in the four-trial radial-arm water maze, and also showed abnormal long-term potentiation. Early-life IISs also resulted in impaired new cell formation and decreased cell counts in the hippocampus, indicating a potential mechanism in which IISs during development can produce cumulative lasting effects in addition to any dynamic disruptions at the time.

STUDIES IN PATIENTS

Animal studies, as described previously, would predict that IISs will result in transitory cognitive impairment in humans. Early work investigating this hypothesis relied on adult patients, because controlled cognitive testing with EEG leads in place was a difficult testing scenario and not easily attained in a pediatric ward. This work showed that IISs in humans could indeed produce brief disturbances in neural processing, resulting in a phenomenon called transitory or transient cognitive impairment (Binnie 2003). In a seminal study, Aarts et al. (1984) found that IISs can briefly disrupt neural processes affecting function within the brain region where they occur. For example, in right-handed individuals, IISs were associated with errors in a nonverbal task. Left hemisphere IISs resulted mainly in errors in verbal tasks, fitting functional lateralization. Similarly, Shewmon and Erwin (1988a; 1988b; 1988c; 1989) found that IISs in the occipital region (i.e. visual cortex) caused transitory deficits with stimuli presented in the contralateral visual field. Deficits were most pronounced when the stimulus was presented during the inhibitory slow wave following the spikes.

The transitory effects of IISs have been studied in patients with epilepsy undergoing intracranial EEG. In a study of 10 adult patients with depth electrodes implanted into their hippocampi for preoperative seizure localization, Kleen et al. (2013) recorded EEG during 2070 total trials of a short-term memory task, with memory processing categorized into encoding, maintenance, and retrieval. The influence of hippocampal IIS on these processes was analyzed and adjusted to account for individual differences between patients. Hippocampal IIS during memory retrieval was related to more error responses when they were contralateral to the seizure focus ($p < 0.05$) or bilateral ($p < 0.001$). Bilateral IIS during the memory maintenance period had a similar effect ($p < 0.01$), particularly with spike–wave complexes of longer duration ($p < 0.01$). The results translated animal data as mentioned previously (Kleen et al. 2010) and strengthened the view that IISs contribute to cognitive impairment in epilepsy depending upon when and where they occur. The results of this study confirmed an earlier study by Krauss et al. (1997) who found declines in working memory due to IISs.

The role of IIS in benign rolandic epilepsy (BRE) has generated considerable interest. The characteristic of interictal EEG abnormality in this syndrome is a high-amplitude, usually diphasic spike with a prominent following slow wave. The spikes (<70ms) or sharp waves (<200ms) appear isolated or in groups at the mid-temporal (T3, T4) and central (rolandic) regions (C3, C4). When assesing with bipolar recording montages, the spikes may be most prominent in the central region or mid-temporal region, and usually occur synchronously in both the regions. There is increasing evidence that the IISs in BRE may reflect an underlying network disorder (Clemens et al. 2013; Besseling et al. 2013a; 2013b; 2013c; 2014). Kavros et al. (2008) reviewed 14 studies dealing with attention in BRE and found that in all controlled studies, there were deficits in three attention systems: alerting, orienting, and executive networks. These systems are impaired in children with active centrotemporal spikes, implying a widespread functional cortical disturbance in BRE. This would argue that IISs are a biomarker of a network abnormality, in addition to likely causing a localized disturbance of nearby neurons.

Children with BRE have a variety of cognitive impairments (Fonseca et al. 2007; Danielsson and Petermann 2009), particularly language defects, revealed by tests measuring phonemic fluency, verbal elaboration of semantic knowledge, and lexical comprehension (Riva et al. 2007; Verrotti et al. 2011). They also often have impairments in nonverbal functions (Metz-Lutz et al. 1999; Metz-Lutz and Filippini 2006). The cognitive profile of the deficits is related to the side of focus, similar to the results of transient cognitive impairment studies described previously. For example, nonverbal deficits significantly correlate with lateralization of the epileptic focus in the right hemisphere. Conversely, verbal deficits can be seen with left hemisphere discharges. Frontal functions such as attention control, response organization, and fine motor speed tend to be impaired in the presence of active discharges independently of the lateralization of the epileptic focus (Metz-Lutz et al. 1999; Metz-Lutz and Filippini 2006). However, not all studies have shown consistent neuropsychological profiles in children with BRE. Variability in functional impairment may be explained by fluctuations in IIS frequency and cognitive performance. In a study of six children with BRE, month-to-month marked fluctuations in cognitive abilities and the frequency and location of IISs have been noted (Ewen et al. 2011).

Transitory cognitive impairment has been studied during IIS in children with BECTS using EEG and computerized neuropsychological testing in a visual discrimination task between words and pseudo-words (Fonseca et al. 2007). Approximately 15% of children made a significantly greater proportion of errors during IIS than during IIS-free periods. Of interest, in this study, the IIS seemed to be suppressed in most children (20 of 33), when they were engaged in the task. This could be due to increased alertness and physiological engagement of underlying neural networks, thus avoiding domination by synchronous activity that could result in epileptiform bursts. However, this interpretation is purely speculative.

Whether there is a relationship between the frequency of IIS and cognition is unclear. Some authors used a simple approach looking at the rate of IISs and cognitive performance. Some showed an inverse relationship (Filippini et al. 2013), whereas others found no such relationship (Fonseca et al. 2007; Goldberg-Stern et al. 2010; Tedrus et al. 2010). In a study of IIS in 182 children with a variety of epilepsy syndromes, including BECTS, Ebus et al. (2012) calculated the IIS index using a 24-hour ambulatory EEG and compared the IIS burden to neuropsychological test performance. The IIS index was calculated in wakefulness and sleep as percentage of time in five categories (0%, <1%, 1%–10%, ≥10%–50%, and ≥50%). The group of patients with diurnal IIS in 10% or more of the EEG record had impaired central information processing speed, short-term verbal memory, and visual motor integration. This was independent from other EEG-related and epilepsy-related characteristics, and from epilepsy syndrome diagnosis. It is important to note that these studies did not take into account the timing of the IISs and it is likely they did not evaluate the full impact of IISs (which can be profound) on specific cognitive faculties (Kleen et al. 2010).

There have been attempts to improve cognitive and behavioral functions by suppressing IIS with antiepileptic drugs. However, a notable obstacle to designing studies to treat IIS is the lack of well-tolerated drugs that effectively suppress IIS. In one randomized study, children with controlled or mild epilepsy were assigned to get lamotrigine add-on therapy either before or after placebo (Pressler et al. 2005). Global behavior rating significantly improved only among those patients with a significant reduction in interictal discharges during active treatment. However, another small study using sulthiame to reduce IIS in BECTS found that children had a significant deterioration in their reading ability, despite a reduction in IIS frequency (Wirrell et al. 2008). Of note, the long-term prognosis in BRE is quite favorable, and it is thus uncertain whether IISs in BRE in particular contribute to the long-term cognitive and behavioral impairment or if they are simply a biomarker of a disrupted neuronal network.

However, there are two other conditions in which the IISs appear to have long-standing adverse effects on behavior and cognition. LKS and CSWS have a substantially worse prognosis (Metz-Lutz and Filippini 2006; Seegmuller et al. 2012) and are both associated with chronic impairment in behavior and cognition.

Acquired epileptic aphasia (LKS) is a childhood epilepsy syndrome that may be heavily influenced by interictal activity. It is characterized by a loss or regression of previously acquired language and prominent epileptiform discharges involving the temporal or parietal regions of the brain (Landau and Kleffner 1957; Cooper and Ferry 1978; Hirsch et al. 1990; Beaumanoir 1992; Deonna and Roulet-Perez 2016). Although a considerable amount of variation exists in the disorder, the typical history is of developing a loss of language ability and inattentiveness to sound. The onset is usually during the first decade of life. This regression of communication skills is closely preceded, accompanied, or followed by the onset of seizures or an abnormal EEG or both (Sawhney et al. 1988; Deonna 1991). In addition, auditory agnosia may be the dominant feature early in the course of the disorder, and many of the children have behavioral and psychomotor disturbances, resembling autistic spectrum disorder.

The signature of EEG in LKS shows repetitive spikes, sharp waves, and spike-and-wave activity occurring in the temporal or parietal–occipital regions. Sleep frequently activates the EEG abnormalities, and, in some cases, the abnormalities are only seen in sleep recordings. Speech deficits in the syndrome may be explained by excessive inhibitory reaction to epileptiform discharges or simply more static disruption of normal network connections. The severity of the aphasia does not have a close correlation with the degree of EEG abnormality (Foerster 1977; Holmes et al. 1981) or clinical seizures (Landau and Kleffner 1957). A number of authors have suggested that the epileptiform activity is an epiphenomenon reflecting underlying cortical abnormalities (Lou et al. 1977; Kellermann 1978; Holmes et al. 1981). As such, if the EEG were to parallel speech recovery, this would not be necessarily causative; rather, the decreased epileptiform activity during speech recovery may reflect resolving injury to the speech areas. Limited data suggest a direct relationship between IIS and language impairment. However, subpial resection, which drastically reduces epileptiform activity in the receptive language cortex, can reduce IISs and also resolve linguistic function in LKS (Grote et al. 1999). Because this intervention would not be expected to alter the underlying etiology of LKS, improvement with an otherwise destructive surgical procedure would suggest that the epileptiform discharges contribute LKS.

A condition related to LKS is CSWS, a disorder also termed electrical status epilepticus during sleep (Tassinari et al. 2000). The distinguishing EEG feature of CSWS is continuous bilateral and diffuse slow spike–wave activity persisting through all of the slow-wave sleep stages. The proportion of time in which spikes and waves occupy the EEG during non-rapid eye movement sleep in this disorder ranges from 85% to 100%. The cause of CSWS is unknown, but early developmental lesions play a major role in approximately half of the patients. Genetic contributions have also recently been described. As would be expected from the discussion previously, children with this disorder can have profound cognitive deficits. It is likely that the pathological epileptiform activity pervades the important periods of memory consolidation during sleep. Clinical, neurophysiological, and cerebral glucose metabolism data support the hypothesis that IISs play a prominent role in the cognitive deficits by interfering with the neuronal networks at the site of the epileptic foci but also at distant connected areas. High-dose benzodiazepines and corticosteroids have been successfully used to treat electroencephalographic features, with some degree of subsequent clinical improvement (Okuyaz et al. 2005; Nickels and Wirrell 2008; Lagae 2009). As with LKS, there are no definitive data that indicate that the EEG abnormalities are responsible for the cognitive impairment. However, improvement often parallels a reduction of spike–wave discharges during sleep (Scholtes et al. 2005).

Conclusion

There is now clear evidence that both seizures and IISs in immature rats and children can result in cognitive impairment. The effects of both IISs and spikes in the immature brain are dependent on brain maturation. In the fully developed brain, seizures and IISs result in temporary impairment and appear to have few long-term effects, whereas in the developing brain, both IISs and seizures have more profound effects. Disentangling the effects of seizures from IISs is difficult. However, considering that IISs occur 24 hours/day 7 days a week, it may be that IISs are more detrimental. It is widely believed that frequent epileptiform events seen in children with epilepsy are capable of causing deleterious alterations in developing brain networks and are therefore associated with the high incidence of cognitive deficits and psychiatric comorbidities in these patients.

REFERENCES

Aarts JH, Binnie CD, Smit AM and Wilkins AJ (1984) Selective cognitive impairment during focal and generalized epileptiform EEG activity. *Brain* 107: 293–308.

Austin JK and Dunn DW (2002) Progressive behavioral changes in children with epilepsy. *Prog Brain Res* 135: 419–427.

Austin JK, Dunn DW, Johnson CS and Perkins SM (2004) Behavioral issues involving children and adolescents with epilepsy and the impact of their families: Recent research data. *Epilepsy Behav* 5: S33–S41.

Bailet LL and Turk WR (2000) The impact of childhood epilepsy on neurocognitive and behavioral performance: A prospective longitudinal study. *Epilepsia* 41: 426–431.

Baumbach HD and Chow KL (1981) Visuocortical epileptiform discharges in rabbits: Differential effects on neuronal development in the lateral geniculate nucleus and superior colliculus. *Brain Res* 209: 61–76.

Beaumanoir A (1992) The Landau-Kleffner syndrome. In: Roger J, Bureau M, Dravet C et al., editors. *Epileptic Syndromes in Infancy, Childhood and Adolescence* (pp. 231–243). John Libbey, London.

Berg AT, Langfitt JT, Testa FM et al. (2008) Global cognitive function in children with epilepsy: A community-based study. *Epilepsia* 49: 608–614.

Berg AT, Zelko FA, Levy SR and Testa FM (2012) Age at onset of epilepsy, pharmacoresistance, and cognitive outcomes: A prospective cohort study. *Neurology* 79: 1384–1391.

Besseling RM, Jansen JF, Overvliet GM et al. (2013a) Reduced structural connectivity between sensorimotor and language areas in rolandic epilepsy. *PLoS ONE* 8: e83568.

Besseling RM, Jansen JF, Overvliet GM et al. (2013b) Reduced functional integration of the sensorimotor and language network in rolandic epilepsy. *Neuroimage Clin* 2: 239–246.

Besseling RM, Overvliet GM, Jansen JF et al. (2013c) Aberrant functional connectivity between motor and language networks in rolandic epilepsy. *Epilepsy Res* 107: 253–262.

Besseling RM, Jansen JF, Overvliet GM et al. (2014) Delayed convergence between brain network structure and function in rolandic epilepsy. *Front Hum Neurosci* 8: 704.

Binnie CD (2003) Cognitive impairment during epileptiform discharges: Is it ever justifiable to treat the EEG? *Lancet Neurol* 2: 725–730.

Bjornaes H, Stabell K, Henriksen O and Loyning Y (2001) The effects of refractory epilepsy on intellectual functioning in children and adults. A longitudinal study. *Seizure* 10: 250–259.

Bourgeois BFD, Prensky AL, Palkes HS, Talent BK and Busch SG (1983) Intelligence in epilepsy: A prospective study in children. *Ann Neurol* 14: 438–444.

Bulteau C, Jambaque I, Viguier D et al. (2000) Epileptic syndromes, cognitive assessment and school placement: a study of 251 children. *Dev Med Child Neurol* 42: 319–327.

Burroughs SA, Morse RP, Mott SH and Holmes GL (2014) Brain connectivity in West syndrome. *Seizure* 23: 576–579.

Campbell BG, Ostrach LH, Crabtree JW and Chow KL (1984) Characterization of penicillin- and bicuculline-induced epileptiform discharges during development of striate cortex in rabbits. *Brain Res* 317: 125–128.

Cavazzuti GB and Nalin A (1990) Psychobehavioral disturbance in epileptic children. *Child's Nerv Syst* 6: 430–433.

Clemens B, Puskas S, Besenyei M et al. (2013) Remission of benign epilepsy with rolandic spikes: An EEG-based connectivity study at the onset of the disease and at remission. *Epilepsy Res* 106: 128–135.

Committee on the Public Health Dimensions of the Epilepsies, Board on Health Sciences Policy, Institute of Medicine (2012) *Epilepsy Across the Spectrum: Promoting Health and Understanding*. The National Academies Press, Washington, DC.

Cooper JA and Ferry PC (1978) Acquired auditory verbal agnosia and seizures in childhood. *J Speech Dis* 43: 176–184.

Cormack F, Helen CJ, Isaacs E et al. (2007) The development of intellectual abilities in pediatric temporal lobe epilepsy. *Epilepsia* 48: 201–204.

Crabtree JW, Chow KL, Ostrach LH and Baumbach HD (1981) Development of receptive field properties in the visual cortex of rabbits subjected to early epileptiform cortical discharges. *Brain Res* 227: 269–281.

Danielsson J and Petermann F (2009) Cognitive deficits in children with benign rolandic epilepsy of childhood or rolandic discharges: A study of children between 4 and 7 years of age with and without seizures compared with healthy controls. *Epilepsy Behav* 16: 646–651.

Deonna T and Roulet-Perez E (2016) *The Epilepsy Aphasia Spectrum: From Landau-Kleffner Syndrome to Rolandic Epilepsy*. Mac Keith Press, London.

Deonna TW (1991) Acquired epileptiform aphasia in children (Landau-Kleffner Syndrome). *J Clin Neurophysiol* 8: 288–298.

Dunn DW, Austin JK and Huster GA (1997) Behaviour problems in children with new-onset epilepsy. *Seizure* 6: 283–287.

Ebus S, Arends J, Hendriksen J et al. (2012) Cognitive effects of interictal epileptiform discharges in children. *Eur J Paediatr Neurol* 16: 697–706.

Ewen JB, Vining EP, Smith CA et al. (2011) Cognitive and EEG fluctuation in benign childhood epilepsy with central-temporal spikes: A case series. *Epilepsy Res* 97: 214–219.

Farwell JR, Dodrill CB and Batzel LW (1985) Neuropsychological abilities of children with epilepsy. *Epilepsia* 26: 395–400.

Fastenau PS, Jianzhao S, Dunn DW and Austin JK (2008) Academic underachievement among children with epilepsy: Proportion exceeding psychometric criteria for learning disability and associated risk factors. *J Learn Disabil* 41: 195–207.

Fastenau PS, Johnson CS, Perkins SM et al. (2009) Neuropsychological status at seizure onset in children: Risk factors for early cognitive deficits. *Neurology* 73: 526–534.

Filippini M, Boni A, Giannotta M and Gobbi G (2013) Neuropsychological development in children belonging to BECTS spectrum: long-term effect of epileptiform activity. *Epilepsy Behav* 28: 504–511.

Foerster C (1977) Aphasia and seizure disorders in childhood. In: Penry JK, editor. *Epilepsy: The Eighth International Symposium* (pp. 305–306). Raven Press, New York.

Fonseca LC, Tedrus GM, Pacheco EM et al. (2007) Benign childhood epilepsy with centro-temporal spikes: Correlation between clinical, cognitive and EEG aspects. *Arq Neuropsiquiatr* 65: 569–575.

Genton P and Dravet C (1997) Lennox-Gastaut and other childhood epileptic encephalopathies. In: Engel J Jr. and Pedley TA, editors. *Epilepsy: A Comprehensive Textbook* (pp. 2355–2366). Lippincott-Raven Publishers, Philadelphia, PA.

Glass HC, Glidden D, Jeremy RJ et al. (2009) Clinical neonatal seizures are independently associated with outcome in infants at risk for hypoxic-ischemic brain injury. *J Pediatr* 155: 318–323.

Glosser G, Cole LC, French JA, Saykin AJ and Sperling MR (1997) Predictors of intellectual performance in adults with intractable temporal lobe epilepsy. *J Int Neuropsychol Soc* 3: 252–259.

Goldberg-Stern H, Gonen OM, Sadeh M et al. (2010) Neuropsychological aspects of benign childhood epilepsy with centrotemporal spikes. *Seizure* 19: 12–16.

Grote CL, Van SP and Hoeppner JA (1999) Language outcome following multiple subpial transection for Landau-Kleffner syndrome. *Brain* 122: 561–566.

Halasz P, Kelemen A, Clemens B et al. (2005) The perisylvian epileptic network. A unifying concept. *Ideggyogy Sz* 58: 21–31.

Hermann B, Seidenberg M and Jones J (2008) The neurobehavioural comorbidities of epilepsy: Can a natural history be developed? *Lancet Neurol* 7: 151–160.

Hermann BP, Seidenberg M and Bell B (2002) The neurodevelopmental impact of childhood onset temporal lobe epilepsy on brain structure and function and the risk of progressive cognitive effects. *Prog Brain Res* 135: 429–438.

Hernan AE, Holmes GL, Isaev D, Scott RC and Isaeva E (2013) Altered short-term plasticity in the prefrontal cortex after early life seizures. *Neurobiol Dis* 50: 120–126.

Hirsch E, Marescaux C, Maquet P et al. (1990) Landau-Kleffner Syndrome: A clinical and EEG study of five cases. *Epilepsia* 31: 756–767.

Holmes GL, Chronopoulos A, Stafstrom CE et al. (1993) Effects of kindling on subsequent learning, memory, behavior, and seizure susceptibility. *Brain Res Dev Brain Res* 73: 71–77.

Holmes GL, Gairsa JL, Chevassus-Au-Louis N and Ben-Ari Y (1998) Consequences of neonatal seizures in the rat: Morphological and behavioral effects. *Ann Neurol* 44: 845–857.

Holmes GL, McKeever M and Saunders Z (1981) Epileptiform activity in aphasia of childhood: An epiphenomenon? *Epilepsia* 22: 631–639.

Huang L, Cilio MR, Silveira DC et al. (1999) Long-term effects of neonatal seizures: A behavioral, electrophysiological, and histological study. *Brain Res Dev Brain Res* 118: 99–107.

Huang LT, Yang SN, Liou CW et al. (2002) Pentylenetetrazol-induced recurrent seizures in rat pups: Time course on spatial learning and long-term effects. *Epilepsia* 43: 567–573.

Huttenlocher PR and Hapke RJ (1990) A follow-up study of intractable seizures in childhood. *Ann Neurol* 28: 699–705.

Isaeva E, Isaev D, Khazipov R and Holmes GL (2006) Selective impairment of GABAergic synaptic transmission in the flurothyl model of neonatal seizures. *Eur J Neurosci* 23: 1559–1566.

Isaeva E, Isaev D, Khazipov R and Holmes GL (2009) Long-term suppression of GABAergic activity by neonatal seizures in rat somatosensory cortex. *Epilepsy Res*.

Isaeva E, Isaev D, Savrasova A, Khazipov R and Holmes GL (2010) Recurrent neonatal seizures result in long-term increases in neuronal network excitability in the rat neocortex. *Eur J Neurosci* 31: 1446–1455.

Karnam HB, Zhao Q, Shatskikh T and Holmes GL (2009a) Effect of age on cognitive sequelae following early life seizures in rats. *Epilepsy Res* 85: 221–230.

Karnam HB, Zhou JL, Huang LT et al. (2009b) Early life seizures cause long-standing impairment of the hippocampal map. *Exp Neurol* 217: 378–387.

Kavros PM, Clarke T, Strug LJ et al. (2008) Attention impairment in rolandic epilepsy: Systematic review. *Epilepsia* 49: 1570–1580.

Kellermann K (1978) Recurrent aphasia with subclinical bioelectric status epilepticus during sleep. *Eur J Pediatr* 128: 207–212.

Khan OI, Zhao Q, Miller F and Holmes GL (2010) Interictal spikes in developing rats cause long-standing cognitive deficits. *Neurobiol Dis* 39: 362–371.

Kleen JK, Scott RC, Holmes GL and Lenck-Santini PP (2010) Hippocampal interictal spikes disrupt cognition in rats. *Ann Neurol* 67: 250–257.

Kleen JK, Scott RC, Holmes GL et al. (2013) Hippocampal interictal epileptiform activity disrupts cognition in humans. *Neurology* 81: 18–24.

Kleen JK, Sesque A, Wu EX et al. (2011a) Early-life seizures produce lasting alterations in the structure and function of the prefrontal cortex. *Epilepsy Behav* 22: 214–219.

Kleen JK, Wu EX, Holmes GL, Scott RC and Lenck-Santini PP (2011b) Enhanced oscillatory activity in the hippocampal-prefrontal network is related to short-term memory function after early-life seizures. *J Neurosci* 31: 15397–15406.

Korman B, Krsek P, Duchowny M et al. (2013) Early seizure onset and dysplastic lesion extent independently disrupt cognitive networks. *Neurology* 81: 745–751.

Krauss GL, Summerfield M, Brandt J, Breiter S and Ruchkin D (1997) Mesial temporal spikes interfere with working memory. *Neurology* 49: 975–980.

Lagae L (2009) Rational treatment options with AEDs and ketogenic diet in Landau-Kleffner syndrome: Still waiting after all these years. *Epilepsia* 50: 59–62.

Landau WM and Kleffner FR (1957) Syndrome of acquired aphasia with convulsive disorder in children. *Neurology* 7: 523–530.

Liu Z, Yang Y, Silveira DC et al. (1999) Consequences of recurrent seizures during early brain development. *Neuroscience* 92: 1443–1454.

Lou HC, Brandt S and Bruhn P (1977) Aphasia and epilepsy in childhood. *Acta Neurol Scand* 56: 46–54.

Lucas MM, Lenck-Santini PP, Holmes GL and Scott RC (2011) Impaired cognition in rats with cortical dysplasia: Additional impact of early-life seizures. *Brain* 134: 1684–1693.

McCabe BK, Silveira DC, Cilio MR et al. (2001) Reduced neurogenesis after neonatal seizures. *J Neurosci* 21: 2094–2103.

Metz-Lutz MN and Filippini M (2006) Neuropsychological findings in Rolandic epilepsy and Landau-Kleffner syndrome. *Epilepsia* 47: 71–75.

Metz-Lutz MN, Kleitz C, de Saint MA et al. (1999) Cognitive development in benign focal epilepsies of childhood. *Dev Neurosci* 21: 182–190.

Montgomery SM and Buzsaki G (2007) Gamma oscillations dynamically couple hippocampal CA3 and CA1 regions during memory task performance. *Proc Natl Acad Sci U S A* 104: 14495–14500.

Nabbout R and Dulac O (2003) Epileptic encephalopathies: a brief overview. *J Clin Neurophysiol* 20: 393–397.

Neill JC, Liu Z, Sarkisian M et al. (1996) Recurrent seizures in immature rats: Effect on auditory and visual discrimination. *Brain Res Dev Brain Res* 95: 283–292.

Neyens LG, Aldenkamp AP and Meinardi HM (1999) Prospective follow-up of intellectual development in children with a recent onset of epilepsy. *Epilepsy Res* 34: 85–90.

Nickels K and Wirrell E (2008) Electrical status epilepticus in sleep. *Semin Pediatr Neurol* 15: 50–60.

Okuyaz C, Aydin K, Gucuyener K and Serdaroglu A (2005) Treatment of electrical status epilepticus during slow-wave sleep with high-dose corticosteroid. *Pediatr Neurol* 32: 64–67.

Ostrach LH, Crabtree JW, Campbell BG and Chow KL (1984) Effects of bicuculline-induced epileptiform activity on development of receptive field properties in striate cortex and lateral geniculate nucleus of the rabbit. *Brain Res* 317: 113–123.

Panayiotopoulos CP (2002) Epileptic encephalopathies in early childhood. In: Panayiotopolous CP, editor. *A Clinical Guide to Epileptic Syndromes and Their Treatment* (pp. 70–88). Bladon Medical Publishing, Oxfordshire, UK.

Payne ET, Zhao XY, Frndova H et al. (2014) Seizure burden is independently associated with short term outcome in critically ill children. *Brain* 137: 1429–1438.

Pellock JM (2004) Understanding co-morbidities affecting children with epilepsy. *Neurology* 62: S17–S23.

Pressler RM, Robinson RO, Wilson GA and Binnie CD (2005) Treatment of interictal epileptiform discharges can improve behavior in children with behavioral problems and epilepsy. *J Pediatr* 146: 112–117.

Riva D, Vago C, Franceschetti S et al. (2007) Intellectual and language findings and their relationship to EEG characteristics in benign childhood epilepsy with centrotemporal spikes. *Epilepsy Behav* 10: 278–285.

Riviello P, de Rogalski Landrot I and Holmes GL (2002) Lack of cell loss following recurrent neonatal seizures. *Brain Res Dev Brain Res* 135: 101–104.

Sawhney IMS, Suresch N, Dhand UK and Chopra JS (1988) Acquired aphasia with epilepsy—Landau-Kleffner Syndrome. *Epilepsia* 29: 283–287.

Scholtes FB, Hendriks MP and Renier WO (2005) Cognitive deterioration and electrical status epilepticus during slow sleep. *Epilepsy Behav* 6: 167–173.

Seegmuller C, Deonna T, Dubois CM et al. (2012) Long-term outcome after cognitive and behavioral regression in nonlesional epilepsy with continuous spike-waves during slow-wave sleep. *Epilepsia* 53: 1067–1076.

Seidenberg M, Beck N, Geisser M et al. (1986) Academic achievement of children with epilepsy. *Epilepsia* 27: 753–759.

Shewmon DA and Erwin RJ (1988a) Focal spike-induced cerebral dysfunction is related to the after-coming slow wave. *Ann Neurol* 23: 131–137.

Shewmon DA and Erwin RJ (1988b) The effect of focal interictal spikes on perception and reaction time. I. General considerations. *Electroencephalogr Clin Neurophysiol* 69: 319–337.

Shewmon DA and Erwin RJ (1988c) The effect of focal interictal spikes on perception and reaction time. II. Neuroanatomic specificity. *Electroencephalogr Clin Neurophysiol* 69: 338–352.

Shewmon DA and Erwin RJ (1989) Transient impairment of visual perception induced by single interictal occipital spikes. *J Clin Exp Neuropsychol* 11: 675–691.

Sillanpaa M, Jalava M, Kaleva O and Shinnar S (1998) Long-term prognosis of seizures with onset in childhood. *N Engl J Med* 338: 1715–1722.

Sogawa Y, Monokoshi M, Silveira DC et al. (2001) Timing of cognitive deficits following neonatal seizures: Relationship to histological changes in the hippocampus. *Brain Res Dev Brain Res* 131: 73–83.

Tassinari CA, Rubboli G, Volpi L et al. (2000) Encephalopathy with electrical status epilepticus during slow sleep or ESES syndrome including the acquired aphasia. *Clin Neurophysiol* 111: S94–S102.

Tedrus GM, Fonseca LC, Castilho DP et al. (2010) Benign childhood epilepsy with centro-temporal spikes: Evolutive clinical, cognitive and EEG aspects. *Arq Neuropsiquiatr* 68: 550–555.

Urrestarazu E, Jirsch JD, Levan P et al. (2006) High-frequency intracerebral EEG activity (100–500 Hz) following interictal spikes. *Epilepsia* 47: 1465–1476.

Verrotti A, D'Egidio C, Agostinelli S et al. (2011) Cognitive and linguistic abnormalities in benign childhood epilepsy with centrotemporal spikes. *Acta Paediatr* 100: 768–772.

Villeneuve N, Ben-Ari Y, Holmes GL and Gaiarsa JL (2000) Neonatal seizures induced persistent changes in intrinsic properties of CA1 rat hippocampal cells. *Ann Neurol* 47: 729–738.

Wakamoto H, Nagao H, Hayashi M and Morimoto T (2000) Long-term medical, educational, and social prognoses of childhood-onset epilepsy: A population-based study in a rural district of Japan. *Brain Dev* 22: 246–255.

Williams J, Griebel ML and Dykman RA (1998) Neuropsychological patterns in pediatric epilepsy. *Seizure* 7: 223–228.

Wirrell E, Sherman EM, Vanmastrigt R and Hamiwka L (2008) Deterioration in cognitive function in children with benign epilepsy of childhood with central temporal spikes treated with sulthiame. *J Child Neurol* 23: 14–21.

Zhou JL, Lenck-Santini PP and Holmes GL (2007a) Postictal single-cell firing patterns in the Hippocampus. *Epilepsia* 48: 713–719.

Zhou JL, Lenck-Santini PP, Zhao Q and Holmes GL (2007b) Effect of interictal spikes on single-cell firing patterns in the hippocampus. *Epilepsia* 48: 720–731.

7
CHRONIC COGNITIVE EFFECTS OF ANTIEPILEPTIC DRUGS IN CHILDHOOD EPILEPSY

Albert P Aldenkamp, Willem Lavrijssen and Dominique Ijff

Introduction

The cognitive side effects of the antiepileptic drugs (AEDs) have emerged as an important aspect in medical decision making in childhood epilepsy (Mandelbaum et al. 2009). Children with epilepsy have a higher risk of learning disabilities and academic weakness because of the epilepsy and the seizures (Helmstaedter et al. 2014). In such a situation, even a modest adverse drug effect may have consequences because it can amplify the already existing weaknesses and ultimately may cause developmental arrest (Mula and Trimble 2009; Cross 2010; IJff and Aldenkamp 2013). Children are potentially more susceptible to the adverse effects of AEDs than adults because of the potential effect of AEDs on brain maturation and hence on neurodevelopment (Cross 2010; Ijff and Aldenkamp 2013). Early identification of AED-induced cognitive impairment in children with epilepsy is, therefore, crucial because those deficits impact on future educational possibilities and eventually the occupational and social outcomes.

The first studies on cognitive side effects of AEDs were published in the early 1970s. However, recently, most studies have focused on adults, which limits the generalization of findings to children. More importantly, most studies have been of limited duration. Most of our knowledge is based on clinical trials lasting on average 12 weeks (Vermeulen and Aldenkamp 1995). This is completely different from normal clinical practice where treatment is assessed over years rather than weeks (Mula and Trimble 2009).

We, therefore, screened the literature for studies on the relationships between chronic AED treatment and cognitive function in children. "Chronic" was here defined as treatment durations of greater than 6 months, preferably in a controlled trial. Studies were evaluated using the U.S. Preventive Services Task Force (USPSTF) evidenced-based classification levels (see Table 1). The discussion of the identified studies was limited to currently used AEDs in the general childhood epilepsy population rather than effects in specific syndromes. For example, we do not discuss the use of vigabatrin in infantile spasms or the use of levetiracetam in continuous spike-waves during slow wave sleep.

79

Also only those studies are discussed that used formal neuropsychological testing. The add-on design studies sometimes showed interpretable and interesting results. Polytherapy studies were not used.

In Box 1, we explain the evaluation strategy, based on an evidence level approach. In Table 7.2, we provide the evaluation of all articles that passed the search strategy.

General comments

In total, 18 studies were identified that met our inclusion criteria. No level 1 studies have been found. A disappointing number of controlled studies allowed us to study chronic effects: level II-1 and—if not available—level II-2 studies. In addition, almost all studies were comparative studies using an active comparator (another AED), which allowed us only to draw relative conclusions in a nonequivalent analysis (not worse than another AED) rather than absolute conclusions (no side effects).

Evaluation per AED

Carbamazepine (CBZ)

Four relatively recently published level II-1 studies are available (Chen et al. 1996; Donati et al. 2006, 2007; Kang et al. 2007; Eun et al. 2012b). These are all comparative studies with an active control revealing no absolute effects (effects against no drug treatment) but only relative effects. The four studies did not show inferior performance compared to lamotrigine (LTG), valproate (VPA), topiramate (TPM), phenobarbitone (PHB), and oxcarbazepine (OXC). Three studies used a 6-month follow-up, and one (Kang et al. 2007) a 12-month follow-up. In total, 156 children had a chronic exposure (28 vs OXC; 35 vs LTG; 43 vs TPM; 25 vs PHB; and 25 vs VPA).

We may conclude that CBZ does not induce more impairment after chronic treatment than other first-line AEDs: VPA, LTG, and OXC and no worse impairment than TPM.

Valproate

Four level II-1 studies were available (Vining et al. 1987; Chen et al. 1996; Donati et al. 2006, 2007; Glauser et al. 2013). No differences with CBZ or VPA were found. Compared to ethosuximide (ETS) and LTG, attentional problems were found. Cognitive global level was higher than PHB in a crossover trial (Vining et al. 1987), but this was not confirmed in the comparative trial of Chen et al. (1996). Long-term data are available for a total of 201 children in the level II-1 studies. All studies used follow-up periods of 12 months except for Donati et al. (2006, 2007) with 6-month follow-up. The study by Glauser et al. (2013) is noteworthy because of the large number of children on VPA (n=147) showing attentional problems relative to those on LTD (n=149) and ETS (n=155). As this study was performed in children with typical absences, one would not expect a confounding seizure effect. We may, therefore, cautiously conclude that VPA may induce attentional problems after 12 months of treatment.

OXCARBAZEPINE

One level II-1 study is available (Donati et al. 2006, 2007) in 55 children on OXC. The study did not reveal differences with 28 children on CBZ and 29 on VPA after 6 months of treatment. No confirmation of this finding is available.

LAMOTRIGINE

Two level II-1 studies are available, showing no impairment relative to ETS and VPA (Glauser et al. 2013) and CBZ (Eun et al. 2012b). Again the study by Glauser has a high power because of the large number of patients included. In total, 181 patients were studied over 6 months (Eun et al. 2012b) and 12 months (Glauser et al. 2013).

LEVETIRACETAM

No interpretable long-term studies are available.

TOPIRAMATE

Only one study is available, a class II-1 study in which TPM is compared with CBZ over a 6-month period (Kang et al. 2007). They found impairment on the arithmetic subscale of the Wechsler Intelligence Scale for Children at higher doses of TPM.

PHENOBARBITONE

A number of studies are available on the long-term effect of PHB. This is possibly due to the use of PHB for febrile seizures in toddlers, raising the issue of later developmental consequences. There are two level II-1 studies (Vining et al. 1987; Chen et al. 1996). In the study by Vining et al. (1987), intelligence and memory scores were lower in the PHB condition in a crossover design with 6-months of treatment in 21 children. However, in the study by Chen et al. (1996), no differences with CBZ or VPA were found after 12 months of treatment in 23 children. Both used the same intelligence test. Vining et al. (1987), however, used in addition a large test battery and used compensation or correction for multiple testing.

PHENYTOIN

No interpretable long-term studies are available.

ETHOSUXIMIDE

Only one level II-1 study is available; however, the well-powered study by Glauser et al. (2013) including 155 children on monotherapy ETS in a comparative design versus VPA and LTG over 12 months revealed no long-term side effects.

ZONISAMIDE

One class II-1 study is available comparing high dose with low dose ZSM in 70 children, revealing cognitive impairment at higher dose concerning language development, or more specifically vocabulary acquisition (Eun et al. 2011) after 6 months of treatment.

TABLE 7.1
Summary of results per antiepileptic drug

AED	No cognitive effects (confirmed)	Probably no cognitive effects (confirmation needed)	Possible cognitive effects (to be confirmed; caution is needed with long-term treatment)	Cognitive effects at long term (confirmed)	Inconclusive (contradictory results)	No data
Carbamazepine	Not inferior to LTG, VPA, TPM and OXC					
Valproate			Attentional problems after 12mo of treatment relative to ETS and LTG			
Oxcarbazepine		Not inferior to VPA and CBZ in one class II-1 study				
Lamotrigine	Not inferior to ETS or CBZ and better outcome compared to VPA					
Levetiracetam						No interpretable studies
Phenytoin						No interpretable studies
Topiramate			Inferior compared to CBZ over a 6mo period at higher doses of TPM			
Zonisamide			Language impairment at higher dose after 6mo treatment			
Phenobarbital					Two studies available with contradictory results	
Ethosuximide		Not inferior to LTG and superior to VPA				

LTG, lamotrigine; VPA, valproate; TPM, topiramate; OXC, oxcarbazepine; ETS, ethosuximide; CBZ, carbamazepine.

Conclusion

The results are summarized in Table 7.1. For none of the AEDs confirmed cognitive adverse effects have been demonstrated after long-term treatment (≥6mo). For CBZ and LTG confirmed evidence is available that they do not impair cognitive function in the long term. This statement must, however, be considered as a relative statement as all the evidence comes from comparative design, implying noninferiority versus a number of other AEDs. For OXC and ETS, evidence is found in the same positive direction, but confirmation is needed. AEDs that seem to increase the risk for cognitive adverse effects after long-term treatment are TPM, zonisamide, and VPA. In all three cases, confirmation has yet to be found. Not surprisingly, for the newer AEDs, such as lacosamide or pregabaline, no long-term data are yet available. However, for important AEDs in current use, phenytoin and LEV, data are also lacking.

The overall conclusion is as follows:

A. Long-term treatment with most of the AEDs does not seem to endanger cognitive development in children.
B. However, because of the lack of long-term data, this conclusion must be drawn with great caution. Clearly, we need more studies, such as the study by Glauser et al. (2013), with a large number of patients, newly diagnosed, in types of epilepsy where seizures are no major confounders and preferably assessed at a no-medication baseline, at a steady state and after 6 months of treatment.

BOX 1 Levels of evidence used based on the US Preventive Services Task Force classification

Level I: Evidence obtained from at least one properly designed randomized controlled trial.

Level II-1: Evidence obtained from well-designed controlled trials without randomization.

Level II-2: Evidence obtained from well-designed cohort or case-control analytic studies, preferably from more than one center or research group.

Level II-3: Evidence obtained from multiple time series designs with or without the intervention. Dramatic results in uncontrolled trials might also be regarded as this type of evidence.

Level III: Opinions of respected authorities, based on clinical experience, descriptive studies, or reports of expert committees.

In addition, we added a level IV class: case reports with a limited number of patients.

Summary of the evaluated studies

The results of studies that used a comparative design may be presented in different parts of Table 7.2.

TABLE 7.2
Summary of the evaluated studies

AED	Study	N	Age	Design	Type of cognitive impairment
Oxcarbazepine (OXC)					
	Donati et al. (2006; 2007)	55 on OXC vs 28 on CBZ and 29 on VPA	9.8y	Open-label randomized active-control three-arm study in newly diagnosed patients on monotherapy	No difference with CBZ or VPA
OXC oral suspension	Eun et al. (2012a)	168	8.4y	Prospective open-label trial comparing intellectually normal children vs intellectually impaired children; all newly diagnosed	No difference between baseline and endpoint and no difference between the two groups based on intelligence
	Tzitiridou et al. (2005)	70	6.5–10.2y	Open study with children with Rolandic epilepsy vs 45 controls; all newly diagnosed	Mild cognitive improvements, correlating with EEG improvements
Carbamazepine (CBZ)					
	Donati et al. (2006; 2007)	28 on CBZ vs 55 on OXC and 29 on VPA	9.8y	Open-label randomized active-control three-arm study in newly diagnosed patients on monotherapy	No difference with OXC or VPA
	Eun et al. (2012 b)	35 (start 41)	8.3–9.2y	Randomized open-label comparative design comparing monotherapy CBZ with LTG in newly diagnosed partial epilepsy	No cognitive differences with LTG over time
	Piccinelli et al. (2010)	8	9.5–9.9y	Open-label study comparing patients with all sorts on epilepsy relative to VPA	Lower attentional function
	Kang et al. (2007)	43 (vs 45 for TPM)	8.7y	Randomized open-label comparative design, comparing TPM with CBZ in Rolandic epilepsy	No impairment
	Mandelbaum and Burack (1997)	43	4–16y	Open-label study with untreated baseline	No impairment
	Chen et al. (1996)	25 on CBZ vs 25 on VPA and 23 on PHB	9.9–10.8	Open randomized comparative design	No impairment vs VPA

Type of measurement	Confounders	Evidence level	Effect size	Length of follow-up
Attention and central processing speed (FePsy) and intelligence (Raven)	None: type of epilepsy, seizure type, and seizure frequency not different among the groups.	Level II-1	Well-powered study (for OXC) showing no cognitive effects relative to CBZ and VPA	6mo
Intelligence (WISC), attention and memory (FePsy)	Seizure effects during the trial; some patients came into remission, others not	Level 11-3	Well-powered study showing no cognitive change vs a nonmedication baseline	6mo
Intelligence (WISC), Gestalt (Bender), psychomotor (ITPA)	Seizure control effects	Level II-3	Well-powered study showing no cognitive change vs a nonmedication baseline	18mo
Attention and central processing speed (FePsy) and intelligence (Raven)	None: type of epilepsy, seizure type, and seizure frequency not different among the groups.	Level II-1	Moderate-powered study (for CBZ) showing no cognitive effects relative to OXC and VPA	6mo
Intelligence (WISC)	None: same types of epilepsy; same treatment effects	Level II-1	Moderate-powered study showing no cognitive effects relative to LTG	6mo
Intelligence (WISC), attention (CPT), memory (TEMA), executive function (WCST)	All kinds of confounders; type of epilepsy, seizure control, underlying etiology	Case study	No conclusions possible	12mo
Gestalt (Bender), intelligence (WISC),	Seizure effect	Level II-1	Moderate-powered design	6mo
Composite index consisting intelligence (WISC), Gestalt (Bender). Learning (WRAT), memory (DTLA-2)	Seizure effects; different types of epilepsy	Case reports	No conclusions possible	6mo (*n* = 12); 12mo (*n* = 5)
Intelligence (WISC) and Gestalt (Bender)	Open study	Level II-1	Reasonable power	12mo

TABLE 7.2 continued

AED	Study	N	Age	Design	Type of cognitive impairment
	Jung et al. (2015)	40 on CBZ vs 41 on LTG	4–16y	Open-label randomized comparative design comparing CBZ to LTG	No impairment
	Stores et al. (1992)	29 on CBZ vs 34 on VPA	10y	Open-label nonrandomized comparative trial	No impairment
	Mandelbaum et al. (2009)	31 (out of 57 at baseline)	Unknown	Open-label trial in children with newly diagnosed idiopathic epilepsy	Impairment only in focal epilepsies, maybe due to CBZ treatment
Valproate (VPA)	Donati et al. (2006; 2007)	29 on VPA vs 28 on CBZ vs 55 on OXC	9.8y	Open-label randomized active-control three-arm study in newly diagnosed patients on monotherapy	No difference with CBZ or VPA
	Piccinelli et al. (2010)	35	9.5–9.9y	Open-label study comparing patients with all sorts on epilepsy relative to CBZ	No cognitive change over time
	Glauser et al. (2013)	147 (vs 149 LTG vs 155 ETS)	7.5y	Randomized comparative study in children with childhood absence epilepsy	Attentional impairment relative to ETS and LTG
	Mandelbaum and Burack (1997)	5 (6 m), 3 (12 m)	4–16y	Open-label study with untreated baseline	No impairment
	Calandre et al. (1990)	26 on VPA (initially 32) vs 23 on PHB (initially 32)	8.9y	Open-label, partly retrospective comparative study comparing VPA to PHB	No impairment
	Chen et al. (1996)	25 on VPA vs 25 on CBZ and 23 on PHB	9.9–10.8	Open randomized comparative design comparing VPA with CBZ and PHB	No impairment
	Stores et al. (1992)	34 on VPA vs 29 on CBZ	10y	Open-label nonrandomized comparative trial	No impairment
	Vining et al. (1987)	21	10.2y	Randomized crossover design	Intelligence and memory lower in the PHB condition

Type of measurement	Confounders	Evidence level	Effect size	Length of follow-up
Intelligence (WISC)	Selection bias before inclusion	Level II-2	Moderate power	12mo
Intelligence (WISC), memory, attention, learning abilities	Treatment bias	Level III	No definitive conclusions	12mo
Intelligence (Kaufman), memory (WRAML; CVLT), attention (Stroop; Tova), executive function (TMT)	All kinds; this is a series of case reports	Case reports	No power; no conclusions possible	12mo
Attention and central processing speed (FePsy) and intelligence (Raven)	None: type of epilepsy, seizure type, and seizure frequency not different among the groups.	Level II-1	Moderate-powered study (for 6mo VPA) showing no cognitive effects relative to OXC and VPA	
Intelligence (WISC),attention (CPT), memory (TEMA), executive function (WCST)	All kinds of confounders; type of epilepsy, seizure control, underlying etiology	Case study	No conclusions possible	12mo
Attention (Conners CPT)	No blinding	Level II-1	High-powered study; results convincing ($p \leq 0.01$)	12mo
Composite index consisting intelligence (WISC), Gestalt (Bender). Learning (WRAT), memory (DTLA-2)	Seizure effects; different types of epilepsy	Case reports	No conclusions possible	6mo ($n = 4$); 12mo ($n = 3$)
Intelligence (WISC)	Selective dropout; treatment bias (treatment assignment non-randomized)	Level II-3	Limited power; limited effects (4 IQ points difference between VPA and PHB)	6–9mo
Intelligence (WISC) and Gestalt (Bender)	Open study	Level II-1	Reasonable power	12mo
Intelligence (WISC), memory, attention, learning abilities	Treatment bias	Level III	No definitive conclusions	12mo
Intelligence (WISC) and large comprehensive battery	Treatment bias	Level II-1	$p < 0.01$, however not corrected for multiple testing	12mo (6mo per drug)

TABLE 7.2 continued

AED	Study	N	Age	Design	Type of cognitive impairment
Zonisamide (ZNS)					
	Eun et al. (2011)	70	7.8–8.3y	Open-label randomized comparative design comparing low dose vs high dose in newly diagnosed	Cognitive impairment at higher dose: language development, especially vocabulary acquisition
Lamotrigine (LTG)					
	Eun et al. (2012 b)	32 (start 43)	8.3–9.2y	Randomized open-label comparative design comparing monotherapy LTG with CBZ in newly diagnosed partial epilepsy	No cognitive differences with CBZ over time
	Glauser et al. (2013)	149 (vs 155 ETS vs 147 VPA)	7.5y	Randomized comparative study in children with childhood absence epilepsy	No impairment relative to ETS and VPA
	Jung et al. (2015)	41 on LTG vs 40 on CBZ	4–16y	Open-label randomized comparative design comparing LTG to CBZ	No impairment
Topiramate (TPM)					
	Kang et al. (2007)	45 (vs 43 for CBZ)	8.7y	Randomized open label comparative design, comparing TPM with CBZ in Rolandic epilepsy	Only impairment on one subtest of WISC arithmetic and only on higher dose of TPM
Phenobarbital (PHB)					
	Camfield et al. (1979)	24 (18 controls)	15–17mo	Randomized placebo controlled in patients with febrile seizures	Memory impairment
	Farwell et al. (1990)	83 (94 placebo)	8–36mo	Randomized Placebo controlled in patients with febrile seizures	Intelligence
	Calandre et al. (1990)	23 on PHB (initially 32) vs 26 on VPA (initially 32)	8.9y	Open-label, partly retrospective comparative study comparing VPA to PHB	Impairment of intelligence
	Chen et al. (1996)	23 on PHB vs 25 on VPA vs 25 on CBZ	9.9–10.8	Open randomized comparative design	No impairment

Type of measurement	Confounders	Evidence level	Effect size	Length of follow-up
Intelligence (WISC)	None: no differences in seizure control (both groups >50% in remission); assignment to dose group randomized	Level II-1	Well-powered study showing risks for language development at higher dose	6mo
Intelligence (WISC)	None: same types of epilepsy; same treatment effects	Level II-1	Moderate-powered study showing no cognitive effects relative to CBZ	6mo
Attention (Conners CPT)	No blinding; seizure effects	Level II-1	High-powered study; results convincing	12mo
Intelligence (WISC)	Selection bias before inclusion	Level II-2	Moderate power	12mo
Gestalt (Bender), intelligence (WISC),	Seizure effect	Level II-1	Moderate effects reported (1 subtest; no Bonferroni correction)	6mo
Intelligence (Bayley or Stanford Binet)	No epilepsy; selective dropout (about 40%)	Level II-2	Low-powered study	8–12mo
Intelligence (Stanford Binet)	Selection bias and selective drop-out	Level 11-2	High-powered study showing a 8-point drop in IQ ($p = 0.006$)	2y
Intelligence (WISC)	Selective dropout; treatment bias (treatment assignment nonrandomized)	Level II-3	Limited power; limited effects (4 IQ points difference between VPA and PHB)	6–9mo
Intelligence (WISC) and Gestalt (Bender)	Open study	Level II-1	Reasonable power	12mo

TABLE 7.2 continued

AED	Study	N	Age	Design	Type of cognitive impairment
	Vining et al. (1987)	21	10.2y	Randomized crossover design	Intelligence and memory lower in the PHB condition
Ethosuximide (ETS)					
	Glauser et al. (2013)	155 (vs 149 LTG vs 147 VPA)	7.5y	Randomized comparative study in children with childhood absence epilepsy	No impairment relative to LTG and VPA
	Mandelbaum and Burack (1997)	7 (6 m), 4 (12 m)	4–16y	Open-label study with untreated baseline	No impairment

REFERENCES

Calandre EP, Dominguez-Granados R, Gomez-Rubio M and Molina-Font JA (1990) Cognitive effects of long-term treatment with phenobarbital and valproic acid in school children. *Acta Neurol Scand* 81: 504–506.

Camfield CS, Chaplin S, Doyle AB et al. (1979) Side effects of phenobarbital in toddlers; behavioral and cognitive aspects. *J Pediatr* 95: 361–365.

Chen YJ, Kang WM and So WC (1996) Comparison of antiepileptic drugs on cognitive function in newly diagnosed epileptic children: A psychometric and neurophysiological study. *Epilepsia* 37: 81–86.

Cross JH (2010) Neurodevelopmental effects of anti-epileptic drugs. *Epilepsy Res* 88: 1–10.

Donati F, Gobbi G, Campistol J et al. (2006) Effects of oxcarbazepine on cognitive function in children and adolescents with partial seizures. *Neurology* 67: 679–682.

Donati F, Gobbi G, Campistol J et al. (2007) The cognitive effects of oxcarbazepine versus carbamazepine or valproate in newly diagnosed children with partial seizures. *Seizure* 16: 670–679.

Eun SH, Eun BL, Lee JS et al. (2012a) Effects of lamotrigine on cognition and behavior compared to carbamazepine as monotherapy for children with partial epilepsy. *Brain Dev* 34: 818–823.

Eun SH, Kim HD, Chung HJ et al. (2012 b) A multicenter trial of oxcarbazepine oral suspension monotherapy in children newly diagnosed with partial seizures: A clinical and cognitive evaluation. *Seizure* 21: 679–684.

Eun SH, Kim HD, Eun BL et al. (2011) Comparative trial of low- and high-dose zonisamide as monotherapy for childhood epilepsy. *Seizure* 20: 558–563.

Farwell JR, Lee YJ, Hirtz DG et al. (1990) Phenobarbital for febrile seizures—Effects on intelligence and on seizure recurrence. *N Engl J Med* 322: 364–369.

Glauser TA, Cnaan A, Shinnar S et al. (2013) Ethosuximide, valproic acid, and lamotrigine in childhood absence epilepsy: Initial monotherapy outcomes at 12 months. *Epilepsia* 54: 141–155.

Helmstaedter C, Aldenkamp AP, Baker GA et al. (2014) Disentangling the relationship between epilepsy and its behavioral comorbidities—The need for prospective studies in new-onset epilepsies. *Epilepsy Behav* 31: 43–47.

Ijff DM and Aldenkamp AP (2013) Chapter 73 - Cognitive side-effects of antiepileptic drugs in children. In: Olivier Dulac ML and Harvey BS, editors. *Handbook of Clinical Neurology* (Vol. 111, pp. 707–718). Oxford: Elsevier Science.

Type of measurement	Confounders	Evidence level	Effect size	Length of follow-up
Intelligence (WISC) and large comprehensive battery	Treatment bias	Level II-1	$p < 0.01$, however not corrected for multiple testing	12mo (6mo per drug)
Attention (Conners CPT)	No blinding; seizure effects	Level II-1	High-powered study; results convincing	12mo
Composite index consisting intelligence (WISC), Gestalt (Bender). Learning (WRAT), memory (DTLA-2)	Seizure effects; different types of epilepsy	Case reports	No conclusions possible	6mo ($n = 7$); 12mo ($n = 4$)

Jung DE, Yu R, Yoon JR et al. (2015) Neuropsychological effects of levetiracetam and carbamazepine in children with focal epilepsy. *Neurology* 84: 2312–2319.

Kang HC, Eun BL, Wu Lee C et al. (2007). The effects on cognitive function and behavioral problems of topiramate compared to carbamazepine as monotherapy for children with benign rolandic epilepsy. *Epilepsia* 48: 1716–1723.

Mandelbaum DE and Burack GD (1997) The effect of seizure type and medication on cognitive and behavioral functioning in children with idiopathic epilepsy. *Dev Med Child Neurol* 39: 731–735.

Mandelbaum DE, Burack GD and Bhise VV (2009) Impact of antiepileptic drugs on cognition, behavior, and motor skills in children with new-onset, idiopathic epilepsy. *Epilepsy Behav* 16: 341–344.

Mula M and Trimble MR (2009) Antiepileptic drug-induced cognitive adverse effects. *CNS Drugs* 23: 121–137.

Piccinelli P, Beghi E, Borgatti R et al. (2010) Neuropsychological and behavioural aspects in children and adolescents with idiopathic epilepsy at diagnosis and after 12 months of treatment. *Seizure* 19: 540–546.

Stores G, Williams PL, Styles E and Zaiwalla Z (1992) Psychological effects of sodium valproate and carbamazepine in epilepsy. *Arch Dis Child* 67: 1330–1337.

Tzitiridou M, Panou T, Ramantani G et al. (2005) Oxcarbazepine monotherapy in benign childhood epilepsy with centrotemporal spikes: A clinical and cognitive evaluation. *Epilepsy Behav* 7: 458–467.

Vermeulen J and Aldenkamp AP (1995) Cognitive side-effects of chronic antiepileptic drug treatment: A review of 25 years of research. *Epilepsy Res* 22: 65–95.

Vining EP, Mellitis ED, Dorsen MM et al. (1987) Psychologic and behavioral effects of antiepileptic drugs in children: A double-blind comparison between phenobarbital and valproic acid. *Pediatrics* 80: 165–174.

8
OUTCOME AFTER NEONATAL SEIZURES

Renée A Shellhaas and Courtney J Wusthoff

Introduction

A child is at his highest lifetime risk of seizure during the first month of life. Neonatal seizures occur in 1–5 per 1000 term newborn infants, with estimates as high as 1 per 20 among preterm or very-low-birth-weight newborn infants (Vasudevan and Levene 2013). Although neonatal seizures can occur at any point up to 4 weeks after term equivalent age, the majority of neonatal seizures occur during the first few days after birth. Seizures in the neonatal period are most often symptomatic of acute brain injury and less commonly reflect an early-onset epilepsy syndrome.

Neonatal seizures are defined electrographically as sudden, evolving, rhythmic discharges lasting longer than 10 seconds. As with seizures in older age groups, neonatal seizures may manifest clinically as a variety of motor signs, automatisms, or autonomic fluctuations. The majority of seizures are subclinical, which is unique to neonatal seizures. These require EEG for diagnosis; as such, the true incidence of neonatal seizures may be higher than previously recognized. Because the majority of neonatal seizures occur in patients with coexisting neurological disorders, it is difficult to disentangle the contribution of seizures to later outcomes from the role of the underlying brain problem that caused the seizures. Furthermore, there are concerns that chronic antiepileptic drug administration to infants may in itself negatively impact brain development. Despite these complexities, a growing body of research has begun to elucidate the relationship between neonatal seizures and neurodevelopmental outcomes.

Diagnosis of neonatal seizures

Neonatal seizures are particularly challenging to diagnose. In contrast to seizures in older children and adults, the large majority of neonatal seizures are subclinical—they have no clear outward signs. Alternately, neonatal seizures are sometimes described as "subtle" or "nonconvulsive." Because there are not reliable outward clinical signs, EEG is required for accurate diagnosis.

Traditionally, neonatal seizures had been diagnosed primarily by clinical observation. They were widely characterized and classified according to the system proposed by Volpe (2008). This system classifies seizures by their motor signs as focal clonic, multifocal clonic, generalized tonic, myoclonic, and subtle. In this classification scheme, subtle seizures include those with smaller, distinctive signs such as eye movements, lip smacking, swimming or pedaling movements, tonic posturing of a single limb, or apnea. Early research in neonatal seizures relied on clinical features for the diagnosis of seizure. However, EEG data have clarified that not all clinically suspicious events are epileptic seizures. For example, in their study of 349 neonates, Mizrahi and Kellaway (1987) reviewed EEG monitoring to correlate the observed clinical signs on video with epileptic seizures recorded on EEG. Of 415 events characterized as seizure on the basis of signs seen on video, 296 (71%) had an inconsistent or no relationship to ictal discharges on EEG. In particular, events of motor automatisms (mouth movements, eye movements) or myoclonus were often found to lack clear EEG correlate. These findings call into question the reliability of clinical observation for the diagnosis of epileptic neonatal seizures. Although it is possible that the events without EEG correlates truly were epileptic seizures, but with foci too deep to record on scalp EEG, the authors suggest that it is more likely that many of the abnormal events diagnosed clinically as seizures were, in fact, not epileptic seizures. These findings have been replicated in other studies using video EEG monitoring to demonstrate poor accuracy of bedside observation for diagnosis of neonatal seizures.

Although clinical observation alone may lead to incorrect diagnosis of abnormal movements as seizures, conversely, many subtle and subclinical seizures are missed when diagnosis is made by clinical observation alone. One study reviewed EEG recordings among 41 patients with neonatal seizures (Clancy and Legido 1988). During the EEG recordings, experienced EEG technologists noted any observed signs suspicious for seizure as they occurred. The authors found that, overall, 79% of seizures had no distinctive clinical signs. More recently, 51 term neonates had continuous video EEG recordings reviewed to define the gap between clinical diagnosis and EEG-based diagnosis of seizure burden (Murray et al. 2008). Two-thirds of captured seizures had no clinical signs on video, whereas only 9% of all seizures were recognized and documented by the bedside nurse or physician. At the same time, 73% of the events documented by the bedside nurse or physician were not associated with electrographic seizures. Again, these findings confirm that clinical diagnosis is unreliable for neonatal seizures. That seizures in neonates are most often subclinical should be intuitive—unless the seizure originates or propagates to the motor cortex, there will be no abnormal movements, and a non-verbal newborn infant will never complain of a stereotyped sensory aura. Because of the preponderance of subclinical seizures, EEG monitoring provides the criterion standard for diagnosis. For this reason, it has been recommended that all neonates at high risk for seizures are assessed using full-array video EEG monitoring (Shellhaas et al. 2011).

More recently, amplitude-integrated EEG (aEEG) has gained popularity as a tool for seizure detection in the intensive care nursery. aEEG is a simplified trend, based on two- or three-channel EEG recording. The recordings are time compressed (6cm per hour) and processed to display a bedside trend for the nurse or neonatologist to interpret in real time. There is a wide variability in the sensitivity of aEEG for seizure detection, with reported sensitivities most often about 25–35%, and rarely as high as 85%, for individual seizure detection (Glass et al. 2013). Given this suboptimal rate of seizure detection, caution must be used in interpreting data regarding seizures diagnosed by aEEG.

Overall, significant evidence supports continuous EEG as the criterion standard for neonatal seizure diagnosis. Clinical observation alone suffers from high rates of both over-diagnosis of clinically suspected seizures and missing common subclinical seizures in these neonates. Similarly, aEEG fails to detect a significant percentage of neonatal seizures. This has implications for research regarding the outcomes following neonatal seizures. Studies that relate only clinical seizures to outcomes may be incomplete, by missing subclinical seizures. Furthermore, they run the risk of including infants with inaccurate diagnoses of neonatal seizure, based on clinical signs alone and/or including infants with only subclinical seizures in the "seizure-free" control group. The best evidence comes from those studies that apply the criterion standard for neonatal seizure diagnosis, continuous video EEG monitoring, but these typically lack long-term follow-up.

Aetiologies and comorbidities of neonatal seizures

When considering neurodevelopmental outcomes following neonatal seizures, there is a complex interplay between the role of the seizures themselves and the contribution of the underlying brain disorder that is causing the seizures. The large majority of neonatal seizures are symptomatic of an underlying acute process (Table 8.1). In North America and Europe, hypoxic-ischemic encephalopathy (HIE) is the most common cause of neonatal seizures, accounting for roughly half of term newborn infants with seizures. The incidence of associated seizures may have declined with a widespread use of therapeutic hypothermia as a neuroprotection strategy for neonates with HIE. Yet, studies using video EEG have demonstrated that about half of neonates receiving hypothermia still have seizures during the first 4 days of life (Glass et al. 2014). In these cases, the hypoxic-ischemic injury confers a risk of impaired development, independent from, and in addition to the risk, from the seizures. Stroke is the next most common aetiology in term newborn infants, causing approximately 10% to 15% of neonatal seizures (Vasudevan and Levene 2013). In preterm neonates, intraventricular hemorrhage is the second most common cause of neonatal seizures. Finally, meningitis, glucose and electrolyte derangements, and maternal drug withdrawal are all potential causes of symptomatic seizures.

Less common are neonatal-onset epilepsy syndromes. Some of these are now known to be the result of genetic mutations, inborn errors of metabolism, or cerebral malformations. Genetic disorders are increasingly identified in patients with neonatal-onset epilepsies. For example, mutations in the potassium channel gene *KCNQ2* are now known to cause the majority of cases of benign familial neonatal seizures. Glucose transporter deficiency syndrome is an example of a metabolic disorder that similarly causes, difficult to control neonatal seizures. Pyridoxine-dependent epilepsy may also present in the neonatal period. Cerebral malformations have been estimated to cause up to 10% of all neonatal seizures.

Finally, because many of these children are critically ill, they often experience comorbidities, which may further affect neurodevelopment. For example, a child with seizures due to HIE is at neurodevelopmental risk due to the primary brain injury, in addition to the seizures, but may also have sepsis in the neonatal period, or feeding difficulties with poor nutritional intake, further elevating the risk of later neurodevelopmental impairment.

TABLE 8.1
Aetiologies of neonatal seizures

Categories of seizure aetiologies	Examples[1]
Reversible causes	Hypoglycemia Hypocalcemia Hypernatremia Neonatal abstinence syndrome
Acute acquired brain injury	Hypoxic ischemic encephalopathy Arterial ischemic stroke Cerebral sinovenous thrombosis Intraventricular hemorrhage
Infection	Meningitis Encephalitis Toxoplasmosis, Rubella, Cytomegalovirus and Herpes simplex virus infections[2]
Congenital brain malformations	Malformations of cortical development (e.g. lissencephaly or focal cortical dysplasia) Disorders of prosencephalic development (e.g. holoprosencephaly)
Genetic epilepsy syndromes or metabolic disorders[3]	Benign familial neonatal seizures Glucose transporter deficiency syndrome Pyridoxine-dependent epilepsy Early myoclonic epilepsy of infancy Ohtahara syndrome Inborn errors of metabolism Urea cycle disorders

[1] These lists are not meant to be exhaustive; rather, they are designed to represent some of the major aetiologies of neonatal seizures.
[2] TORCH infections include toxoplasmosis, rubella, cytomegalovirus, and herpes simplex virus.
[3] These are *far* less common than the other aetiologies listed in this table.

Barriers to long-term developmental follow-up

Neonatal seizures are common and consequential, but alarmingly large knowledge gaps remain. Although neonatal seizures, as a group, occur quite commonly, their causes are manifold and individually rare. Because of this, even large-scale cohort studies lack power to assess outcomes according to subgroups. Many of the published longitudinal follow-up studies have not included, for example, any patients with the (benign or refractory) neonatal epilepsy syndromes. Similarly, infants with major congenital anomalies and chromosomal abnormalities are virtually always excluded. Therefore, of necessity, overall conclusions and case-by-case predictions about long-term outcomes are challenging.

Long-term follow-up studies for neonates with seizures do, however, provide clues regarding risk factors for adverse (or favorable) outcomes. The literature must be interpreted carefully, as there are various potential pitfalls and nuances. There may be bias in loss to follow-up. For example, neonates who appear normal as toddlers may not present for formal developmental follow-up assessments. Conversely, some parents of survivors with poor outcomes choose not to quantify the adverse development or need to prioritize multiple specialist appointments and so do not present for follow-up. Distance to follow-up centers, cost of developmental assessment, and short-term grant funding cycles are all barriers to high-quality, objective neurodevelopmental follow-up studies.

The source of patients is also a key factor. Neonates selected from neurology clinics are, perhaps, more likely to be followed due to epilepsy. Infants enrolled from a high-level intensive care nursery may not be representative of the entire population of neonates with seizures because of a referral bias that enriches the neonatal intensive care unit (NICU) population for severe aetiologies and therefore high risk for adverse outcomes.

There are a multitude of options for developmental outcomes assessments. Some require intensive in-person evaluations and provide detailed and reproducible data regarding various developmental domains. Others are screening questionnaires administered by mail or by telephone, and provide an overall assessment without the details. Many studies have relied on a neurologist's personal impression of a "good" or "unfavourable" outcome, without any validated assessment measure. Few provide truly long-term outcome assessments. The standard for neonatal intensive care follow-up studies at present is an evaluation at 18–22 months. From a societal perspective, understanding outcomes as survivors enter adulthood would be valuable, but have not typically been feasible.

As discussed previously, another consideration as one interprets the literature is the criteria for neonatal seizure diagnosis. Most of the longer term (beyond 2 years) follow-up studies are based on clinical diagnosis of seizures. Because seizure diagnosis in newborn infants is notoriously difficult, studies of clinical seizures are potentially problematic (seizures may be both under- and overdiagnosed). Similarly, treatment is not often discussed in long-term follow-up studies, but duration of treatment and selection of antiseizure medication regimens are potentially relevant considerations.

Animal models of neonatal seizures

Distinguishing the impact of seizures in human neonates on long-term outcomes from their underlying aetiologies and treatments is extremely challenging. However, a robust body of experimental literature provides clues regarding the contributions of seizures and their treatments to long-term clinical outcomes. The evidence suggests that these seizures adversely affect the developing brain.

Rather than inducing neuronal cell loss, the reported abnormalities include aberrant synaptogenesis, synaptic plasticity, and synaptic reorganization, particularly in the hippocampus. Neurogenesis is also affected, as are gamma-aminobutyric acid and glutamate physiology. Otherwise, healthy rats subjected to early-life seizures have repeatedly been shown to exhibit cognitive deficits when tested during adolescence or adulthood, as demonstrated by poor performance in Morris water maze experiments and aberrant hippocampal place cell firing patterns (reviewed in [Holmes 2009]). Early-life status epilepticus has been associated with alterations in social behaviors and anxiety in rat models (e.g. Castelhano et al. 2013).

Conversely, treatment with phenobarbital is reported to induce abnormal neuronal apoptosis (Bittigau et al. 2002) and may result in long-term functional deficits in rats. In particular, spatial memory is impaired (Morris water maze test) in phenobarbital-exposed neonatal rats when they are tested as adults. Others have demonstrated impaired learning and/or recall using passive avoidance tests in adult rats that were treated with phenobarbital on P7–P10 (Gutherz et al. 2014).

Range of outcomes after neonatal seizures

Cognitive and behavioral outcomes are enmeshed in multiple medical and social factors for survivors of neonatal seizures. For the most part, outcomes are driven by the aetiology of the seizures. It is difficult to distinguish the effects of neonatal seizures from the cerebral disturbance(s) causing them. Neonates with seizures due to epilepsy (e.g. associated with a structural brain malformation or a severe genetic channelopathy) nearly always have severe lifelong neurodevelopmental disability. Conversely, newborn infants with transient acute symptomatic seizures related to easily reversible causes, such as moderate hypoglycemia or hypocalcemia, typically do very well and are not usually followed longitudinally in any study. However, for many affected neonates, the prognosis is not so clear.

Mortality after neonatal seizures ranges between approximately 10% and 30% in the neonatal period and is highest among preterm infants. The broad range may reflect changes in clinical NICU practice over time, as well as cultural differences regarding the practice of withdrawal of intensive care for neonates with very poor prognosis. Some survivors, typically those with comorbid severe developmental disabilities, die during childhood.

Adverse neurodevelopmental outcomes occur in approximately 50% of survivors. This figure includes 15–30% of those who develop post-neonatal epilepsy (acute symptomatic seizures subside, but recurrent unprovoked seizures develop later). Most often, epilepsy develops in the first 1 to 4 years of life (median = 9 months in [Ronen et al. 2007]), and many of these infants and children develop severe epilepsy syndromes, such as West syndrome (10–16%). Many survivors with epilepsy have comorbid cerebral palsy and intellectual disability. Approximately 25–45% of all neonates with seizures go on to develop some degree of cerebral palsy (Uria-Avellanal et al. 2013). Having cerebral palsy is a significant risk factor for post-neonatal epilepsy and neurocognitive disability.

Developmental and cognitive outcomes are variable, but there is no doubt that a history of neonatal seizures is a major risk factor for intellectual disability and global developmental delay. Precise definitions of the cognitive outcomes vary across published studies. Some have used standardized, validated neurodevelopmental testing, such as the Bayley Scales of Infant and Toddler Development, but others employ a more global assessment of "good" or "adverse" outcomes. Most often, cognitive and behavioral outcomes are not reported separately from neuromotor deficits. NICU follow-up studies are typically powered for a combined outcome of death or moderate-to-severe disability, which is defined as a mental development index less than two standard deviations below the mean, and/or cerebral palsy, and/or epilepsy, and/or blindness, and/or requirement for assistive hearing devices.

Several studies have reported outcomes for unselected populations of neonates with clinical seizures. A population-based study of 90 neonates (any gestational age) born in 1990–1994 in Newfoundland, Canada, and followed-up 10 years later reported that 21% died (median age at death was 13mo), whereas 35% had normal outcomes (defined as the absence of physical or intellectual impairment), and 41% survived with neurodevelopmental impairment (cerebral palsy, cognitive impairment, learning disability at school age, other neurological impairments, and/or post-neonatal epilepsy) (Ronen et al. 2007).

Another study, of 120 term neonates with clinical seizures due to various causes, who were all followed by a single child neurologist, reported that by 1–2 years of age, 9% had

TABLE 8.2
Risk factors for adverse outcomes after neonatal seizures

Categories of risk factors	Examples
Clinical risk factors	Abnormal neurological examination (especially severe encephalopathy)
	Prematurity
	Abnormal neuroimaging
	Need for multiple anticonvulsant medications
	Increased seizure burden (clinical or EEG)
	Status epilepticus
	Socioeconomic status
EEG risk factors	Multifocal seizure onset
	Status epilepticus
	Persistently abnormal interictal EEG (especially burst suppression)
Risk factors for post-neonatal epilepsy	Burst suppression on neonatal EEG
	Multifocal seizures; ictal spread to contralateral hemisphere
	Neonatal status epilepticus
	Structural brain abnormality (acquired or developmental)
	Cerebral palsy
	Intellectual disability

died, 44% had a normal and 47% an abnormal outcome. Cerebral palsy was diagnosed in 28% of survivors, 38% had global developmental delay, and 27% had epilepsy (infantile spasms in three individuals) (Garfinkle and Shevell 2011).

About one-third of neonates with seizures go on to develop epilepsy, and many of these individuals have comorbid global developmental delay and/or cerebral palsy. Among people with epilepsy, a history of clinical neonatal seizures is a clear risk factor for non-remission of the epilepsy (Sillanpää et al.1995). By extension, because treatment-resistant epilepsy syndromes are associated with array cognitive and behavioral challenges, early-life seizures may predispose to long-term intellectual and behavioral difficulties.

Risk factors for adverse outcomes
Even though neonatal seizures are relatively common, they arise from such a diverse range of aetiologies that it remains difficult to apply many of the published data to individual patients. Nonetheless, some specific risk factors and subgroups are commonly studied (Table 8.2).

Data regarding electrographic seizures among preterm infants are sparse. However, studies that evaluate clinically diagnosed seizures among preterm and term infants consistently identify prematurity as a risk factor for adverse outcomes, including death, cerebral palsy, and developmental delays. Additionally, studies of extremely low-birth-weight neonates report clinical neonatal seizures as one of the most robust predictors of abnormal 18- to 22-month outcomes, along with intracranial hemorrhage, and male sex (Teune et al. 2011). Although no published study has explicitly evaluated sex as a risk factor for adverse outcomes after human neonatal seizures, male sex has repeatedly been highlighted as a risk factor for abnormal neurodevelopment among preterm infants and in animal models of hypoxia-ischemia.

A high seizure burden, especially status epilepticus, appears to augment the risk for unfavorable outcomes. The risk of post-neonatal epilepsy is substantially higher among those with electrographic status epilepticus than those with isolated neonatal seizures, even after adjustment for MRI-detected brain injury and severity of encephalopathy (~50% to 80% of the adverse outcome after status epilepticus vs 15% to 30% after isolated seizures, e.g., [Glass et al. 2011]).

Beyond status epilepticus, electrographic features of the seizures, especially multifocal onset and ictal spread to the contralateral hemisphere, are predictive of post-neonatal epilepsy. Persistently abnormal interictal EEG abnormalities, including lack of sleep–wake cycling, confer the risk of unfavorable neurodevelopmental outcomes. The presence of burst suppression, at any time point, is also an ominous sign.

About half of survivors have clinically significant global developmental delays. Just as increasing neonatal seizure burden is associated with later epilepsy, it is also associated with later neurocognitive deficits. Among neonates with HIE who were evaluated at the age of 4 years, those with the highest electrographic seizure burden were reported to have an average full-scale IQ 33 points (two standard deviations) lower than those without neonatal seizures, even after adjusting for injury on brain MRI (Glass et al. 2009). Those with milder seizure burden still scored one full standard deviation lower, on average, than their seizure-free peers. These startling results suggest that neonatal seizures augment the adverse effects of acute neonatal encephalopathy.

Newborn infants with congenital heart disease form a particularly well-studied subgroup. Among the longest term follow-up studies of neonates with EEG-confirmed seizures, the Boston Circulatory Arrest Study results indicate that perioperative seizures are associated with 12.6 (clinical seizures) and 7.7 (EEG seizures) points lower than the full-scale IQ scores at an age of 4 years, compared with seizure-free neonates with transposition of the great arteries. When these children were reexamined at the age of 16 years, neonatal seizures were reported to predict worse scores across cognitive domains, including tests of reading and math, general memory, executive function, visual–spatial, and social awareness (Bellinger et al. 2011). In a separate cohort, postoperative EEG seizures were associated with measurable impairment in executive functioning and social behavior 4 years after congenital heart surgery (Gaynor et al. 2013).

Potentially modifiable risk factors

Most of the risk factors for adverse cognitive and medical outcomes after neonatal seizures are fixed from the time of diagnosis. However, a few are potentially modifiable and warrant consideration. The environment of rearing has a meaningful impact on the development after acquired neonatal brain injury in animal models (Chou et al. 2001). Among preterm infants and those with presumed perinatal unilateral arterial ischemic stroke, maternal education is a leading influence on long-term cognitive development (Wickremasinghe et al. 2012; van Buuren et al. 2013). Support of families of neonates with seizures, including social and financial resources, could optimize long-term outcomes.

The impact of neonatal seizure treatment is the most elusive, but potentially influential, modifiable factor. Medical treatments for neonatal seizures are inadequately efficacious, with seizure resolution in approximately 50% with initial doses of phenobarbital or phenytoin (Painter et al. 1999), and the ideal dose and duration of treatment remain uncertain. A trial of short versus moderate duration phenobarbital therapy for acute symptomatic neonatal seizures (PROPHENO, NCT01089504) failed because of challenges with enrollment. Although adequate numbers of potential participants were identified, a high proportion of parents refused to consent and many clinicians refused to enrol their patients. Future studies of neonatal seizure treatments must evaluate not only short-term efficacy but also the most appropriate duration of therapy.

Implications for clinical care

Because neonatal seizures are associated with impaired neurodevelopmental outcome, it is appropriate to pursue accurate diagnosis and treatment. In neonates with clinical events suspicious for seizure, or at high risk for subclinical seizures, EEG monitoring should be employed for diagnosis whenever possible (Shellhaas et al. 2011). Indeed, the 2011 World Health Organization guideline on neonatal seizures makes a strong recommendation that where available, all clinical seizures in the neonatal period should be confirmed by EEG (WHO/ILAE/IRCCS 2011). Similarly, because higher seizure burden has been associated with worse outcomes, all EEG-confirmed seizures should be treated. This includes subclinical seizures. In counselling families regarding neurodevelopmental prognosis following neonatal seizures, we focus on the underlying aetiology of the neonatal seizures, as this has the largest influence on outcome. Given the high risk of developmental impairment and epilepsy following neonatal seizures, we plan neurodevelopmental follow-up after hospital discharge to facilitate early identification of sequelae. This includes a full developmental assessment by 24 months of age to evaluate for cognitive or behavioral problems.

Future research directions

Despite robust basic science literature that indicates neonatal seizures have adverse effects on the developing brain, and observational studies that demonstrate the high risk of death, neuromotor impairment, and a broad-array of cognitive disabilities associated with early-life seizures, substantial knowledge gaps remain. Heterogeneity across the studies of neonatal seizures, including diagnosis by clinical observation versus EEG criteria, duration, quality, and quantity of follow-up data, and a lack of multicenter studies are consequential limitations to the clinical research knowledge base. Perhaps most importantly, treatments for neonatal seizures are incompletely effective and are known to have independent consequences on the developing brain. Large-scale multicenter studies with standardized EEG criteria for seizure diagnosis and high-quality follow-up are needed to further elucidate the relationship between neonatal seizures and outcomes, and to identify interventions to reduce neurodevelopmental risk.

REFERENCES

Bellinger DC, Wypij D, Rivkin MJ et al. (2011) Adolescents with d-transposition of the great arteries corrected with the arterial switch procedure: Neuropsychological assessment and structural brain imaging. *Circulation* 124: 1361–1369.

Bittigau P, Sifringer M, Genz K et al. (2002) Antiepileptic drugs and apoptotic neurodegeneration in the developing brain. *Proc Natl Acad Sci USA* 99: 15089–15094.

Castelhano ASS, Cassane GST, Scorza FA and Cysneiros RM (2013) Altered anxiety-related and abnormal social behaviors in rats exposed to early life seizures. *Front Behav Neurosci* 7: 36.

Chou IC, Trakht T, Signori C et al. (2001) Behavioral/environmental intervention imrpoves learning after cerebral hypoxia-ischemia in rats. *Stroke* 32: 2192–2197.

Clancy RR and Legido ADL (1988) Occult neonatal seizures. *Epilepsia* 29: 256–261.

Garfinkle J and Shevell MI (2011) Cerebral palsy, developmental delay, and epilepsy after neonatal seizures. *Pediatr Neurol* 44: 88–96.

Gaynor JW, Jarvik GP, Gerdes M et al. (2013) Postoperative elecencephalographic seizures are associated with deficits in executive function and social behaviors at 4 years of age following cardiac surgery in infancy. *J Thorac Cardiovasc Surg* 146: 132–137.

Glass HC, Glidden D, Jeremy RJ et al. (2009) Clinical neonatal seizures are independently associated with outcome in infants at risk for hypoxic-ischemic brain injury. *J Pediatr* 155: 318–323.

Glass HC, Hong KJ, Rogers EE et al. (2011) Risk factors for epilepsy in children with neonatal encephalopathy. *Pediatr Res* 70: 535–540.

Glass HC, Wusthoff CJ and Shellhaas RA (2013) Amplitude integrated EEG: The child neurologist's perspective. *J Child Neurol* 28: 1342–1350.

Glass HC, Wusthoff CJ, Shellhaas RA et al. (2014) Risk factors for EEG seizures in neonates treated with hypothermia: A multi-center cohort study. *Neurology* 82: 1239–1244.

Gutherz SB, Kulick CV, Soper C et al. (2014) Brief postnatal exposure to phenobarbital impairs passive avoidance learning and sensorimotor gating in rats. *Epilepsy Behav* 37: 265–269.

Holmes GL (2009) The Long-term effects of neonatal seizures. *Clin Perinatol* 36: 901–914.

Mizrahi EM and Kellaway P (1987) Characterization and classification of neonatal seizures. *Neurology* 37: 1837–1844.

Murray DM, Boylan GB, Ali I et al. (2008) Defining the gap between electrographic seizure burden, clinical expression and staff recognition of neonatal seizures. *Arch Dis Child Fetal Neonatal Ed* 93: F187–F191.

Painter MJ, Scher MS, Stein AD et al. (1999) Phenobarbital compared with phenytoin for the treatment of neonatal seizures. *N Engl J Med* 341: 485–489.

Ronen GM, Buckley D, Penney S and Streiner DL (2007) Long-term prognosis in children with neonatal seizures: A population based study. *Neurology* 69: 1816–1822.

Shellhaas RA, Chang T, Tsuchida T et al. (2011) The American clinical neurophysiology society's guideline on continuous electroencephalography monitoring in neonates. *J Clin Neurophysiol* 28: 611–617.

Sillanpää M, Camfield P and Camfield C (1995) Predicting long-term outcome of childhood epilepsy in Nova Scotia, Canada, and Turku, Finland. Validation of a simple scoring system. *Arch Neurol* 52: 589–592.

Teune MJ, van Wassenaer AG, van Dommelen P, Mol BWJ and Opmeer BC (2011) for the Dutch POPS-19 collaborative study group. Perinatal risk indicators for long-term neurological morbidity among preterm neonates. *Am J Obstet Gynecol* 204: e1–e14.

Uria-Avellanal C, Marlow N and Rennie JM (2013) Outcome following neonatal seizures. *Semin Fetal Neonatal Med* 18: 224–232.

van Buuren LM, van der Aa NE, Dekker HC et al. (2013) Cognitive outcome in childhood after unilateral perinatal brain injury. *Dev Med Child Neurol* 55: 934–940.

Vasudevan C and Levene M (2013) Epidemiology and aetiology of neonatal seizures. *Semin Fetal Neonatal Med* 18: 185–191.

Volpe JJ (2008) Chapter 5: Neonatal Seizures. In: Volpe JJ editor. *Neurology of the Newborn* (5th ed., pp. 203–244). Saunders Elsevier, Philadephia, PA.

WHO/ILAE/IRCCS (2011) Guidelines on Neonatal Seizures. Accessed September 29, 2014, at http://www.who.int/mental_health/publications/guidelines_neonatal_seizures/en/.

Wickremasinghe AC, Hartman TK, Voight RG et al. (2012) Evaluation of the ability of neurobiological, neurodevelopmental, and socio-economic variables to predict cognitive outcome in premature infants. *Child Care Health Dev* 38: 683–689.

9
'BENIGN' CHILDHOOD EPILEPSY SYNDROMES: WHY DO SOME PRESENT WITH LEARNING PROBLEMS?

Stéphane Auvin

What is a 'benign' childhood epilepsy?

There are several childhood epilepsy syndromes that were reported as benign. The term 'benign' was used to characterize epilepsy syndromes of childhood with an expected remission without significant neurological sequelae in almost all affected patients. These syndromes also include childhood absence epilepsy (CAE), benign childhood epilepsy with centrotemporal spikes (BECTS), and Panayiotopoulos syndrome. Some other syndromes were also called benign, but these syndromes are less frequent (e.g. benign myoclonic epilepsy of infancy, now called myoclonic epilepsy of infancy).

The Report of the International League Against Epilepsy (ILAE) Commission on Classification and Terminology, 2005–2009, proposed to avoid using the term 'benign' to characterize any epilepsy syndrome. This is based on the better understanding and the data from research on comorbidities (cognition, psychiatric, and behavior comorbidities) showing that patients with these syndromes also exhibit a higher risk for cognitive and/or psychiatric involvement (Berg et al. 2010). This is also based on the long-term outcome. The proposal from the ILAE to define the epilepsy syndromes that tend to resolve spontaneously with time is to use the term "self-limited."

Even if an ILAE report strongly suggests avoiding the word 'benign' to define any group of epilepsy, the same published report include the name 'benign' epilepsy with centrotemporal spikes for the rolandic epilepsy syndrome. However, the work on terminology and classification of the ILAE is an ongoing process; this point might be clarified when a new classification of seizures and epilepsy syndrome will be adapted by ILAE.

Beyond the discussion around terminology to define epilepsy syndrome, it might be helpful in clinical practice to avoid the term 'benign.' The health care professional might then pay more attention to finding patients with cognitive or psychiatric comorbidities leading to early recognition and management. This might have a significant impact on the risk of academic underachievement.

Self-limited childhood epilepsies: are they benign?

BENIGN EPILEPSY WITH CENTROTEMPORAL SPIKES

BECTS or rolandic epilepsy is the most frequent epilepsy syndrome in children (Shinnar et al. 1999; Zarrelli et al. 1999). These are sensorimotor seizures (warming/paresthesia perioral; clonic involvement of the face/upper limb; speech arrest) that occur most frequently after falling asleep or before awakening. In some patients, a bilateral involvement happens shortly after the start of the seizure. Most of the patients experience very few seizures. The ictal recording of a seizure in this syndrome is very rare. Interictal EEG shows spikes of the centrotemporal area (Wirrell 1998).

BECTS should be considered as a self-limited epilepsy syndrome because in mid-adolescence, the seizures disappear in 100% of cases (Bouma et al. 1997; Peters et al. 2001). The good outcome regarding the remission of seizure does should not imply that BECTS is 'benign;' treatment with antiepileptic drugs (AEDs) is not usual. In a review of the literature on the treatment of BECTS by AEDs, Hughes (2010) reported that two-thirds of 96 studies generally favored and one-third generally did not favor AED treatment for BECTS. Only two studies favored treatment for all patients with BECTS; many other investigations were in favor, with some restrictions such as treating only patients with early onset, multiple seizures at onset, or large numbers of seizures, especially generalized tonic–clonic seizures, and limiting treatment to 1 year (Hughes 2010).

In BECTS, the evaluation of IQ is usually normal (Pinton et al. 2006; Riva et al. 2007; Piccinelli et al. 2008; Tedrus et al. 2009). However, specific cognitive deficits are prevalent in BECTS. These deficits are the major concerns because they result in a risk of academic underachievement explaining why this syndrome is not always 'benign.' Indeed, detailed studies have reported the problems in specific cognitive domains, particularly in language and verbal memory (Piccinelli et al. 2008; Danielsson and Petermann 2009; Overvliet et al. 2011). Some studies report language deficits and normal nonverbal abilities (Riva et al. 2007; Goldberg-Stern et al. 2010), but more frequently, the nonverbal performance is also found to be lower in patients with BECTS than in controls (Piccinelli et al. 2008; Danielsson and Petermann 2009).

An attention deficit as well as inhibition problems are also frequently reported (Kim et al. 2014). These have been shown in several studies with poorer performance on auditory attention and inhibition subtests (Deltour et al. 2007; Verrotti et al. 2013). These types of cognitive/behavior problems are prevalent in BECTS. They are also common in childhood epilepsy more generally (Hermann et al. 2006).

These specific cognitive deficits are subtle differences shown by comparing a group of patients matched to controls. Children and adolescents with BECTS are also at a higher risk of poorer academic performance. In a study comparing 20 patients with BECTS to 21 controls, 45% of children with epilepsy had specific difficulties in reading or writing compared with 9% of controls, and 31% of patients had specific difficulties in mathematics compared with 6% of controls (Piccinelli et al. 2008). Overvliet et al. (2011) noted that 23% of 48 children with BECTS had a history of speech therapy.

Finally, the global psychosocial outcome of BECTS raises more concern about the benignity of this epilepsy syndrome. Using adverse social outcomes, Camfield and Camfield (2014) report mitigated long-term outcome (37±3.4y follow-up). They used the following criteria to evaluate the social outcomes: failure to complete high school, pregnancy outside of a stable relationship (<6mo), depression or another psychiatric diagnosis, unemployment, living alone, never in a romantic relationship for more than 3 months, and poverty. In BECTS, they reported 41% with one criterion or more and 22% with two criteria or more (Camfield and Camfield 2014).

CHILDHOOD ABSENCE EPILEPSY

Childhood absence epilepsy begins usually between 4 and 12 years of age with a peak onset at 6 years. This syndrome represents up to 10% of the pediatric epilepsies (Shinnar et al. 1999; Zarrelli et al. 1999). In this syndrome, only one type of seizure is observed: typical absence seizure. A history of febrile seizures is possible, but any other type of seizures rules out the diagnosis. Absences occur very frequently, often 20 to 100 times per day. Absence seizures are brief seizures (mean duration of 8s) clinically characterized by impairment of consciousness with automatisms in some patients, concomitant to a typical EEG pattern of generalized, bilateral, synchronous, symmetrical 3Hz spike–wave discharges (Matricardi et al. 2014).

Recently, a double-blind, randomized, controlled clinical trial (RCT) has compared ethosuximide, valproate, and lamotrigine in children with newly diagnosed CAE. Four hundred and fifty-three children were randomly assigned to treatment with ethosuximide (ESM; $n = 156$), lamotrigine (LTG; $n = 149$), or valproic acid (VPA; $n = 148$) (Glauser et al. 2010). After 16 weeks of therapy, the freedom-from-failure rates for ESM and VPA were similar (53% and 58%, respectively; $p = 0.35$) and were higher than the rate for LTG (29%; $p < 0.001$ for comparisons of ESM to LTG and VPA to LTG). During the RCT, there was no significant difference among the three drugs with regard to discontinuation because of adverse events. Pretreatment evaluation demonstrated that 36% of the included patients exhibited attention deficits. Notably, attention deficits persisted at 16 to 20 weeks even if seizure freedom was achieved (Masur et al. 2013). However, attention dysfunction was more common after the treatment with VPA than with ESM (49% of the children vs 33%; $p = 0.03$) (Glauser et al. 2010; 2013). A recent prospective study reports the long-term prognosis of CAE (Berg et al. 2014). The epilepsy remission seems to be linked to the initial treatment (Berg et al. 2014). Seventy-three children were initially diagnosed with CAE. The initial treatment was ESM in 41 and VPA in 18 children. Initial success rates were identical in these two groups (59% for ESM and 56% for VPA). Using a multivariate analysis, only the initial treatment predicts the long-term outcome. At the time of last follow-up contact, 38 (64%) of 59 participants were in complete remission (5y seizure free and 5y off medication), 31 (76%) of those first treated with ESM and 7 (39%) of those treated with VPA ($p = 0.007$). In 53 children followed for 10 years or more, 10-year remission was also higher in the ESM (76%) versus VPA (44%) group ($p = 0.06$) (Berg et al. 2014).

These data are in line with our view that CAE should be considered as possibly self-limited because only a proportion of the patients (about 60%) will have complete remission

(Matricardi et al. 2014). Some patients seem to develop a lifelong epilepsy syndrome such as juvenile myoclonic epilepsy (Wirrell et al. 1996). In an additional study reporting the long-term outcome of the patients included in the large RCT conducted by Glauser et al. (median of follow-up: 7y), the occurrence of at least generalized tonic–clonic seizure was reported in 12% (n = 53) at a median age of 13.1 years (Shinnar et al. 2015).

Cognitive concerns in CAE have been raised by the very few available studies (Caplan et al. 2008). Most of the studies have evaluated a group of patients with various childhood epilepsy syndromes, and some of them focused on idiopathic generalized epilepsy. In a large group of children with epilepsy including 12 patients with CAE, Jambaque et al. (1993) reported that children with idiopathic generalized epilepsy performed poorly relative to controls on visual memory, while verbal memory was unaffected. The finding that general intellectual functioning is lowered in children with generalized idiopathic epilepsy syndromes is consistent with the results of later work (Nolan et al. 2003). In most of the studies, CAE was not a selectively studied group but was studied in the group of idiopathic generalized epilepsy syndromes, thereby restricting the ability to draw any conclusion restricted to only one syndrome. In a case–control study with CAE patients matched for sex and socioeconomic status, it has been shown that four-fifths of the patients had normal IQ scores (Pavone et al. 2001). However, patients had lower IQ than matched controls. In a more detailed evaluation, a lower level of general cognition, visual spatial skills, nonverbal memory, and delayed recall have been identified in children with CAE. While investigating the particular cases of early-onset CAE (onset before 3y of age), Chaix et al. (2003) suggested that the overall prognosis for children with early-onset absence epilepsy is poorer than a more typical CAE.

The pretreatment cognitive evaluation of 450 patients from the large RCT found 36% of children with attention troubles, whereas global cognition as well as specific cognitive domain were normal (Masur et al. 2013). This attention disturbance results in memory and executive function involvement and academic underachievement (Masur et al. 2013).

Comparing patients with CAE (n = 56) to patients with juvenile arthritis (n = 61), it has been shown that the patients with prior CAE were more likely to require special educational help (p < 0.02), to have below average academic performance (p < 0.01), or to repeat a grade (p < 0.005) (Wirrell et al. 1997).

Finally, the psychosocial outcome further suggests that CAE should not be considered as a 'benign' epilepsy. Comparing patients with CAE (n = 56) to patients with juvenile arthritis (n = 61), it has been shown that the patients with prior CAE were more likely to have an unplanned pregnancy (p < 0.001) and were less likely to graduate from high school (p < 0.005) or attend college/university (p < 0.001) (Wirrell et al. 1997).

Why do some patients present with learning problems?

There are multiple factors that might contribute to the learning problems reported in childhood self-limited epilepsy syndromes (Fig 9.1). It remains currently unclear what is the contribution of each factors. Learning problems represent more than cognitive involvement. Psychiatric comorbidities and behavior disturbances could also play a role by modifying the interactions during learning processes.

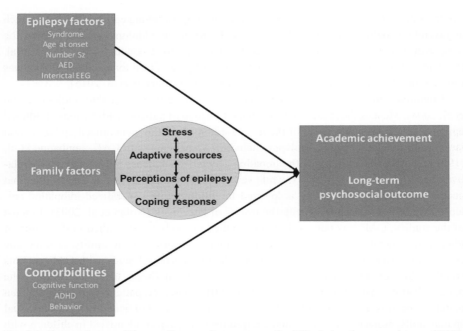

Fig. 9.1. Factors that possibly contribute to the outcome of self-limited epilepsy syndrome. ADHD, attention-deficit–hyperactivity disorder; AED, antiepileptic drug; EEG, electroencephalogram; Sz, seizure.

EPILEPSY FACTORS

Among the childhood epilepsy syndromes, even BECTS and CAE, the severity differs from one patient to another. The number of seizures and the number of AEDs are the major factors that could impact both cognition and psychiatric comorbidities that can contribute to learning difficulties. Looking at the epilepsy parameters, it is difficult to have a clear view of the role of each factor because these are frequently interrelated; early onset, poor seizure control, and antiepileptic polytherapy that are interrelated. Some studies have pointed out the role of the age at onset as a predictive factor for achievement (Piccinelli et al. 2008; Fastenau et al. 2009).

The role of interictal abnormalities is frequently discussed in childhood epilepsy syndromes, particularly BECTS. Few studies correlated particular cognitive profiles observed in BECTS to the most affected hemisphere. The left-side centrotemporal spikes would lead to speech disturbance, whereas the right-side centrotemporal spikes would lead to visuospatial skills and some language processes. However, most studies did not find any correlation between the side of the spike discharge and the cognitive outcome (Vannest et al. 2015). The inconsistency in these findings might be attributable to small sample sizes, variability in assessment tools, and the focus on a specific cognitive process. Both the reports of the frequency of speech therapy before the diagnosis of rolandic epilepsy and the occurrence of literacy and language impairment in the family members of children with rolandic epilepsy suggest that these difficulties might not be related to the epileptiform activity (Clarke et al. 2007; Overvliet et al. 2011; Smith et al. 2012). Further studies are still needed to better delineate the relationship between seizures, interictal discharge particularly during sleep, and the cognitive involvement in BECTS.

As mentioned previously, it is established that children and adolescents with self-limited epilepsy have a higher risk of exhibiting some deficits in a particular area of cognition. However, there are limited data on the possible influence of specific neuropsychological deficits on academic underachievement. This would be of great interest to develop and evaluate new rehabilitation strategies.

Even if the exact causes of cognitive impairment in children and adolescents with epilepsy are not fully understood, the effects of AED should be considered (Fastenau et al. 2009). Even if some AEDs have been particularly reported as having effects on cognition (Ijff and Aldenkamp 2013; Eddy et al. 2011), all AEDs might have some effects on cognitive functions. In a prospective study comparing 282 children with the first recognized seizure to 147 healthy siblings, the use of AED was identified as an increased risk for neuropsychological deficit (odds ratio = 2.27) (Fastenau et al. 2009). A recent study also stressed the effect of AEDs on cognition. This was shown by a cognitive assessment after drug withdrawal in a group of 301 children operated for epilepsy (Boshuisen et al. 2015). Pre- and postoperative IQ scores were analyzed taking into account the reduction of AED dose or the AED withdrawal. After epilepsy surgery in children, the start of AED withdrawal, the number of AEDs reduced, and complete AED withdrawal were associated with improved postoperative IQ scores and gain in IQ, independent of other determinants of cognitive outcome (Boshuisen et al. 2015). As already established, a study further pointed out a stronger cognitive impact of AEDs when they are combined. In a population of school-aged children with active epilepsy, IQ evaluation revealed that 24% of 85 children were functioning below IQ 50, and 40% had IQ scores below 70. Polytherapy was a significant risk factor for global cognitive impairment ($\beta = -13.0$; 95% confidence interval $= -19.3$, -6.6; $p = 0.0001$) (Anderson et al. 2015). Anderson et al. (2015) also pointed out the risk of polytherapy in a prospective study of 180 children. Adverse events were reported in 31% consisting more frequently behavioral problems and somnolence (21% of adverse events in monotherapy vs 60% of adverse events in polytherapy). The occurrence of adverse event was linked to polytherapy (Anderson et al. 2015).

Most of the studies assessing cognitive impairment in BECTS have included patients receiving antiepileptic drugs. The variability of treatment regimen in these studies makes it difficult to draw any conclusion on the role of AED, or any particular AED, in cognitive function (Vannest et al. 2015). A study showed that VPA improved language skills, whereas sulthiame monotherapy had an impact on language and verbal memory ability despite its reduction of interictal abnormalities (Baglietto et al. 2001; Wirrell et al. 2008).

In case of CAE, some AEDs may result in a negative change of attention deficit as shown with VPA despite its ability to control absence seizure was similar to ESM (Glauser et al. 2010).

FAMILIAL FACTORS

The family factors including parent–child relationship are well-known factors that can contribute to the child psychopathology (Rodenburg et al. 2006). It is also highly probable that these factors play a role in the academic achievement. Some studies have highlighted this issue. Using a scale assessing educational materials in the household and family involvement in stimulating activities, the Home Observation for Measurement of the Environment scale, a correlation between the score on this scale and academic achievement has been reported (Mitchell et al. 1991). This has also been suggested by Fastenau reporting that disorganized home environments or unsupportive home environments were risk factors for lower academic achievement (Fastenau et al. 2009). In addition to family environmental factors, parental mental health is also an important component. Academic difficulties have been identified as a possible consequence of high parental anxiety (Dunn et al. 2010). Maternal depression symptoms have also been associated with more child behavior problems in children with epilepsy (Hoare and Kerley 1991).

Among family factors, stress, adaptive resources, perceptions of childhood epilepsy, and coping response are possible factors that might change child behavior and academic performance.

The involvement of stress has been identified in behavior problems of children with epilepsy for a while (Hoare and Kerley 1991). Epilepsy in children is also stressful for their parents. This seems particularly true at the onset of the disease with an increase of parental anxiety (Save-Pedebos et al. 2014). It might be linked to the fear that some parents have that their child might die during a seizure (Besag et al. 2005). In addition, the unpredictable and paroxystic nature of the seizures are probably the factors that increase stress for the family. It is also highly possible that an interplay between parental and children anxiety/stress exists; however, this has not been established in children with epilepsy and their family.

It is also possible that familial adaptive resources might be a contributing factor. In families of children with epilepsy, lower parent education and poverty status were associated with more behavior problems (Hoare and Kerley 1991). Lower financial well-being was reported to be associated with more behavior/depression problems (Austin 1988). However, another study did not confirm these findings.

Family members' beliefs about epilepsy seem also highly relevant because of the stigma commonly associated with epilepsy. It would be possible that more parental negative attitudes and greater perceived stigma related to epilepsy are associated with greater child psychopathology (Sbarra et al. 2002). The type of studies has shown a mutual influence of parental perception and child behavior problems. It is, therefore, difficult to draw any conclusion from the direction of the influence of these two parameters.

Coping responses could also contribute to behavioral changes and academic achievement of the patients. Parental acceptance was described as negatively associated with behavior problems, and psychological control was positively associated with child behavior problems (Sbarra et al. 2002). Lower family esteem, poor communication and less extended family support have also been associated with more child behavior problems (Austin 1988; Austin et al. 1992). Difficulties continuing their habitual parenting style were identified as a contributor to poorer academic scores (Oostrom et al. 2003).

SELF-ESTEEM AND STIGMA

Lower self-esteem has been more frequently observed in children with epilepsy compared to children with other chronic disease such as diabetes (Hoare and Mann 1994). Stigma might contribute to this high frequency of low self-esteem in children with epilepsy (Oostrom et al. 2000). It is still controversial that self-esteem might modify academic performance because the available studies display conflicting results (Austin et al. 2008). In adolescents with epilepsy, a higher level of perceived stigma was correlated with poorer self-esteem (Westbrook et al. 1992). Seizure type, seizure frequency, seizure duration, sex, and racial or ethnic identity were not significantly related to perceived stigma (Westbrook et al. 1992). Goffman et al. (1986) proposed to distinguish enacted stigma (i.e. actual instances of discrimination because of the diagnosis of epilepsy) from felt stigma (i.e. the embarrassment/ disgrace of having epilepsy or the fear of being discriminated against). The diagnosis of epilepsy is frequently hidden from close friends, and even some family members (Jacoby 1994). Some authors suggested that this atmosphere of secrecy can be very socially disabling and isolating (Bandstra et al. 2008). Peter Camfield and Carol Camfield (2002) reported that BECTS disrupts the development in childhood only if it interferes with the child's chances for normal friendships. In their experience, the biggest issue arises when the child wishes to sleep overnight at a friend's house (Camfield and Camfield 2002). Finally, it has been suggested that children's attitude toward epilepsy mediated the relationships between stigma and self-concept and behavior problems, respectively (Funderburk et al. 2007). In contrast, attitude did not mediate the relationship between stigma and social competence (Funderburk et al. 2007). This led to the idea that some intervention promoting a more positive attitude toward having epilepsy might be of interest.

Conclusion

This overview illustrates the risk of cognitive and behavior disturbances in childhood epilepsy syndrome that are considered self-limited. BECTS and CAE are still frequently considered as benign compared to other epilepsy syndromes associated with pharmacoresistance or epilepsy syndrome with lifelong course. However, the long-term psychosocial outcome also seems to be a concern with some patients having problem even if they are no longer exposed to an active epilepsy syndrome.

The current management of the children with self-limited epilepsy syndromes should include an early screening for cognitive and psychiatric comorbidities. It is also probably important to provide to the parents a full description of these risks. By warning them, they may pay more attention to any difficulties promoting early intervention.

The underlying mechanisms of cognitive deficits and attention deficits are not fully understood. Moreover, the contribution of various factors to the academic achievement and the long-term psychosocial outcome remains to be dissected. To change this, we must begin to understand the role of multiple factors. It is most likely that this is the result of the accumulation of several factors such as epilepsy factors, cognitive deficits, behavior difficulties, family factors, self-esteem, and stigma (Fig 9.1). The impact of these factors probably varies from child to child, and some may have an independent positive/negative effect and some may act in combination.

At the individual level, the effort to identify any risk factor may remain elusive, given the heterogeneous nature of childhood epilepsy syndrome and the multiplicity of the factors. However, it might be of interest to explain to the parents and the caregivers, as well as to the patients, which is our current understanding of what might influence the outcome in childhood epilepsy syndrome.

The development and the use of educational programs for children and adolescents with epilepsy as well as their parents might be of interest. Some studies already suggest the improvement of quality of life, self-esteem, or social confidence with such programs (MacLeod and Austin 2003; Snead et al. 2004; Connolly et al. 2006). This kind of program might also avoid misconceptions about epilepsy by the parents and the caregivers, and maybe limit inappropriate restrictive educational attitudes.

REFERENCES

Anderson M, Egunsola O, Cherrill J et al. (2015) A prospective study of adverse drug reactions to antiepileptic drugs in children. *BMJ Open* 5: e008298.

Austin JK (1988) Childhood epilepsy: Child adaptation and family resources. *J Child Adolesc Psychiatr Nurs* 1: 18–24.

Austin JK, Risinger MW and Beckett LA (1992) Correlates of behavior problems in children with epilepsy. *Epilepsia* 33: 1115–1122.

Austin JK, Shore CP, Dunn DW et al. (2008) Development of the parent response to child illness (PRO) scale. *Epilepsy Behav* 13: 662–669.

Baglietto MG, Battaglia FM, Nobili L et al. (2001) Neuropsychological disorders related to interictal epileptic discharges during sleep in benign epilepsy of childhood with centrotemporal or rolandic spikes. *Dev Med Child Neurol* 43: 407–412.

Bandstra NF, Camfield CS, Camfield PR (2008) Stigma of epilepsy. *Can J Neurol Sci* 35: 436–440.

Berg AT, Berkovic SF, Brodie MJ et al. (2010) Revised terminology and concepts for organization of seizures and epilepsies: Report of the ILAE Commission on Classification and Terminology, 2005–2009. *Epilepsia* 51: 676–685.

Berg AT, Levy SR, Testa FM and Blumenfeld H (2014) Long-term seizure remission in childhood absence epilepsy: Might initial treatment matter? *Epilepsia* 55: 551–557.

Besag FMC, Nomayo A and Pool F (2005) The reactions of parents who think that a child is dying in a seizure - In their own words. *Epilepsy Behav* 7: 517–523.

Boshuisen K, van Schooneveld MMJ, Uiterwaal CSPM et al. (2015) Intelligence quotient improves after antiepileptic drug withdrawal following pediatric epilepsy surgery. *Ann Neurol* 78: 104–114.

Bouma PAD, Bovenkerk AC, Westendorp RGJ and Brouwer OF (1997) The course of benign partial epilepsy of childhood with centrotemporal spikes: A meta-analysis. *Neurology* 48: 430–437.

Camfield CS and Camfield PR (2014) Rolandic epilepsy has little effect on adult life 30 years later. *Neurology* 82: 1162–1166.

Camfield P and Camfield C (2002) Epileptic syndromes in childhood: Clinical features, outcomes, and treatment. *Epilepsia* 43: 27–32.

Caplan R, Siddarth P, Stahl L et al. (2008) Childhood absence epilepsy: Behavioral, cognitive, and linguistic comorbidities. *Epilepsia* 49: 1838–1846.

Chaix Y, Daquin G, Monteiro F et al. (2003) Absence epilepsy with onset before age three years: A heterogeneous and often severe condition. *Epilepsia* 44: 944–949.

Clarke T, Strug LJ, Murphy PL et al. (2007) High risk of reading disability and speech sound disorder in rolandic epilepsy families: Case-control study. *Epilepsia* 48: 2258–2265.

Connolly AM, Northcott E, Cairns DR et al. (2006) Quality of life of children with benign rolandic epilepsy. *Pediatr Neurol* 35: 240–245.

Danielsson J and Petermann F (2009) Cognitive deficits in children with benign rolandic epilepsy of childhood or rolandic discharges: A study of children between 4 and 7 years of age with and without seizures compared with healthy controls. *Epilepsy Behav* 16: 646–651.

Deltour L, Quaglino W, Barathon M, de Broca A and Berquin P (2007) Clinical evaluation of attentional processes in children with benign childhood epilepsy with centrotemporal spikes (BCECTS). *Epileptic Disord* 9: 424–431.

Dunn DW, Johnson CS, Perkins SM et al. (2010) Academic problems in children with seizures: Relationships with neuropsychological functioning and family variables during the 3 years after onset. *Epilepsy Behav* 19: 455–461.

Eddy CM, Rickards HE and Cavanna AE (2011) The cognitive impact of antiepileptic drugs. *Ther Adv Neurol Disord* 4: 385–407.

Fastenau PS, Johnson CS, Perkins SM et al. (2009) Neuropsychological status at seizure onset in children Risk factors for early cognitive deficits. *Neurology* 73: 526–534.

Funderburk JA, McCormick BP and Austin JK (2007). Does attitude toward epilepsy mediate the relationship between perceived stigma and mental health outcomes in children with epilepsy? *Epilepsy Behav* 11: 71–76.

Glauser TA, Cnaan A, Shinnar S et al. (2010) Ethosuximide, valproic acid, and lamotrigine in childhood absence epilepsy. *N Engl J Med* 362: 790–799.

Glauser TA, Cnaan A, Shinnar S et al. (2013) Ethosuximide, valproic acid, and lamotrigine in childhood absence epilepsy: Initial monotherapy outcomes at 12 months. *Epilepsia* 54: 141–155.

Goffman E (1986). *Stigma: Notes on the Management of Spoiled Identity*. New York: Simon & Schuster.

Goldberg-Stern H, Gonen OM, Sadeh M et al. (2010) Neuropsychological aspects of benign childhood epilepsy with centrotemporal spikes. *Seizure-Eur J Epilepsy* 19: 12–16.

Hermann B, Jones J, Sheth R et al. (2006) Children with new-onset epilepsy: Neuropsychological status and brain structure. *Brain* 129: 2609–2619.

Hoare P and Kerley S (1991) Psychosocial adjustment of children with chronic epilepsy and their families. *Dev Med Child Neurol* 33: 201–215.

Hoare P and Mann H (1994) Self-esteem and behavioral-adjustment in children with epilepsy and children with diabetes. *J Psychosom Res* 38: 859–869.

Hughes JR (2010) Benign epilepsy of childhood with centrotemporal spikes (BECTS): To treat or not to treat, that is the question. *Epilepsy Behav* 19: 197–203.

Ijff DM and Aldenkamp AP (2013) Cognitive side-effects of antiepileptic drugs in children. *Handb Clin Neurol* 111: 707–718.

Jambaque I, Dellatolas G, Dulac O, Ponsot G and Signoret JL (1993) Verbal and visual memory impairment in children with epilepsy. *Neuropsychologia* 31: 1321–1337.

Jacoby A (1994) Felt versus enacted stigma: A concept revisited. Evidence from a study of people with epilepsy in remission. *Soc Sci Med* 38: 269–274.

Kim E-H, Yum M-S, Kim H-W and Ko T-S (2014) Attention-deficit/hyperactivity disorder and attention impairment in children with benign childhood epilepsy with centrotemporal spikes. *Epilepsy Behav* 37: 54–58.

MacLeod JS and Austin JK (2003). Stigma in the lives of adolescents with epilepsy: A review of the literature. *Epilepsy Behav* 4: 112–117.

Masur D, Shinnar S, Cnaan A et al. (2013) Pretreatment cognitive deficits and treatment effects on attention in childhood absence epilepsy. *Neurology* 81: 1572–1580.

Matricardi S, Verrotti A, Chiarelli F, Cerminara C and Curatolo P (2014) Current advances in childhood absence epilepsy. *Pediatr Neurol* 50: 205–212.

Mitchell WG, Chavez JM, Lee H and Guzman BL (1991) Academic underachievement in children with epilepsy. *J Child Neurol* 6: 65–72.

Nolan MA, Redoblado MA, Lah S et al. (2003) Intelligence in childhood epilepsy syndromes. *Epilepsy Res* 53: 139–150.

Oostrom KJ, Schouten A, Kruitwagen CL et al. (2003) Behavioral problems in children with newly diagnosed idiopathic or cryptogenic epilepsy attending normal schools are in majority not persistent. *Epilepsia* 44: 97–106.

Oostrom KJ, Schouten A, Olthof T, Peters ACB and Jennekens-Schinkel A (2000) Negative emotions in children with newly diagnosed epilepsy. *Epilepsia* 41: 326–331.

Overvliet GM, Aldenkamp AP, Klinkenberg S, Vles JSH and Hendriksen J (2011) Impaired language performance as a precursor or consequence of Rolandic epilepsy? *J Neurol Sci* 304: 71–74.

Pavone P, Bianchini R, Trifiletti RR et al. (2001) Neuropsychological assessment in children with absence epilepsy. *Neurology* 56: 1047–1051.

Peters JM, Camfield CS and Camfield PR (2001) Population study of benign rolandic epilepsy: Is treatment needed? *Neurology* 57: 537–539.

Piccinelli P, Borgatti R, Aldini A et al. (2008) Academic performance in children with rolandic epilepsy. *Dev Med Child Neurol* 50: 353–356.

Pinton F, Ducot A, Motte J et al. (2006) Cognitive functions in children with benign childhood epilepsy with centrotemporal spikes (BECTS). *Epileptic Disord* 8: 11–23.

Riva D, Vago C, Franceschetti S et al. (2007) Intellectual and language findings and their relationship to EEG characteristics in benign childhood epilepsy with centrotemporal spikes. *Epilepsy Behav* 10: 278–285.

Rodenburg R, Meijer AM, Dekovic M and Aldenkamp AP (2006) Family predictors of psychopathology in children with epilepsy. *Epilepsia* 47: 601–614.

Save-Pedebos J, Bellavoine V, Goujon E et al. (2014) Difference in anxiety symptoms between children and their parents facing a first seizure or epilepsy. *Epilepsy Behav* 31: 97–101.

Sbarra DA, Rimm-Kaufman SE and Pianta RC (2002) The behavioral and emotional correlates of epilepsy in adolescence: A 7-year follow-up study. *Epilepsy Behav* 3: 358–367.

Shinnar S, Cnaan A, Hu F et al. (2015) Long-term outcomes of generalized tonic-clonic seizures in a childhood absence epilepsy trial. *Neurology* 85: 1108–1114.

Shinnar S, O'Dell C and Berg AT (1999) Distribution of epilepsy syndromes in a cohort of children prospectively monitored from the time of their first unprovoked seizure. *Epilepsia* 40: 1378–1383.

Smith AB, Kavros PM, Clarke T et al. (2012) A neurocognitive endophenotype associated with rolandic epilepsy. *Epilepsia* 53: 705–711.

Snead K, Ackerson J, Bailey K et al. (2004). Taking charge of epilepsy: The development of a structured psychoeducationalgroup intervention for adolescents with epilepsy and their parents. *Epilepsy Behav* 5: 547–556.

Tedrus GMAS, Fonseca LC, Melo EMV and Ximenes VL (2009) Educational problems related to quantitative EEG changes in benign childhood epilepsy with centrotemporal spikes. *Epilepsy Behav* 15: 486–490.

Vannest J, Tenney JR, Gelineau-Morel R, Maloney T and Glauser TA (2015) Cognitive and behavioral outcomes in benign childhood epilepsy with centrotemporal spikes. *Epilepsy Behav* 45: 85–91.

Verrotti A, Matricardi S, Di Giacomo DL et al. (2013) Neuropsychological impairment in children with Rolandic epilepsy and in their siblings. *Epilepsy Behav* 28: 108–112.

Westbrook LE, Bauman LJ and Shinnar S (1992). Applying stigma theory to epilepsy: A test of a conceptual model. *J Pediatr Psychol* 17: 633–649.

Wirrell EC (1998) Benign epilepsy of childhood with centrotemporal spikes. *Epilepsia* 39: S32–S41.

Wirrell EC, Camfield CS, Camfield PR et al. (1997) Long-term psychosocial outcome in typical absence epilepsy - Sometimes a wolf in sheeps' clothing. *Arch Pediatr Adolesc Med* 151: 152–158.

Wirrell EC, Camfield CS, Camfield PR, Gordon KE and Dooley JM (1996) Long-term prognosis of typical childhood absence epilepsy: Remission or progression to juvenile myoclonic epilepsy. *Neurology* 47: 912–918.

Wirrell E, Sherman EM, Vanmastrigt R and Hamiwka L (2008) Deterioration in cognitive function in children with benign epilepsy of childhood with central temporal spikes treated with sulthiame. *J Child Neurol* 23: 14–21.

Zarrelli MM, Beghi E, Rocca WA and Hauser WA (1999) Incidence of epileptic syndromes in Rochester, Minnesota: 1980–1984. *Epilepsia* 40: 1708–1714.

10
'BENIGN' INFANTILE EPILEPSIES: IMPACT ON LATER COGNITION AND BEHAVIOR

Federico Vigevano and Romina Moavero

Early-onset seizures have always been regarded with great caution and suspicion due to the possibility of long-term neurological and neurodevelopment sequelae. This was particularly true for focal forms of epilepsies, because a symptomatic etiology was always presumed. However, since 1963, this conception has progressively changed, thanks to the first description of infantile seizures with a benign evolution by Fukuyama (1963). Nowadays, benign infantile seizures are a well-described entity, also recognized by the International League against Epilepsy (ILAE) classification (Engel and International League against Epilepsy 2001). However, the appropriateness of the term 'benign' has been the object of long debates in the past few decades. A common thought, in fact, is that this term could only be appropriately used retrospectively, after a long-term follow-up witnessing seizure freedom and normal neurodevelopment. The word 'benign' literally means "to do good" or "gifted of natural goodness", and this term is widely used in the medical literature, clearly opposed to "malignant" or "severe", to define clinical entities in which the prognosis has a favorable outcome (Capovilla et al. 2009). The first ILAE explanation of the meaning of 'benign' comes in the 2001 classification, defining a "benign epilepsy syndrome" as "a syndrome characterized by epileptic seizures that are easily treated or require no treatment, and remit without sequelae" (Engel and International League against Epilepsy 2001). However, the meaning of the terms "no sequelae" and "seizure remission" was not clearly established. In the past few decades, most of the attention in infantile seizures was paid to the epilepsy outcome, with less data regarding the neurodevelopment outcome. However, recent studies using neuropsychological evaluations have demonstrated that in some 'benign' syndromes, a spectrum of neuropsychological sequelae can be present (Capovilla et al. 2009). Although it is not always possible nor simple, establishing since its onset whether an epilepsy could be considered as 'benign' is of crucial importance to make a definite plan for adequate management. The main goal in using the term 'benign' is to try to give early (at seizure onset or after a short follow-up) reliable information on the prognosis of the disease, thus reassuring and decreasing anxiety for patients and caregivers (Capovilla et al. 2009). Furthermore, by knowing *a priori* the possibility of a benign evolution, overtreatment and unnecessary procedures might be avoided. An Expert Meeting held in Italy in 2008 proposed that an epilepsy can be considered benign when characterized by clinical and/or EEG features that predict, with low risk of error, at onset or soon after, remission of seizures (with or without treatment) and without significant, permanent impact on the patient's potential (Capovilla et al. 2009).

In the group of epilepsies with onset during infancy, the term 'benign' is only used for idiopathic/genetic epilepsy syndromes, both with focal seizures, such as the so-called "benign focal infantile seizures," and with generalized seizures, such as the so-called benign myoclonic epilepsy. However, this latter form is actually known as "myoclonic epilepsy in infancy" because the term 'benign' was no more considered appropriate.

Benign focal infantile seizures
ELECTROCLINICAL FEATURES
Benign familial and non-familial infantile seizures
This epileptic syndrome is characterized by the onset of seizures in otherwise healthy infants between 3 and 20 months of age. The benign familial infantile seizures (BFIS) present an autosomal dominant transmission with a slightly earlier onset than sporadic forms, usually between the fourth and the eighth month of life with a peak around the sixth month (Vigevano et al. 1992). In BFIS, first- or second-degree relatives presented convulsions in infancy without subsequent development of other seizure types. The first series of five infants affected by this epileptic syndrome was described more than 20 years ago by Vigevano et al. (1992). The authors stressed that none of the children or their relatives presented seizures in the neonatal age or after the eighth month of life. However, a similar form with seizure onset occurring between neonatal and infantile ages was reported by Kaplan and Lacey (1983). In this form, age at seizure onset ranged from 2 days to 3.5 months, thus partially overlapping with BFIS. The authors proposed to use the term "benign familial neonatal–infantile seizure" (BFNIS), and nearly 20 years later, two other families with onset between 1.9 and 3.8 months of life and a clear autosomal dominant inheritance have been described (Heron et al. 2002). Similar cases without a familial history of seizures, called benign non-familial infantile seizures (BNFIS) have been described.

In both the familial and non-familial cases, seizures are focal and often present in clusters of 8–10 seizures per day, with the cluster lasting 1 to 3 days. When examined in the interictal phase, infants appear to be completely normal, without any neurological deficits (Vigevano et al. 2012). Seizure semiology does not appear to differ between sporadic and familial forms. It is usually characterized by motor arrest, impaired consciousness, staring, head and eye deviation, and convulsions (Vigevano et al. 2012). The side of head and eye deviation might change from seizure to seizure in the same infant (Vigevano et al. 1992). Watanabe underlined the presence of limb and/or oral automatisms in the cases described as "benign partial epilepsy with complex partial seizures" and of prompt generalization with tonic–clonic manifestations in the so-called benign partial epilepsy with secondarily generalized seizures (Watanabe et al. 1990; 1993). Untreated children might present the recurrence of clusters of seizures, while a prompt antiepileptic treatment (i.e. with carbamazepine, valproate, phenobarbital, or zonisamide) is usually able to make seizures cease, and in almost all cases, no more seizures are observed throughout the life course. The interictal EEG is usually normal; lateralized slow waves and spikes in the occipito-parietal areas in the interictal EEG performed during a cluster of seizures have been reported (Vigevano et al. 2012).

Infantile convulsions with choreoathetosis

In 1997, four French families with autosomal inherited benign infantile convulsions and paroxysmal choreoathetosis were described, thus leading to the identification of a new syndrome called infantile convulsions and choreoathetosis (Szepetowski et al. 1997). Several subsequent reports confirmed the existence of this association, with paroxysmal choreoathetosis usually appearing at a later stage than seizures (Lee et al. 1998; Sadamatsu et al. 1999; Tomita et al. 1999; Bennett et al. 2000; Hattori et al. 2000; Swoboda et al. 2000; Thiriaux et al. 2002; Kato et al. 2006; Striano et al. 2006b; Rochette et al. 2010). Seizure characteristics widely overlap with the familial form of benign infantile seizures; therefore, this syndrome is considered as its variant, being characterized by the association of other neurological symptoms.

GENETIC ASPECTS

In familial cases of infantile seizures, autosomal dominant transmission appears to be evident; therefore, different studies tried to find a genetic substrate for this hereditary epilepsy syndrome. A linkage has been demonstrated on chromosome 19q (Guipponi et al. 1997) but also on chromosome 16p (Szepetowski et al. 1997; Caraballo et al. 2001) and 2q (Malacarne et al. 2001). In 1998, genetic mutations *KCNQ2* and *KCNQ3* were described in benign seizures with onset in the neonatal period, thus leading to the consideration of benign neonatal seizures as a channelopathy (Charlier et al. 1998; Singh et al. 1998), and later this concept also extended to BFIS and BFNIS. In fact, in 2002, the two families described by Heron et al. (2002) with BFNIS were found to present a missense mutation of *SCN2A* gene, which was later confirmed in other families with the same phenotype (Berkovic et al. 2004). Missense mutations of *SCN2A* have later been described even in classic cases of BFIS (Striano et al. 2006a), underlying that BNFIS and BFIS might share both clinical and genetic features.

More recently, *PRRT2* gene mutations have been described in BFIS (Schubert et al. 2012; Specchio et al. 2013). Mutations in this gene have been recognized to be involved in paroxysmal choreoathetosis, with or without benign infantile seizures (Heron et al. 2012; Specchio et al. 2013).

LATER COGNITION AND BEHAVIOR

A core feature of this epileptic entity is normal psychomotor development both before epilepsy onset and during the entire follow-up; also affected relatives exhibit normal development. However, it is worth noting that all long-term studies on benign infantile convulsions excluded patients with an evidence of developmental delay because this comorbidity was considered to exclude the diagnosis of benign partial epilepsy of infancy. Therefore, this makes it difficult to ascertain how many children with an "apparent" benign infantile epilepsy later presented some degree of learning disability. However, Okumura et al. (2006) proposed the existence of marginal syndromes of benign partial epilepsy of infancy, in which developmental outcome is not perfect. In their series of 48 children with a possible diagnosis of benign partial epilepsy of infancy at the age of 2 years, they found that 10% of them (four children) presented with learning disability or pervasive developmental disorder after the age of 8 years. In one of them, seizure recurrence was also present, but in the other three, low cognitive level was the only exclusion criterion for the diagnosis of benign partial epilepsy of infancy. When retrospectively reviewed, all their clinical, electrophysiological, and neuroimaging characteristics were absolutely overlapping with those of other children with a more favorable outcome, thus making it difficult to distinguish them since the onset and therefore highlighting the importance of a long-term follow-up even in these syndromes universally recognized as 'benign' (Okumura et al. 2000).

Also in infantile convulsions and choreoathetosis, neurodevelopmental outcome has been described as excellent in all reported cases, although a specific assessment of psychomotor/cognitive abilities is missing.

DIFFERENTIAL DIAGNOSIS

There are other focal epileptic syndromes of infancy that may present in the same age range of benign infantile seizures; therefore, clinicians should carefully consider electroclinical features and family history to achieve the correct diagnosis.

Benign infantile focal epilepsy with midline spikes and waves during sleep

This focal benign epilepsy was initially proposed in 1998 (Bureau and Maton 1998), and it was later characterized as an epileptic syndrome pointing out its homogeneous clinical features and the benign outcome (Capovilla and Beccaria 2000; Capovilla et al. 2006). Seizure onset is usually between 4 and 30 months, and although, rarely, at onset they can present in clusters, they are usually isolated and sporadic thereafter (Capovilla et al. 2006). These infants present with very characteristic seizures of psychomotor arrest, staring or ocular revulsion, loss of contact, hypotonia or stiffening of the arms, and autonomic signs with cyanosis (Bureau and Maton 1998; Capovilla et al. 2006). Sleep EEG reveals the presence, throughout all the sleep stages, of low-voltage spikes in the fronto-central and vertex regions; these abnormalities are constantly present during sleep but might be also observed during awake. Seizures usually remit by the age of 3 to 4 years, even without pharmacological treatment. Neurological examinations and neurodevelopment appear to be normal and remain normal in all described children. Electroclinical features, also including the rarity of seizures during follow-up, and multifactorial genetic susceptibility, makes this epileptic syndrome more similar to other focal "idiopathic" epilepsies seen in later childhood, such as benign epilepsy with centrotemporal spikes or Panayiotopoulos syndrome.

Benign infantile convulsions associated with gastroenteritis

Benign convulsions associated with gastroenteritis have been recognized as a distinct clinical entity and usually occur in previously healthy children between 6 months and 3 years of age (Komori et al. 1995). The infants usually present with brief afebrile seizures associated with a mild gastroenteritis without dehydration, electrolytic derangement, or hypoglycemia, and without signs of meningitis, encephalitis, or encephalopathy (Verrotti et al. 2014). Seizures usually cluster in 24–48 hours appearing quite resistant to common rescue antiepileptic drugs such as benzodiazepines and barbiturates (Uemura et al. 2002). The stormy onset of this entity with repetitive seizures and the frequent need for intensive care might raise some concerns about the long-term sequelae of convulsions associated with gastroenteritis and the risk of recurrence (Verrotti et al. 2014). Recovery is usually complete, although some cases of relapse have been described. Neurodevelopmental outcome is usually excellent, with normal cognitive level and only very rare reports of mild attention deficit (Verrotti et al. 2014). Few familial cases have been described, and the *PRRT2* mutation has been found, thus underlining the close relationship with benign familial infantile seizures (Ishii et al. 2013).

'Benign' myoclonic epilepsy of infancy/myoclonic epilepsy in infancy

ELECTROCLINICAL FEATURES

Benign myoclonic epilepsy of infancy (BMEI) was first described as a distinct epileptic syndrome in 1981 (Dravet and Bureau 1981), and later included in the ILAE classification only in 2001 (Engel and International League against Epilepsy 2001). Seizures usually begin between 6 months and 3 years of age in otherwise healthy children, in the form of several myoclonic jerks per day, mainly involving the head, trunk, and upper limbs, and not resulting in a fall (Dravet and Bureau 1981; Zuberi and O'Regan 2006). A family history for epilepsy or febrile convulsions is described in ~30% of affected children (Mangano et al. 2005; Zuberi and O'Regan 2006); myoclonic jerks at onset might rarely be preceded by febrile convulsions. The myoclonic jerks at onset are usually brief and rare, but they tend to become much more frequent up to several per day; they usually involve the head and the upper limbs rather than the lower limbs, and might cause head drops. When more severe, they might also involve the legs and determine a fall (Guerrini et al. 2012). Although interictal EEG might be normal, generalized epileptiform abnormalities are usually observed during sleep and awake, and myoclonic jerks are always associated with a generalized spike–wave or polyspike–wave complex (Guerrini et al. 2012). A similar but distinct entity is the reflex myoclonic epilepsy of infancy (RMEI), in which myoclonic jerks are usually triggered by auditory or tactile stimuli (Ricci et al. 1995). An overlap between these two syndromes is however present, because some infants with BMEI might have their seizures triggered by sensory stimuli (Zuberi and O'Regan 2006). Children with RMEI might also be untreated, and when an antiepileptic drug is administered, the response is usually excellent.

Although seizure freedom has been reported even in untreated patients, an antiepileptic treatment is usually established, above all due to the high daily frequency of the episodes. There are no specific trials assessing the effectiveness of different antiepileptic drugs in this syndrome; however, these seizures are well responsive to sodium valproate, which can usually be withdrawn prior to school entry (Zuberi and O'Regan 2006).

LATER COGNITION AND BEHAVIOR

Although considered as a benign entity, a long-term follow-up is warranted, because there are some reports of relapse in adolescence as well as possible evolution in different and even refractory epilepsy syndromes (Zuberi and O'Regan 2006; Moutaouakil et al. 2010; Mangano et al. 2011; Auvin et al. 2012). Because of the possibility of less favorable outcome, the term 'benign' should only be used retrospectively, and in the new ILAE classification, this epilepsy syndrome is now recognized as "myoclonic epilepsy in infancy" (Engel 2006), although it is usually referred to as "idiopathic myoclonic epilepsy in infancy" to differentiate it from other myoclonic epilepsies such as Dravet syndrome or myoclonic astatic epilepsy (Guerrini et al. 2012).

Several studies of long-term outcome of BMEI also mention neurodevelopmental outcome, although assessments were not always standardized. Surprisingly, considering that we are speaking of a 'benign' epileptic syndrome with a very high remission rate, 5% to 60% of assessed children presented with neurocognitive problems during follow-up (Dravet and Bureau 1981; Todt and Muller 1992; Rossi et al. 1997; Lin et al. 1998; Darra et al. 2006; Zuberi and O'Regan 2006; Caraballo et al. 2013; Dominguez-Carral et al. 2014). Such difficulties usually presented after the onset of epilepsy and ranged from mild disturbances to more severe conditions, including intellectual disability, specific learning difficulties, language impairment, fine motor skill deficits, and attention deficit/hyperactivity disorder (Rossi et al. 1997; Mangano et al. 2005; Zuberi and O'Regan 2006). Neurocognitive outcome did not appear to be strictly related to epilepsy evolution, because most of these children presented an easy-to-control epilepsy without subsequent relapses or they experienced an epileptic encephalopathy. Mangano et al. (2005) hypothesized that the more immature brain was more vulnerable to "damage" from the epilepsy, perhaps interfering with the growth of developing functions, which results in long-term neuropsychological disabilities (Zuberi and O'Regan 2006). However, children with RMEI usually presented a better long-term cognitive outcome (Verrotti et al. 2013); therefore, a distinction between idiopathic myoclonic epilepsy in infancy and RMEI at the time of diagnosis could have some important prognostic significance.

Conclusion

Although no prognostic factors can be identified for a negative neurocognitive outcome, an earlier seizure onset (before 2y of age) has been suggested to be associated with a higher risk (Mangano et al. 2005). Also delayed treatment has been hypothesized to play a role, but there is still insufficient evidence to make definite conclusions.

REFERENCES

Auvin S, Lamblin MD, Cuvellier JC and Vallee L (2012) A patient with myoclonic epilepsy in infancy followed by myoclonic astatic epilepsy. *Seizure* 21: 300–303.

Bennett LB, Roach ES and Bowcock AM (2000) A locus for paroxysmal kinesigenic dyskinesia maps to human chromosome 16. *Neurology* 54: 125–130.

Berkovic SF, Heron SE, Giordano L et al. (2004) Benign familial neonatal-infantile seizures: Characterization of a new sodium channelopathy. *Ann Neurol* 55: 550–557.

Bureau M and Maton B (1998) Valeur de l'EEG dans le prognostic précoce des epilepsies partielles non-idiopathiques de l'enfant. In: Bureau M, Kahane P and Munari C, editors. *Epilepsies Partielles Graves Pharmacorésistantes de l'enfant: Stratégies Diagnostiques et Traitements Chirurgicaux* (pp. 67–78). John Libbey Eurotext, Montrouge, France.

Capovilla G and Beccaria F (2000) Benign partial epilepsy in infancy and early childhood with vertex spikes and waves during sleep: A new epileptic form. *Brain Dev* 22: 93–98.

Capovilla G, Beccaria F and Montagnini A (2006). "Benign focal epilepsy in infancy with vertex spikes and waves during sleep". Delineation of the syndrome and recalling as "benign infantile focal epilepsy with midline spikes and waves during sleep" (BIMSE). *Brain Dev* 28: 85–91.

Capovilla G, Berg AT, Cross JH et al. (2009). Conceptual dichotomies in classifying epilepsies: Partial versus generalized and idiopathic versus symptomatic (April 18–20, 2008, Monreale, Italy). *Epilepsia* 50: 1645 Monr.

Caraballo R, Pavek S, Lemainque A et al. (2001) Linkage of benign familial infantile convulsions to chromosome 16p12-q12 suggests allelism to the infantile convulsions and choreoathetosis syndrome. *Am J Hum Genet* 68: 788–794.

Caraballo RH, Flesler S, Pasteris MC et al. (2013) Myoclonic epilepsy in infancy: An electroclinical study and long-term follow-up of 38 patients. *Epilepsia* 54: 1605–1612.

Charlier C, Singh NA, Ryan SG et al. (1998). A pore mutation in a novel KQT-like potassium channel gene in an idiopathic epilepsy family. *Nat Genet* 18: 53–55.

Darra F, Fiorini E, Zoccante L et al. (2006). Benign myoclonic epilepsy in infancy (BMEI): a longitudinal electroclinical study of 22 cases. *Epilepsia* 47: 31–35.

Dominguez-Carral J, Garcia-Penas JJ, Perez-Jimenez MA et al. (2014) [Benign myoclonic epilepsy in infancy: natural history and behavioral and cognitive outcome]. *Rev Neurol* 58: 97–102.

Dravet C and Bureau M (1981). [The benign myoclonic epilepsy of infancy (author's transl)]. *Rev Electro-encephalogr Neurophysiol Clin* 11: 438–444.

Engel J Jr. and International League against Epilepsy (2001) A proposed diagnostic scheme for people with epileptic seizures and with epilepsy: Report of the ILAE Task Force on Classification and Terminology. *Epilepsia* 42: 796–803.

Engel J Jr. (2006) Report of the ILAE classification core group. *Epilepsia* 47: 1558–1568.

Fukuyama Y (1963) Borderland of epilepsy with special reference to febrile convulsion and so-called infantile convulsions. *Clin Psychiatry* 5: 211–213.

Guerrini R, Mari F and Dravet C (2012) Idiopathic myoclonic epilepsies in infancy and early childhood. In: Bureau M, Genton P, Dravet C et al., editors. *Epilepsy Syndromes in Infancy, Childhood and Adolescence* (5th edition). John Libbey Eurotext, Montrouge, France.

Guipponi M, Rivier F, Vigevano F et al. (1997). Linkage mapping of benign familial infantile convulsions (BFIC) to chromosome 19q. *Hum Mol Genet* 6: 473–477.

Hattori H, Fujii T, Nigami H et al. (2000) Co-segregation of benign infantile convulsions and paroxysmal kinesigenic choreoathetosis. *Brain Dev* 22: 432–435.

Heron SE, Crossland KM, Andermann E et al. (2002) Sodium-channel defects in benign familial neonatal-infantile seizures. *Lancet* 360: 851–852.

Heron SE, Grinton BE, Kivity S et al. (2012) PRRT2 mutations cause benign familial infantile epilepsy and infantile convulsions with choreoathetosis syndrome. *Am J Hum Genet* 90: 152–160.

Ishii A, Yasumoto S, Ihara Y et al. (2013) Genetic analysis of PRRT2 for benign infantile epilepsy, infantile convulsions with choreoathetosis syndrome, and benign convulsions with mild gastroenteritis. *Brain Dev* 35: 524–530.

Kaplan RE and Lacey DJ (1983) Benign familial neonatal-infantile seizures. *Am J Med Genet* 16: 595–599.

Kato N, Sadamatsu M, Kikuchi T, Niikawa N and Fukuyama Y (2006) Paroxysmal kinesigenic choreoathetosis: From first discovery in 1892 to genetic linkage with benign familial infantile convulsions. *Epilepsy Res* 70: S174–S184.

Komori H, Wada M, Eto M et al. (1995) Benign convulsions with mild gastroenteritis: A report of 10 recent cases detailing clinical varieties. *Brain Dev* 17: 334–337.

Lee WL, Tay A, Ong HT et al. (1998) Association of infantile convulsions with paroxysmal dyskinesias (ICCA syndrome): Confirmation of linkage to human chromosome 16p12-q12 in a Chinese family. *Hum Genet* 103: 608–612.

Lin Y, Itomi K, Takada H et al. (1998) Benign myoclonic epilepsy in infants: Video-EEG features and long-term follow-up. *Neuropediatrics* 29: 268–271.

Malacarne M, Gennaro E, Madia F et al. (2001) Benign familial infantile convulsions: mapping of a novel locus on chromosome 2q24 and evidence for genetic heterogeneity. *Am J Hum Genet* 68: 1521–1526.

Mangano S, Fontana A and Cusumano L (2005) Benign myoclonic epilepsy in infancy: Neuropsychological and behavioural outcome. *Brain Dev* 27: 218–223.

Mangano S, Fontana A, Spitaleri C et al. (2011) Benign myoclonic epilepsy in infancy followed by childhood absence epilepsy. *Seizure* 20: 727–730.

Moutaouakil F, El Otmani H, Fadel H, El Moutawakkil B and Slassi I (2010). Benign myoclonic epilepsy of infancy evolving to Jeavons syndrome. *Pediatr Neurol* 43: 213–216.

Okumura A, Hayakawa F, Kato T et al. (2000) Early recognition of benign partial epilepsy in infancy. *Epilepsia* 41: 714–717.

Okumura A, Watanabe K and Negoro T (2006) Benign partial epilepsy in infancy long-term outcome and marginal syndromes. *Epilepsy Res* 70: S168–S173.

Ricci S, Cusmai R, Fusco L and Vigevano F (1995) Reflex myoclonic epilepsy in infancy: A new age-dependent idiopathic epileptic syndrome related to startle reaction. *Epilepsia* 36: 342–348.

Rochette J, Roll P, Fu YH et al. (2010) Novel familial cases of ICCA (infantile convulsions with paroxysmal choreoathetosis) syndrome. *Epileptic Disord* 12: 199–204.

Rossi PG, Parmeggiani A, Posar A, Santi A and Santucci M (1997). Benign myoclonic epilepsy: Long-term follow-up of 11 new cases. *Brain Dev* 19: 473–479.

Sadamatsu M, Masui A, Sakai T et al. (1999) Familial paroxysmal kinesigenic choreoathetosis: An electrophysiologic and genotypic analysis. *Epilepsia* 40: 942–949.

Schubert J, Paravidino R, Becker F et al. (2012). PRRT2 mutations are the major cause of benign familial infantile seizures. *Hum Mutat* 33: 1439–1443.

Singh NA, Charlier C, Stauffer D et al. (1998) A novel potassium channel gene, KCNQ2, is mutated in an inherited epilepsy of newborns. *Nat Genet* 18: 25–29.

Specchio N, Terracciano A, Trivisano M et al. (2013) PRRT2 is mutated in familial and non-familial benign infantile seizures. *Eur J Paediatr Neurol* 17: 77–81.

Striano P, Bordo L, Lispi ML et al. (2006a). A novel SCN2A mutation in family with benign familial infantile seizures. *Epilepsia* 47: 218–220.

Striano P, Lispi ML, Gennaro E et al. (2006b) Linkage analysis and disease models in benign familial infantile seizures: a study of 16 families. *Epilepsia* 47: 1029–1034.

Swoboda KJ, Soong B, McKenna C et al. (2000) Paroxysmal kinesigenic dyskinesia and infantile convulsions: Clinical and linkage studies. *Neurology* 55: 224–230.

Szepetowski P, Rochette J, Berquin P et al. (1997) Familial infantile convulsions and paroxysmal choreoathetosis: A new neurological syndrome linked to the pericentromeric region of human chromosome 16. *Am J Hum Genet* 61: 889–898.

Thiriaux A, de St Martin A, Vercueil L et al. (2002) Co-occurrence of infantile epileptic seizures and childhood paroxysmal choreoathetosis in one family: Clinical, EEG, and SPECT characterization of episodic events. *Mov Disord* 17: 98–104.

Todt H and Muller D (1992) The therapy of benign myoclonic epilepsy in infants. *Epilepsy Res* Suppl 6: 137–139.

Tomita H, Nagamitsu S, Wakui K et al. (1999) Paroxysmal kinesigenic choreoathetosis locus maps to chromosome 16p11.2-q12.1. *Am J Hum Genet* 65: 1688–1697.

Uemura N, Okumura A, Negoro T and Watanabe K (2002) Clinical features of benign convulsions with mild gastroenteritis. *Brain Dev* 24: 745–749.

Verrotti A, Matricardi S, Capovilla G et al. (2013) Reflex myoclonic epilepsy in infancy: A multicenter clinical study. *Epilepsy Res* 103: 237–244.

Verrotti A, Moavero R, Vigevano F et al. (2014) Long-term follow-up in children with benign convulsions associated with gastroenteritis. *Eur J Paediatr Neurol* 18: 572–577.

Vigevano F, Bureau M and Watanabe K (2012) Idiopathic focal epilepsies in infants. In: Bureau M, Genton P, Dravet C et al., editors. *Epileptic Syndromes in Infancy, Childhood and Adolescence* (5th edition). John Libbey Eurotext, Montrouge, France.

Vigevano F, Fusco L, Di Capua M et al. (1992). Benign infantile familial convulsions. *Eur J Pediatr* 151: 608–612.

Watanabe K, Negoro T and Aso K (1993) Benign partial epilepsy with secondarily generalized seizures in infancy. *Epilepsia* 34: 635–638.

Watanabe K, Yamamoto N, Negoro T et al. (1990). Benign infantile epilepsy with complex partial seizures. *J Clin Neurophysiol* 7: 409–416.

Zuberi SM and O'Regan ME (2006) Developmental outcome in benign myoclonic epilepsy in infancy and reflex myoclonic epilepsy in infancy: A literature review and six new cases. *Epilepsy Res* 70: S110–S115.

11
INFANTILE SPASMS: EARLY TREATMENT MAY IMPROVE NEURODEVELOPMENTAL OUTCOMES

Andrew Lux

Introduction

Infantile spasms is the term given to the most common epilepsy syndrome with onset in infancy. It has been the focus of many studies, in part because of the high probability of children with infantile spasms having poor neurodevelopmental outcomes. In considering the possible effects of infantile spasms upon cognition and behaviour, both during the period in which clinical epileptic spasms are occurring and during subsequent life, it is essential to consider several factors and relationships related to their pathophysiology. The most important of these are (1) the nature of the probable underlying cause (or *aetiology*) for the infantile spasms; (2) the effects that any identified aetiology might have upon the proneness to infantile spasms or other forms of epilepsy, and upon longer term prospects for development; and (3) the causal relationships that are known to exist or might exist between aetiology, the epileptic spasms, and neurodevelopmental outcomes. It is also important to consider questions related to treatment interventions, the key questions being (1) which treatment interventions are most likely to lead to the best cognitive and behavioural outcomes and (2) what is the optimal timing for these interventions.

Classification, terminology and key epidemiological concepts

Because we need to consider the concepts and data gathered from studies over several decades, we also need to appreciate some of the variation and evolution that have occurred in the concepts, classification and terminology relating to infantile spasms. Two issues merit specific emphasis: (1) terms relating to the case definition of infantile spasms and West syndrome and (2) terms relating to aetiological categories.

Since the 1960s, the International League Against Epilepsy (ILAE) has produced several proposals and recommendations on the classification of seizures and epilepsies (Gastaut 1969; Gastaut 1970; Scheffer 2012). These proposals have evolved over time, with substantial additions in the 1980s (Anon 1981; 1989), and the development of a clear five-axis diagnostic framework and glossary in 2001 (Blume et al. 2001; Engel and International League Against Epilepsy 2001). In 2010, there were modifications suggesting a more multidimensional approach to classification and a revised terminology for aetiological categories (Berg et al. 2010; Berg and Scheffer 2011; Scheffer 2012).

CASE DEFINITIONS OF INFANTILE SPASMS AND WEST SYNDROME

It was long considered that arrest or regression of development at the time of onset of *infantile spasms* was one feature of a triad that constituted the epilepsy syndrome called *West syndrome*. However, in 2004, a consensus group of 30 clinicians from 15 countries presented the West Delphi consensus statement on case definitions and outcome measures for use in clinical trials of infantile spasms, and stated the argument that, even though regression of development was common and usual in this condition, it was also difficult to assess reliably in young infants and ought not to be a necessary defining feature of the epilepsy syndrome (Lux and Osborne 2004). The group recommended that the term *West syndrome* is reserved for cases where infantile spasms – that is, the seizure type that can be more generically referred to as *epileptic spasms* – is associated with hypsarrhythmia.

Hypsarrhythmia is an EEG pattern consisting of a combination of a very high-amplitude and asynchronous background and associated frequent, multifocal epileptiform discharges. It is a pattern that is usually found between, rather than during, seizure attacks, and because of its chaotic nature, it is generally considered to be a manifestation of severely disordered brain function. Although it is a very distinctive EEG finding, it is subject to an appreciable degree of inter-rater unreliability (Hussain et al. 2015). During the epileptic spasms in a particular infant, one or more of several different EEG patterns may occur (Kellaway et al. 1979; Fusco and Vigevano 1993).

Given that the terms *infantile spasms* and *West syndrome* have been used inconsistently over the years, and that there are practical problems with reliably identifying EEGs as hypsarrhythmic, this review will use the more generic term *infantile spasms* to refer to both situations unless otherwise specified.

AETIOLOGICAL CLASSIFICATION OF INFANTILE SPASMS

Studies and clinical reports have also been inconsistent in their use of long-established terms applied in epileptology to categories of aetiology – the terms *symptomatic, idiopathic* and *cryptogenic* (Lux and Osborne 2006). More recent ILAE recommendations are that these terms should be replaced by the categories *genetic, structural/metabolic,* and *unknown cause* (Berg et al. 2010), but use of these categories can also lead to ambiguity and uncertainty. When analysing and interpreting aetiological data from studies of infantile spasms, however, it is usually possible to map cases with such labels onto the categories of *proven aetiology* and *unknown aetiology,* which are the terms that will be used in this review unless otherwise specified. It should be borne in mind that, as diagnostic capabilities improve, we would expect a period effect of proportionately more cases falling into the category of *proven aetiology*.

CAUSAL PATHWAYS WITH INFANTILE SPASMS AND NEURODEVELOPMENT

In considering the causal relationships between any identified underlying aetiology, infantile spasms, and neurodevelopmental outcomes that include cognitive and behavioural outcomes, we need to consider the factors that might bias, confound, or modify these relationships. Such factors might include the sex of the child, the age at onset of the spasms, the age at which treatment is first started, the nature of the treatment or the educational attainment of the parents.

Some of these factors, such as the effectiveness of any treatment intervention, are of significant interest in the interpretation of clinical studies. Other factors, such as age at onset of spasms and educational attainment of parents, are unlikely to be the prime focus of attention in clinical studies but can be used to assess the robustness of any identified association that might be potentially causal. As such, data about such factors can be used to assess the potential bias, confounding, or effect modification by such variables by including them in an appropriate data analysis. For example, if the variables of interest were thought to contribute to the effects of a measure of cognitive outcome at the age of 5 years, they might be included as a predictor variable in a linear regression analysis with cognitive outcome as the dependent variable, perhaps identifying them as significant independent predictors of cognitive outcome, or adjusting for their effects.

THE INFLUENCE OF AETIOLOGY UPON NEURODEVELOPMENTAL OUTCOMES

There are many underlying causes of infantile spasms. A review of causes of epileptic encephalopathy by a group in Australia has suggested the classification of genetic causes into structural abnormalities, metabolic conditions, recognisable clinical syndromes, and specific genes (Kamien et al. 2012). Non-genetic causes include hypoxic-ischaemic encephalopathy, arterial ischaemic stroke, central nervous system infections, autoimmune conditions, tumours and trauma.

In the United Kingdom Infantile Spasms Study (UKISS), 207 infants were considered for enrolment in the randomised controlled trial (Osborne et al. 2010). Of those infants, 127 (61%) had a *proven aetiology*, 68 (33%) had *unknown aetiology*, and 12 (6%) were considered to have been insufficiently investigated to permit reliable categorisation.

Given that many neurological conditions are associated with infantile spasms, and that the incidence of infantile spasms is relatively high, there is an argument that any identified genetic, metabolic, or structural condition that is identified in a specific clinical case might in fact be coincidental and not directly involved in the development of infantile spasms. There is also an argument that, just because one aetiology – Down syndrome, say – has been identified, there might be a good reason to seek other potential aetiologies.

These are reasonable considerations in clinical practice, and posing such questions would help us to avoid the clinical risks associated with cognitive biases such as premature diagnostic closure. However, it is reasonable to assume that, in most cases, there is at least a contribution from any identified aetiology to both the risk of developing infantile spasms and the risk of longer term cognitive or behavioural problems. It is also reasonable to assume that studies presenting information relating to aetiology and neurodevelopmental outcomes are, in general, studying a valid relationship that is amenable to statistical analysis and scientific inference.

Cases with *unknown aetiology* are important in clinical practice and in the context of trial methodology because it is generally considered that there is greater potential to influence their neurodevelopmental trajectory than with cases that have severe genetic, structural or metabolic causes of infantile spasms. Therefore, it is in the group with *unknown aetiology* that we are most likely to identify the beneficial effects upon neurodevelopment of novel treatment interventions.

Improving cognitive outcomes following infantile spasms

In order to gain a perspective on our current practice, it is useful to consider the natural history of infantile spasms reported in earlier studies. In the early 1970s, Jeavons et al. (1973) assessed the outcomes for 150 children at the age of 12 years and found that 33 (22%) had died. A study from Nagoya, Japan, during the 1960s and 1970s investigated the outcomes at the age of 6 years or more in 200 children with infantile spasms (Matsumoto et al. 1981). Forty-eight (24%) had died and only 19 (9.5%) were considered to have normal physical and psychological development.

SYSTEMATIC REVIEW OF NEURODEVELOPMENTAL OUTCOMES

The heterogeneity of study design and the focus in earlier studies upon cessation of spasms rather than neurodevelopmental outcomes have led to a relative paucity of data relating to cognitive and behavioural outcomes with infantile spasms. However, investigators in Toronto have made a strong effort to collate data from earlier studies and to provide summary estimates (Widjaja et al. 2015). They aimed to address three main questions: (1) the proportion of cases with good neurodevelopmental outcomes; (2) whether that proportion had changed significantly when comparing studies published before or during 2004 with studies published after 2004 and (3) whether any effects on neurodevelopment might be attributable to differences in lead time to treatment. They also presented a pooled analysis of the proportions with good neurodevelopmental outcome according to whether or not cases had identified aetiologies.

In October 2013, they screened a range of medical databases – Medline, Embase, Cochrane, PsycINFO, Web of Science and Scopus – and identified 1436 studies, either observational or with randomised design elements, of possible relevance. Studies were included in their final analysis if they (1) included five or more participants with infantile spasms; (2) reported outcomes after a median or mean duration of follow-up of more than 6 months and (3) reported neurodevelopmental outcomes. Fifty-five of the articles met those criteria and were analysed further, and all but eight of them had a retrospective study design.

There was no evidence of publication bias (Egger's test: $t = 1.378$; $p = 0.174$). However, there was evidence of significant heterogeneity between studies (Cochran's Q value = 366.849; $p < 0.001$), and thus, the pooled estimate was calculated using a random-effects model. The analysis included 2967 patients and the overall proportion with good neurodevelopmental outcome was 23.6% (95% confidence interval [CI]: 19.3% to 28.6%). There were 34 studies published before or during 2004, and 21 studies published after 2004. The proportion with good neurodevelopmental outcome in the earlier study period was 22.0% (95% CI: 16.8% to 28.3%), and in the later study period, it was 26.4% (95% CI: 19.7% to 34.4%). Comparing the estimates from those two periods showed no significant difference in effect size (Q value = 0.862, $p = 0.353$).

Of the studies included in the systematic review and where aetiological categories were evident, 25 reported outcomes on cases with both *proven aetiology* and *unknown aetiology*, 10 studies reported outcomes solely on cases with *proven aetiology* and 7 studies reported solely on cases with *unknown aetiology*. Pooled estimates of the proportions with good

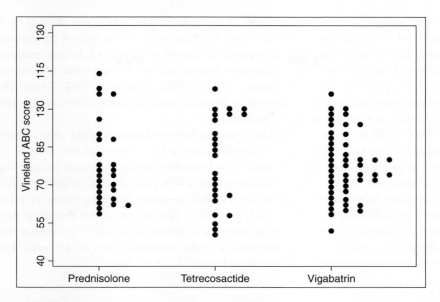

Fig. 11.1 Distribution of Vineland Adaptive Behavior Scale scores at age 14 months in United Kingdom Infantile Spasms Study (UKISS) according to randomly allocated treatment.

neurodevelopmental outcome showed significant differences between cases with *proven aetiology*, where the proportion was 12.5% (95% CI: 9.1% to 17.1%), and cases with *unknown aetiology*, where the proportion was 54.3% (95% CI: 45.8% to 62.5%) (Q value 69.724, $p < 0.001$). For the period to the end of the year 2004, a Forrest plot provided a clear illustration of how the proportion with good outcome was consistently higher in four studies where cases had *unknown aetiology* (Dulac et al. 1993; Vigevano et al. 1993; Gaily et al. 1999; Kivity et al. 2004).

Effects of treatment interventions on neurodevelopment
Given that infantile spasms have such a strong relationship with poor neurodevelopment, probably the most important question facing clinicians and parents of a child with infantile spasms is whether there is an available treatment intervention that is likely to have a positive effect upon subsequent cognition and behaviour.

The UKISS reported neurodevelopmental outcomes at 14 months of age, and for patients where follow-up data could be collected, at the age of 4 years (Lux et al. 2005; Darke et al. 2010). These neurodevelopmental outcomes were related to other potential prognostic factors, and of prime interest was whether the randomised treatment choice of either vigabatrin (a GABA transaminase inhibitor) or a hormonal treatment (tetracosactide depot, a form of synthetic corticotropin, or prednisolone, a synthetic oral corticosteroid) would be associated with greater effects upon both cessation of spasms and better neurodevelopmental scores (Figure 11.1).

The primary outcome measure was *cessation of spasms*, which was defined as the absence of witnessed spasms on days 13 and 14 of the study. On the basis of the intention-to-treat analysis of this outcome, the response rate was 40/55 (73%) for hormonal treatments and 28/52 (54%) for vigabatrin, a difference that was statistically significant (difference = 19% (95% CI 1% to 36%); chi-square = 4.1, p = 0.043) (Lux et al. 2004). These effect estimates were similar to those obtained for a similar comparison of treatments in an earlier but smaller study (Vigevano and Cilio 1997).

The UKISS investigators tested the argument that any treatment effect upon cognitive outcomes would be seen more readily in patients with *unknown aetiology* than in cases with *a proven aetiology*. They found evidence of an interaction between treatment and aetiological category after formal testing of this hypothesis within an analysis of variance model for the Vineland Adaptive Behaviour Scales (VABS) composite score by means of a least significant difference test $t(95)$ = 2.28, p = 0.025. The data suggested that there was a significant benefit related to receiving hormonal treatment rather than vigabatrin in cases with *unknown aetiology*. Box-whisker plots of VABS composite scores at 14 months of age stratified by various variables are shown in Figure 11.2 (Lux 2006).

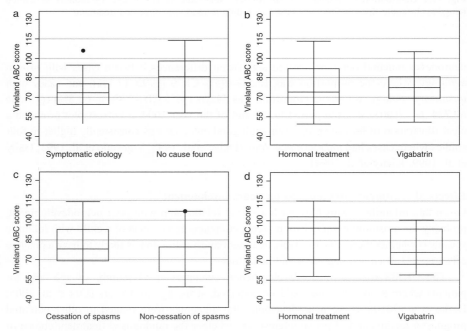

Fig. 11.2. Box-and-whisker plots of Vineland Adaptive Behavior Scale composite scores at age 14 months for children enrolled in the United Kingdom Infantile Spasms Study (UKISS). VABS score (a) by aetiological category, (b) by randomly allocated treatment for all cases, (c) by cessation or non-cessation of spasms by day 13 of study and (d) in cases with *unknown* aetiology. (From Lux 2006.)

TABLE 11.1

Main cognitive and behavioural outcomes with apparent effects related to lead-time to treatment from the studies by Eisermann et al. (2003) and Kivity et al. (2004).

Retrospective study of 18 children with infantile spasms where the sole identified aetiology was Down syndrome (Eisermann et al. 2003)

	Lead-time to treatment		
	<2 months	≥2 months	
Number of cases	8	18	
DQ score (range)	37 (8–56)	14 (5–32)	$p < 0.004$[a]
Autism score (range)	5 (0–22)	23 (10–37)	$p < 0.006$[a]
Persistent epilepsy	None	5	$p = 0.03$[b]

Retrospective study of 37 children with infantile spasms and no identified aetiology (Kivity et al. 2004)

	Lead-time to treatment		
	<1 month	≥1 month	
Number of cases	22	15	
DQ normal[c]	22	6	$p < 0.001$[b]
DQ abnormal	0	9	

[a]Wilcoxon rank-sum test
[b]Fisher exact test
[c]Normal DQ defined as XXX

Effects of lead time to treatment

Delay in diagnosis is common (Auvin et al. 2012). The study by Widjaja et al. (2015) identified 12 studies reporting lead time to treatment but focused on studies that made the comparison between a lead time of less than or greater than 4 weeks (Table 11.1). There were eight studies that made this comparison or the very similar comparison with lead time to treatment of 1 month (Jeavons et al. 1973; Singer et al. 1982; Lombroso 1983; Koo et al. 1993; Holden et al. 1997; Kivity et al. 2004; Cohen-Sadan et al. 2009; Auvin et al. 2012). From these studies, the pooled effect estimate for good neurodevelopment associated with the shorter lead time to treatment was a risk ratio of 1.519 (95% CI: 1.064 to 2.169), which was interpreted by the authors as indicating a 51.9% improvement in neurodevelopmental outcome for those treated within 4 weeks.

The study by Kivity et al. (2004) used detailed neurodevelopmental assessments on 37 children after the age of 6 years, using a Hebrew version of the Wechsler Intelligence Scale for Children . All cases were assessed to have *unknown aetiology* for their infantile spasms and had received treatment with high-dose corticotropin followed by oral prednisone. Participants who were old enough to have completed high school at the time of assessment were also assessed, where such information was available, on the basis of national high-school matriculation records.

Two other important studies assessed neurodevelopmental outcomes on the basis of different thresholds of duration of lead time to treatment (Eisermann et al. 2003; O'Callaghan et al. 2011).

Eisermann et al. (2003) reported a retrospective study of 18 children with Down syndrome and no identified competing or contributory cause of infantile spasms. (Five potential study participants were excluded because of factors such as perinatal hypoglycaemia or previous surgery or treatment in an intensive care setting.) They used a comparison threshold for lead times to treatment of less than or greater than 2 months.

Fourteen of the children were amenable to neurodevelopmental testing and were scored using the Brunet-Lézine test for developmental quotient (DQ) and using a scale that assesses autism spectrum behaviour. The results of an analysis using Spearman's rank correlation coefficient suggested that longer lead time to treatment, total duration of epileptic spasms, and time to cessation of spasms after initiation of treatment were statistically significant factors associated with lower DQ scores. With the exception of time to cessation of spasms following treatment intervention, where the effect was borderline at traditional thresholds of statistical significance (the p-value was 0.06), those factors also had statistically significant associations with scores of autism spectrum behaviour.

Widjaja et al. (2015) pooled the data from the study by Eisermann et al. (2003) with those from a Japanese study reporting the same lead time to treatment threshold of 8 weeks, obtaining a risk ratio of 1.821 (95% CI: 0.944 to 3.513) (Matsumoto et al. 1981). They found that there was no statistical difference in this risk estimate and that obtained from the eight studies with the 4-week threshold (Q value = 0.226; p = 0.634).

Data from the UKISS were collected prospectively as part of a randomised controlled trial and supported the hypothesis that lead time to treatment has a significant influence on cognitive outcomes (O'Callaghan et al. 2011). Using data from the 78 infants who had neurodevelopmental assessments at the age of 4 years and whose aetiological status was clear, the UKISS team assessed whether there was a 'dose–response effect' associated with successively longer categories of lead time to treatment: 7 days or less, between 8 and 14 days, between 15 days and 1 month, between 1 and 2 months, and longer than 2 months. The strongest focus of attention was upon cases in which there was *unknown aetiology* because it was considered that they were more likely to have outcomes amenable to modification by treatment interventions or the duration of epileptic spasms. Data relating to development, assessed by means of VABS, stratified by the presence or absence of a proven aetiology, are shown in Table 11.2. The study showed that, after controlling for the effects of treatment intervention and aetiological category, movement between one category of duration to the adjacent shorter category one was associated with an average increase in VABS score of 3.9 points (95% CI: 0.4 to 7.3 points).

Autism spectrum disorder: an outcome of specific interest
It has long been recognised that there is an association between autism spectrum behaviour and a history of infantile spasms. A study in Finland assessed the outcomes between 3 and 19 years after infantile spasms (Riikonen and Amnell 1981). Of the 192 ascertained cases, 53 (28%) were assessed to have psychiatric problems, with 24 (13%) having autism, although the autism was described as transient in 14 cases.

TABLE 11.2
**Developmental scores at age 4 years in the United Kingdom Infantile Spasms Study (UKISS)
according to aetiological category and duration of spasms.**

Lead-time to treatment	Proven aetiology		No identified aetiology	
	Number	VABS score[a]	Number	VABS score[a]
Less than 8 days	5	55 (13)	6	93 (26)
8–14 days	10	50 (13)	6	85 (30)
15 days to 1 month	3	51 (14)	5	74 (35)
1–2 months	8	60 (27)	7	71 (23)
More than 2 months	10	44 (9)	11	66 (29)
Not known	3		2	
Total number	39		37	

[a]Vineland Adaptive Behavior Scale score (standard deviation)
Modified from O'Callaghan et al. (2011) with score and SD rounded to nearest whole number

Investigators in Iceland identified 20 children with previous infantile spasms and enrolled 17 of them into a study examining autism behaviour using the Social Communication Questionnaire and the Autism Diagnostic Interview (Revised), and either the Autism Diagnostic Observation Schedule or the Childhood Autism Rating Scale (Saemundsen et al. 2007). They reported that 14 children had at least one identified neurodevelopmental disorder, and that six children had features consistent with autism spectrum disorder, of whom four also had very low DQ (<20).

Investigators in Turkey studied 90 children with a history of infantile spasms and found that 21 cases had features of autism on the basis of the Autism Behavior Checklist and the Childhood Autism Rating Scale (Dilber et al. 2013). They performed 18F-fluorodeoxyglucose positron emission tomography (FDG-PET) scans on 17 cases with autism, although 2 scans were of low quality and were excluded from analysis. Nine cases of previous infantile spasms but no features of autism were used as a control group.

Of the 15 cases with autism who had FDG-PET scans, 7 (47%) also had very low DQs. All of the nine control participants had developmental impairment, considered moderate in six particpants and mild in three. Of the 15 children with autism, 11 had an identified aetiology and four were considered to have *cryptogenic* infantile spasms. One problem with interpretation of regional differences in glucose metabolism assessed by FDG-PET is that they may have no independent functional significance in the context of focal or multifocal brain injury or structural abnormality. However, the authors described the changes in glucose metabolism in the temporal and frontal lobes as being more strongly correlated with autism than the changes in glucose metabolism in the parietal and occipital lobes.

Another Turkish study examined the relationship between previous infantile spasms and subsequent autism spectrum disorder, focusing specifically on potential EEG markers indicating an increased risk of autism (Kayaalp et al. 2007). This study compared 14 children with autism with a control group of 14 infants who had also had infantile spasms but who subsequently had not developed autism. The diagnosis of autism was determined by means of the Autism Behavior Checklist and the criteria from the DSM-IV.

The investigators reviewed 108 EEGs in the autism group and 123 EEGs in the control group, and found that a factor that seemed to indicate an increased risk of autism was the persistence of a pattern of hypsarrhythmia beyond the age of 12 months (12 vs 4 children; Fisher's exact test, $p = 0.006$). The same assessment for persistent hypsarrhythmia at the age of 3 years showed respective numbers of 11 and 3 children, which was also statistically significant (Fisher's exact test, $p = 0.007$). (The original paper reported chi-square tests on these data, but given the small number of observed data, the more conservative Fisher's exact test is more appropriate.)

The authors also suggested that the presence of epileptogenic foci in the frontal areas is another biomarker of risk for autism. However, their statistical analysis of those data used the EEG, rather than the enrolled child, as the unit of randomisation, and the validity of those analyses can be questioned because sequential EEGs from any one individual are likely to have correlated features and cannot be assumed to have a random distribution. However, this study suggests that the EEG has potential value as a biomarker of possible future behavioural morbidity.

There have been several studies of cognition and behaviour from California in the challenging context of infantile spasms treated surgically. One of these studies suggested that drug-resistant infantile spasms are associated with reduced facial expression of positive affect and impaired use of facial expression during social interactions (Caplan et al. 1999a). Another study by the same group used the Early Social Communication Scale to assess 29 children who underwent multilobar resective surgery or hemispherectomy for drug-resistant infantile spasms. They reported that children whose surgical interventions were in the right hemisphere showed a statistically significant average increase in social interaction but not in other gestural behaviours (Caplan et al. 1999b). These observations may relate to the risks of autism spectrum disorder and where this propensity might be modified by surgical intervention.

The potential value of biomarkers

There are two fairly controversial and slightly ephemeral electroclinical concepts that influence our thinking about infantile spasms as an epilepsy syndrome: the concept of the epileptic encephalopathy and the concept of nonconvulsive status epilepticus. In particular, there is the question of whether hypsarrhythmia, the interictal EEG pattern seen in West syndrome, is in effect a form of nonconvulsive status epilepticus (Lux 2007). Several studies have explored in some detail the relationships between EEG and the development of infantile spasms in children who are at increased risk.

Endoh et al. (2007, 2011) performed a retrospective study of 67 children who had infantile spasms, more specifically stated as having 'symptomatic West syndrome'. They identified 25 children in which there had been EEGs performed prior to the onset of infantile spasms and before a corrected age of 6 months.

Philippi et al. (2008) performed a retrospective study on 39 children and identified 18 children who had had at least 2 non-REM sleep EEGs with a duration of at least 10 minutes prior to the onset of infantile spasms. There were various aetiologies, including previous hypoxia-ischaemia, cortical malformations, meningoencephalitis, non-ketotic hyperglycinaemia, hypoglycaemia associated with deficiency of growth hormone and pyruvate dehydrogenase deficiency.

Kato et al. (2010) studied 17 infants who had been born after 34 weeks' gestation and who had suffered hypoxic-ischaemic encephalopathy. They found that infantile spasms developed in the four infants who had an EEG pattern categorised as depressed beyond 21 days compared with only one of the 13 infants whose EEG pattern was no longer depressed at that age.

EEG biomarkers provide a potential mechanism for secondary prevention of the longer term harm that can be associated with infantile spasms, and in some cases may prevent even the occurrence of infantile spasms. Studies of presymptomatic treatment intervention require methodological care with the selection of control groups.

Randò et al. (2004) studied the relationship between EEG patterns and visual behaviour in cases of infantile spasms, using Griffiths Mental Development Scales to assess neurodevelopment at the time of diagnosis of spasms and 2 months later (Randò et al. 2005). They reported that the most affected domain of the Griffiths Mental Development Scales related to eye–hand coordination, that this tended to recover during the 2 months between assessments in the cases that were least affected, and that there seemed to be an EEG correlation not, as might be expected, with hypsarrhythmia in the awake state, but rather with the degree to which there were normally organised EEG sleep patterns.

PRESYMPTOMATIC SEIZURE TREATMENT IN TUBEROUS SCLEROSIS COMPLEX

It has been reported that the occurrence of infantile spasms in children with tuberous sclerosis complex (TSC) is associated with a poorer neurodevelopmental outcome (O'Callaghan et al. 2004), leading to the suggestion that treatment with antiepileptic drugs before the onset of epilepsy might have a beneficial long-term effect upon cognitive and behavioural outcomes (Jóźwiak et al. 2011). This depends, at least in part, upon the predictive value of EEG changes and the degree of warning that they give. In a study from Warsaw of five infants with presymptomatic EEGs in TSC, epileptiform discharges were between 1 and 8 days before the onset of seizures (Domańska-Pakieła et al. 2014). This same group has reported a study of 45 infants with TSC, 14 of whom were given presymptomatic treatment with vigabatrin in a non-randomised, open-label study. At the age of 48 months, cognitive outcomes were reported to be better in the intervention group, as was the current seizure status (Jóźwiak et al. 2011).

Another focus of attention in TSC is the mechanistic target of rapamycin pathway. One animal study, in which epileptic spasms were precipitated in normal Sprague–Dawley rats by a combination of dexamethasone and *N*-methyl-D-aspartate, reported that presymptomatic treatment with methylprednisolone or vigabatrin had a significant effect on suppressing infantile spasms, but that such suppression of infantile spasms was not found following treatment with rapamycin (sirolimus), a drug that has an inhibitory effect on the mechanistic target of rapamycin complex 1 (mTORC1) (Chachua et al. 2011).

Conclusion

Even though cognitive and behavioural outcomes are the key concerns with infantile spasms, there are many limitations with studies in this area to date. Most studies have been very small and have focused on spasm and other seizure outcomes rather than capturing data about later neurodevelopmental outcomes.

A systematic review of studies reporting neurodevelopmental outcomes, some of which were obtained with greater rigour and methodological reliability than others, reported pooled analyses suggesting the good neurodevelopmental outcomes in approximately half of cases with *unknown aetiology* compared with only one-eighth of cases with *proven aetiology* (Widjaja et al. 2015). Overall, one-quarter of cases were considered to have good neurodevelopmental outcomes, and this proportion has not changed significantly between the periods before and since the end of 2004, a date that was chosen because it coincides with the first substantive U.S. expert consensus statement on the management of infantile spasms (Mackay et al. 2004).

There were significant limitations to the studies included in the systematic review, including the fact that most of them have used development or intelligence quotients as surrogate measures of cognition rather than conducting a comprehensive panel of cognitive assessments, which ideally would include detailed measures of memory, language, motor and executive function. Indeed, 27 of the 55 studies included in the systematic review failed to define the instruments used for the measurement of neurodevelopmental outcome. A fuller assessment of neurodevelopment would also employ tools to assess behavioural and emotional functioning, and social communication skills.

There is now some empirical information that supports the broadly held view that neurodevelopmental outcomes are more amenable to improvement by treatment intervention for cases with *unknown aetiology*, and in particular the evidence of effect modification reported in the UKISS study. Although we continue the search for the best initial or combined treatments, we should bear in mind the growing body of evidence that the timeliness of treatment is also extremely important. Strategies for earlier and more effective treatment intervention might be informed by such factors as better understanding by health care workers in primary and secondary care settings of the prodromal and seizure features, and secondary prophylaxis in high-risk groups – such as infants who have suffered previous hypoxic-ischaemic encephalopathy or who have been identified to have TSC – using EEG biomarkers. With further study, the EEG may also prove to be a reliable biomarker of risks, in children who have had infantile spasms, for future cognitive and behavioural morbidity.

The challenge is to test and implement these improved insights in order to preserve and improve cognitive and behavioural outcomes for any child who has, or who is at high risk of having, infantile spasms.

REFERENCES

Anon (1989) Proposal for revised classification of epilepsies and epileptic syndromes. Commission on classification and terminology of the international league against epilepsy. *Epilepsia* 30: 389–399.

Anon (1981) Proposal for revised clinical and electroencephalographic classification of epileptic seizures. From the commission on classification and terminology of the international league against epilepsy. *Epilepsia* 22: 489–501.

Auvin S, Hartman AL, Desnous B et al. (2012) Diagnosis delay in West syndrome: Misdiagnosis and consequences. *Eur J Pediatr* 171: 1695–1701.

Berg AT and Scheffer IE (2011) New concepts in classification of the epilepsies: Entering the 21st century. *Epilepsia* 52: 1058–1062.

Berg AT, Berkovic SF, Brodie MJ et al. (2010) Revised terminology and concepts for organization of seizures and epilepsies: Report of the ILAE commission on classification and terminology, 2005–2009. *Epilepsia* 51: 676–685.

Blume WT, Lüders HO, Mizrahi E et al. (2001) Glossary of descriptive terminology for ictal semiology: Report of the ILAE task force on classification and terminology. *Epilepsia* 42: 1212–1218.

Caplan R, Guthrie D, Komo S et al. (1999a) Infantile spasms: Facial expression of affect before and after epilepsy surgery. *Brain Cogn* 39: 116–132.

Caplan R, Guthrie, D, Komo S et al. (1999b) Infantile spasms: The development of nonverbal communication after epilepsy surgery. *Dev Neurosci* 21: 165–173.

Chachua T, Yum MS, Velíšková J et al. (2011) Validation of the rat model of cryptogenic infantile spasms. *Epilepsia* 52: 1666–1677.

Cohen-Sadan S, Kramer U, Ben-Zeev B et al. (2009) Multicenter long-term follow-up of children with idiopathic West syndrome: ACTH versus vigabatrin. *Eur J Neurol* 16: 482–487.

Darke K, Edwards SW, Hancock E et al. (2010) Developmental and epilepsy outcomes at age 4 years in the UKISS trial comparing hormonal treatments to vigabatrin for infantile spasms: A multi-centre randomised trial. *Arch Dis Child* 95: 382–386.

Dilber C, Çalışkan M, Sönmezoğlu K et al. (2013) Positron emission tomography findings in children with infantile spasms and autism. *J Clin Neurosci* 20: 373–376.

Domańska-Pakieła D, Kaczorowska M, Jurkiewicz E et al. (2014) EEG abnormalities preceding the epilepsy onset in tuberous sclerosis complex patients–A prospective study of 5 patients. *Eur J Paediatr Neurol* 18: 458–468.

Dulac O, Plouin P and Jambaqué I (1993) Predicting favorable outcome in idiopathic West syndrome. *Epilepsia* 34: 747–756.

Eisermann MM, DeLaRaillere A, Dellatolas G et al. (2003) Infantile spasms in Down syndrome—Effects of delayed anticonvulsive treatment. *Epilepsy Res* 55: 21–27.

Endoh F, Yoshinaga H, Ishizaki Y et al. (2011) Abnormal fast activity before the onset of West syndrome. *Neuropediatrics* 42: 51–54.

Endoh F, Yoshinaga H, Kobayashi K et al. (2007) Electroencephalographic changes before the onset of symptomatic West syndrome. *Brain Dev* 29: 630–638.

Engel J and International League Against Epilepsy (ILAE)(2001) A proposed diagnostic scheme for people with epileptic seizures and with epilepsy: Report of the ILAE task force on classification and terminology. *Epilepsia* 42: 796–803.

Fusco L and Vigevano F (1993) Ictal clinical electroencephalographic findings of spasms in West syndrome. *Epilepsia* 34: 671–678.

Gaily E, Appelqvist K, Kantola-Sorsa E et al. (1999) Cognitive deficits after cryptogenic infantile spasms with benign seizure evolution. *Dev Med Child Neurol* 41: 660–664.

Gastaut H (1969) Classification of the epilepsies. Proposal for an international classification. *Epilepsia* 10: 14–21.

Gastaut H (1970) Clinical and electroencephalographical classification of epileptic seizures. *Epilepsia* 11: 102–113.

Holden KR, Clarke SL and Griesemer DA (1997) Long-term outcomes of conventional therapy for infantile spasms. *Seizure* 6: 201–205.

Hussain SA, Kwong G, Millichap JJ et al. (2015) Hypsarrhythmia assessment exhibits poor interrater reliability: A threat to clinical trial validity. *Epilepsia* 56: 77–81.

Jeavons PM, Bower BD and Dimitrakoudi M (1973) Long-term prognosis of 150 cases of 'West syndrome'. *Epilepsia* 14: 153–164.

Jóźwiak S, Kotulska K, Domańska-Pakieła D et al. (2011) Antiepileptic treatment before the onset of seizures reduces epilepsy severity and risk of mental retardation in infants with tuberous sclerosis complex. *Eur J Paediatr Neurol* 15: 424–431.

Kamien BA Cardamone M, Lawson JA et al. (2012) A genetic diagnostic approach to infantile epileptic encephalopathies. *J Clin Neurosci* 19: 934–941.

Kato T, Okumura A, Hayakawa F et al. (2010) Prolonged EEG depression in term and near-term infants with hypoxic ischemic encephalopathy and later development of West syndrome. *Epilepsia* 51: 2392–2396.

Kayaalp L, Dervent A, Saltik S et al. (2007) EEG abnormalities in West syndrome: Correlation with the emergence of autistic features. *Brain Dev* 29: 336–345.

Kellaway P, Hrachovy RA, Frost JD et al. (1979) Precise characterization and quantification of infantile spasms. *Ann Neurol* 6: 214–218.

Kivity S, Lerman P, Ariel R et al. (2004) Long-term cognitive outcomes of a cohort of children with cryptogenic infantile spasms treated with high-dose adrenocorticotropic hormone. *Epilepsia* 45: 255–262.

Koo B, Hwang PA and Logan WJ (1993) Infantile spasms: Outcome and prognostic factors of cryptogenic and symptomatic groups. *Neurology* 43: 2322–2327.

Lombroso CT (1983) A prospective study of infantile spasms: Clinical and therapeutic correlations. *Epilepsia* 24: 135–158.

Lux AL (2006) *The Epidemiology and Treatment of Infantile Spasms*. (PhD Thesis) University of Bath.

Lux AL (2007) Is hypsarrhythmia a form of non-convulsive status epilepticus in infants? *Acta Neurol Scand* 115: 37–44.

Lux AL and Osborne JP (2004) A proposal for case definitions and outcome measures in studies of infantile spasms and West syndrome: Consensus statement of the West Delphi group. *Epilepsia* 45: 1416–1428.

Lux AL and Osborne JP (2006) The influence of etiology upon ictal semiology, treatment decisions and long-term outcomes in infantile spasms and West syndrome. *Epilepsy Res* 70: S77–S86.

Lux AL, Edwards SW, Hancock E et al. (2004) The United Kingdom Infantile Spasms Study comparing vigabatrin with prednisolone or tetracosactide at 14 days: A multicentre, randomised controlled trial. *Lancet* 364: 1773–1778.

Lux AL, Edwards SW, Hancock E et al. (2005) The United Kingdom Infantile Spasms Study (UKISS) comparing hormone treatment with vigabatrin on developmental and epilepsy outcomes to age 14 months: A multicentre randomised trial. *Lancet Neurol* 4: 712–717.

Mackay MT, Weiss SK, Adams-Webber T et al. (2004) Practice parameter: Medical treatment of infantile spasms: Report of the American academy of neurology and the child neurology society. *Neurology* 62: 1668–1681.

Matsumoto A, Watanabe K, Negoro T et al. (1981) Long-term prognosis after infantile spasms: A statistical study of prognostic factors in 200 cases. *Dev Med Child Neurol* 23: 51–65.

O'Callaghan FJK, Lux AL, Darke K et al. (2011) The effect of lead time to treatment and of age of onset on developmental outcome at 4 years in infantile spasms: Evidence from the United Kingdom Infantile Spasms Study. *Epilepsia* 52: 1359–1364.

O'Callaghan FJK, Harris T, Joinson C et al. (2004) The relation of infantile spasms, tubers, and intelligence in tuberous sclerosis complex. *Arch Dis Child* 89: 530–533.

Osborne JP, Lux AL, Edwards SW et al. (2010) The underlying etiology of infantile spasms (West syndrome): Information from the United Kingdom Infantile Spasms Study (UKISS) on contemporary causes and their classification. *Epilepsia* 51: 2168–2174.

Philippi H, Wohlrab G, Bettendorf U et al. (2008) Electroencephalographic evolution of hypsarrhythmia: Toward an early treatment option. *Epilepsia* 49: 1859–1864.

Randò T, Baranello G, Ricci D et al. (2005) Cognitive competence at the onset of West syndrome: Correlation with EEG patterns and visual function. *Dev Med Child Neurol* 47: 760–765.

Randò T, Bancale A, Baranello G et al. (2004) Visual function in infants with West syndrome: Correlation with EEG patterns. *Epilepsia* 45: 781–786.

Riikonen R and Amnell G (1981) Psychiatric disorders in children with earlier infantile spasms. *Dev Med Child Neurol* 23: 747–760.

Infantile Spasms: Early Treatment May Improve Neurodevelopmental Outcomes

Saemundsen E, Ludvigsson P and Rafnsson V (2007) Autism spectrum disorders in children with a history of infantile spasms: A population-based study. *J Child Neurol* 22: 1102–1107.

Scheffer IE (2012) Epilepsy: A classification for all seasons? *Epilepsia* 53: 6–9.

Singer WD, Haller JS, Sullivan LR et al. (1982) The value of neuroradiology in infantile spasms. *J Pediatr* 100: 47–50.

Vigevano F and Cilio MR (1997) Vigabatrin versus ACTH as first-line treatment for infantile spasms: A randomized, prospective study. *Epilepsia* 38: 1270–1274.

Vigevano F, Fusco L, Cusmai R et al. (1993) The idiopathic form of West syndrome. *Epilepsia* 34: 743–746.

Widjaja E, Go C, McCoy B et al. (2015) Neurodevelopmental outcome of infantile spasms: A systematic review and meta-analysis. *Epilepsy Res* 109: 155–162.

12
DRAVET SYNDROME: MORE THAN SEIZURES

Emma Losito and Rima Nabbout

Introduction

Dravet syndrome is classified in the group of epileptic encephalopathies (Berg et al. 2010), where the epileptic activity itself contributes to the final cognitive and behavioural impairment (Nabbout and Dulac 2003). Up to 80% of patients with Dravet syndrome present a genetic basis (Depienne et al. 2009; Marini et al. 2011). However, as for many of genetic epileptic encephalopathies, the impact of seizures, EEG abnormalities, treatments and genetic mutations on the global outcome is not clear.

Dravet syndrome was first described by Charlotte Dravet in 1978 under the terminology of severe myoclonic epilepsy in infancy (Dravet 1978). It was recognized as an epileptic syndrome in 1989 by the Commission on Classification and Terminology of the International League Against Epilepsy (ILAE) (1989). Typical Dravet syndrome is characterised by 'febrile and afebrile generalised and unilateral, clonic or tonic-clonic, seizures, that occur in the first year of life in an otherwise normal infant and are later associated with myoclonus, atypical absences and partial seizures. Seizures are resistant to antiepileptic drugs (AEDs). Developmental delay becomes apparent within the second year of life and is followed by definite cognitive impairment and personality disorders' (Commission on Classification and Terminology of the International League Against Epilepsy 1989).

The course of the epilepsy in Dravet syndrome can be divided into three stages (Bureau and Dalla Bernardina 2011; Dravet and Guerrini 2011). The first or "febrile stage" is characterized by the occurrence of the first seizure at the age of less than 1 year and mainly between the ages 3 and 9 months in a previously normal infant. The first seizure is usually febrile (70% of patients), convulsive and related to fever due to febrile illness or vaccination. Typically, the seizure is clonic with a focal onset and invading one side of the body (hemiclonic). It can generalize secondarily. The seizure usually lasts for longer than15 minutes, and can evolve into status epilepticus if not treated. Neurological examination is normal and might reveal transient unilateral motor deficit on the same side of the hemiclonic seizure. EEG and MRI are normal at this stage. This first seizure is often considered as a complicated febrile seizure (in opposition to simple febrile seizures because of the focal onset and the long duration) and the diagnosis of Dravet syndrome is rarely suspected. Shortly after, often within a few weeks, other seizures occur despite the initiation of therapy with AEDs. Seizures can be febrile or not, brief or long lasting. At this stage, the diagnosis should be highly suspected especially in case of alternating hemiclonic seizures. This sequence is highly pathognomonic and should not be wrongly considered as complicated febrile seizures.

The second stage (18mo to 5y) is characterized by the onset of various seizure types, the beginning of cognitive slowing and the appearance of gait disturbance. The syndrome becomes evident and the diagnosis cannot be missed at this stage. Fever sensitivity remains frequent; in addition, exercise and external heat can be the major trigger factors. Pattern sensitivity can also occur at this stage. Various seizure types appear between 18 months and 4–5 years: atypical absences, focal seizures, brief myoclonic seizures or myoclonic non-convulsive status described as "obtundation status" (status with consciousness impairment of variable intensity) (Yakoub et al. 1992; Dravet et al. 2005a).

At this stage, neurological signs are observed in some of the patients: gait delay and gait disturbances in almost 60% of patients resembling ataxia but with no signs of cerebellar involvement, such as nystagmus or dysmetria, and moderate pyramidal signs.

The third stage is reported in the literature as 'stabilization stage'. This stabilization is not synonymous with improvement but with the chronicity of the ongoing symptoms. Seizures remain pharmacoresistant, and although they tend to decrease in some patients, they can remain active in many others, and only a few patients became seizure free despite polytherapies. Nocturnal seizures might become predominant with a decrease in convulsive diurnal seizures (Dravet et al. 2005b). Fever sensitivity persists at this stage.

More than 800 mutations have been associated with Dravet syndrome, randomly distributed across the SCN1A protein. Most mutations are *de novo*, and approximately 5%–10% are inherited from an unaffected parent (Depienne et al. 2009; Ragona et al. 2010; Marini et al. 2011; Caraballo et al. 2013).

The cognitive and behavioural outcome

The *cognitive outcome* in patients with Dravet syndrome is usually considered poor (Giovanardi-Rossi et al. 1991; Yakoub et al. 1992; Wang et al. 1996; Caraballo and Fejerman 2006) (Table 12.1). Few papers described the time course of psychomotor and cognitive development (Fig 12.1) (Cassé-Perrot et al. 2001; Wolff et al. 2006; Ragona et al. 2010; 2011; Nabbout et al. 2013).

The development is reported as normal before the onset of seizures and during the first months after seizures (Dravet et al. 2002; 2005a; 2005b). In one paper focusing on the early developmental profile, Chieffo et al. (2011b) suggested, on a small series of five patients, that some slight abnormalities might be present when patients are tested during the first months after onset. Five patients, with a diagnosis of Dravet syndrome, were longitudinally followed up from the clinical onset (follow-up between 24mo and 42mo) and underwent a full assessment, including global development, visual functions and behaviour. Four of them showed an early impairment of visual functions, preceding the cognitive decline, appearing between 6 and 30 months.

A progressive stagnation of acquisitions is observed from the age of 18 months to 2 years until the instauration of an intellectual disability, generally reported after the age of

TABLE 12.1

Articles in scientific literature describing the cognitive outcome of Dravet syndrome patients

Authors	Year	R/P	N	Age range	Test	Cognitive	Neurypsychiatric comorbidities	Comments
Yakoub et al.	1992	R	20	3y 2mo to 9y 4mo	Brunet-Lezine scales, clinical observation	Twelve patients tested at approximately 5y: all intellectual disability	All patients with behavioural disorder	Poor cognitive and behavioural outcome
Caraballo and Fejerman	2006	R	53	4y to 14y	Wechsler Preschool and Primary Scale of Intelligence WIPPSI, Wechsler Intelligence Scale for Children WISC, clinical observation	All patients mild to severe mental delay; expressive and receptive dysphasia in eight patients	hyperactivity in 45 patients; autism in 2 patients	Poor cognitive and epileptic outcome
Buoni et al.	2006	R	1	13y	WISC-R	IQ 125 at 13y		Good outcome attributed to progressive seizure reduction after the age of 4 years
Wolff et al.	2006	P	20	11mo to 16y	Brunet-Lezine scales, clinical observation	Slowing or stagnation of psychomotor development between 1y and 4y; stabilisation below normal at 5y to 16y	All patients with behavioural disorders	Negative prognostic factors on cognition: frequency of convulsive seizures greater than five per month
Riva et al.	2009	P	2	11mo to 8y6mo	Griffiths scales, Child Behaviour Checklist	Two patients with truncating SCN1A mutations; two different epilepsy phenotypes, similar cognitive progressive decline		Role of SCN1A mutation in the cognitive impairement

	Year		N	Tests	Cognitive	Behavioural	Comments
Ragona et al.	2010	R	37	6mo to 28y	Griffiths scales, Wechsler scales, clinical observations	Cognitive disability in 33 patients	Behavioural disorders in 21 patients	No true deterioration: slowing or stagnation befor the age of 5y and stabilisation thereafter
Ragona et al.	2011	R	26	12mo to 5y	Griffiths scales, Brunet-Lezine scales	Correlation between cognitive outcome and epileptic data		Negative prognostic factors on cognition: early appearance of myoclonus and/or absences
Chieffo et al.	2011a	P	5	6mo to 51mo	Griffiths scales, visual functions, Achenbach Child Behaviour Checklist	Cognitive deterioration slightly later than previously reported; abnormalities of visual functions in four of five patients	Behavioural problems appeared later than developmental problems; absent in one of five patients	Abnormalities of visual functions can precede the beginning of neurocognitive involvement
Chieffo et al.	2011b	R and P	12	3y to 9y	Griffiths scales, WPPSI, WISC-R, specific cognitive skills, Achenbach Child Behaviour Checklist	The global development less affected than in previous studies (two patients having normal IQ during the follow-up); impairment of specific cognitive skills (language attention, visuospatial organisation, working memory and executive function)	Behavioural disorders disappeared at outcome	Hypothesis of a cerebellar disorder; no significant correlation between cognitive and epileptic data

TABLE 12.1 *continued*

Authors	Year	R/P	N	Age range	Test	Cognitive	Neurypsychiatric comorbidities	Comments
Li et al.	2011	P	41	2y to 6y	DSM-IV Diagnostic and Statistical Manual of Mental Disorders, fourth edition, International Classification of Diseases ICD-10, Autism Behavior Checklist, Childhood Autism Rating Scale, Autism Diagnostic Interview, Autism Diagnostic Observation Schedule, Diagnostic Interview for Social Communication Disorders, Chinese WISC	Thirty-seven patients tested: all with intellectual disability (two—borderline)	Nine patients met the criteria for autism; most of the remaining showed some autistic spectrum symptoms.	No significant difference in epileptic phenotype between patients with autism and those without autism
Brunklaus et al.	2012	P	241	6mo to 42y	Developmental status: Likert scale, motor disorders and behavioural problems assessed by clinical observation	Identifying the predictors of developmental outcome	Behavioural disorders in 98 of 213 patients; motor disorders in 77 of 214 patients	Prognostic negative factors on cogniticon: status epilepticus, interictal electroencephalography abnormalities in the first year of life, motor disrders
Nabbout et al.	2013	R and P	67	1y 8mo to 24y	General intelligence scale (Brunet-Lezine, WPPSI, WISC-IV), semi-quantitative psychomotor scale Behavioral evaluation: clinical observation, parent's interview, Achenbach Child Behaviour Checklist and Conners Rating Scale	Progressive decrease of DQ/IQ from 2y up to 6y, but without regressions; hand—eye coordination significantly lower than language, posture and sociability	Highest pathological hyperactivity score between 2y and 5y	No significant correlation between cognitive and epileptic data, except for myoclonus, focal seizures and mutation-positive patients

Takayama et al.	2014	R	64	11y to 34y 5mo	Intellectual level determined by clinical assessment	Intellectual disability in all patients		Negative prognostic factors on cognition: typical Dravet syndrome, high frequency of GTCS daily to weekly; positive prognostic factors on cognition: presence of an alpha occipital rythm
Villeneuve et al.	2014	R and P	21	6y to 10y	General intelligence scale (WISC-III, WISC-IV), adaptive development (Vineland Adaptive Behavioural Scale)	After 6y, none had a normal IQ; cognitive profile: dysexecutive syndrome	Socialisation skills more preserved than communication ones	Hypothesis of dysexecutive syndrome; no significant correlation between cognitive and epileptic data
Ricci et al.	2015	P	5	4y to 8y	General intelligence scales (Griffiths scales, WPPSI, WISC III), specific visual function assessments	A continuity of visual function deterioration from basic abilities toward a specific impairment of visuomotor dorsal pathways skills		Hypothesis of a dorsal pathway vulnerability; no significant correlation between cognitive and epileptic data

R, retrospective; P, prospective.

First stage or "febrile stage" (1–12 months)

- Convulsive and mainly febrile. Hemiclonic and long lasting are characteristics of Dravet syndrome.
- Normal EEG and MRI.
- **Normal psychomotor development and early visual functions impairment.**

Second stage (12–15 months–5 years)

- Polymorphous pharmacoresistant seizures: myoclonia, atypical absences, tonic–clonic and focal seizures.
- Gait disturbances.
- Normal EEG or showing a slowing in the background activity and multifocal abnormalities.
- **Cognitive slowing with attention deficit, behaviour disorders and ASD in some patients.**

Third stage (>6 years)

- Pharmacoresistant seizures persisting with a few seizure free patients.
- Nocturnal seizures might be more frequent than diurnal.
- Persistance of fever sensitivity.
- **Definite intellectual disability, stagnation without regression.**
- **Executive functions deficit.**
- **Language output more impaired than comprehension.**
- **Persistent deterioration of visual functions.**

Fig. 12.1 The course of Dravet syndrome in three stages with the clinical and **cognitive** states at each stage.

4 years followed by a stabilisation after the age of 6–7 years. The decline in the developmental quotient is constant although variable in different studies (Wolff et al. 2006; Ragona et al. 2011; Nabbout et al. 2013). This delay is often heterogeneous and might affect differently the specific skills (Wolff et al. 2006; Nabbout et al. 2013).This decline results from the stagnation of the psychomotor development and is not due to a regression as in neurodegenerative diseases (Ragona et al. 2011; Nabbout et al. 2013).

Some variability has been reported with the onset of the stagnation of acquisitions later up to the fourth year (Guzzetta 2011; Nabbout et al. 2013).

Nonetheless, a few patients corresponding to the diagnostic criteria for Dravet syndrome had preserved intellectual abilities over 6 years of life. Buoni et al. (2006) reported a 13-year-old boy with a normal IQ (125 at the Wechsler Intelligence Scale for Children-Revised). He presented a *de novo* frameshift mutation in the exon 14 causing a premature termination (c.2528delG). The authors attributed the normal cognitive development to the reduction in the frequency of seizures. Chieffo et al. (2011a), in a longitudinal clinical and neuropsychological evaluation of 12 patients with Dravet syndrome, reported 1 patient presenting a borderline IQ score at 6 years, who reached again the normal range in the last evaluation at 9 years. This was the only patient who was seizure free in their small series.

Nabbout et al. (2013) reported 4 patients with normal IQ aged more than 5 years in a large series of 67 patients. They all presented *SCN1A* mutation, three received the tritherapy (Valproate, stiripentol, Clobazam) and two were almost seizure free.

Patients with Dravet syndrome often present characteristic neuropsychiatric comorbidities, in particular hyperactivity, attention deficit, opposing and provocative behaviours, anxiety-like behaviours, impaired social interactions, restricted interests and poor danger awareness (Giovanardi-Rossi et al. 1991; Yakoub 1992; Wang et al. 1996; Caraballo and Fejerman 2006; Wolff et al. 2006; Genton et al. 2011; Brunklaus et al. 2012; Li et al. 2011; Nabbout et al. 2013; Villeneuve et al. 2014).

Wolff et al. (2006), in their prospective study, have clinically observed hyperactivity, poor relational capacities and gestural stereotypies in 18 of 20 patients.

Through the Achenbach and Conners scales, Nabbout et al. (2013) have observed attention deficit and hyperactivity, reaching the highest pathological scores (Conners test hyperactivity score >70) between 2 and 5 years.

In adulthood, these behavioural disorders tend to change, in particular with an improvement in attention deficit and hyperactivity replaced by extreme slowness and perseveration in movement, thinking and verbal expression (Scheffer and Dravet 2014).

Patients with Dravet syndrome might present some traits within the spectrum of autism spectrum disorders but without the involvement of the three main domains: stereotypical behaviours, social interactions and verbal and non-verbal communication. Li et al. (2011) have evaluated 37 Dravet syndrome patients with the DSM-IV, criteria, the Autism Behaviour Checklist and the Childhood Autism Rating Scale. Patients were aged from 2 to 6 years, and 9 of 37 patients had a diagnosis of autism, and most of the remaining showed some traits without fulfilling the criteria for autism. The mostly affected domains were verbal communication, narrow interests and emotional reciprocity (Li et al. 2011). There was no difference in the clinical characteristics of epilepsy between patients with and without autism. In another series of 21 patients aged 6 to 10 years assessed by the Vineland Adaptive Behaviour Scale, communication was significantly more affected than socialisation (Villeneuve et al. 2014). The authors also suggested that patients can present some autistic traits, but they do not fulfil all the criteria of autism.

Cognitive profiles in Dravet syndrome

In an attempt to better define the cognitive profile, three main domains of intellectual abilities have been reported as compromised: (1) executive functions, (2) the output of the language more than its comprehension and (3) visual functions.

In a prospective and retrospective study, Nabbout et al. (2013) have reported 67 patients with typical Dravet syndrome and described their cognitive development using the Brunet-Lezine scale (Joose 1997). They have observed that developmental quotient DQ/IQ decreased with age (in all except for four patients), from a normal score before 2 years to below the normal score after 4 years. Comparing the four tested domains in this scale (hand–eye coordination, language, posture and sociability), they observed that hand–eye coordination sub-scores (oculomotor abilities) were significantly lower than the three others. Villeneuve et al. (2014) have evaluated the

IQ (Wechsler Intelligence Scale) and adaptive scores (Vineland Adaptive Behavioural Scale) in 21 patients aged 6 to 10 years. They have observed a significant deficit in executive functions (verbal planning, auditory and working memory, visuomotor abilities, visuospatial organisation and fine motor skills), and they have related it to a possible 'dysexecutive syndrome'.

They have also observed, in line with this idea, that the communication and autonomy capacities were lower than the socialisation ones, considering the weakness in expressive language as part of an underling executive deficit.

Chieffo et al. (2011a) had previously reported, in a longitudinal study on 12 patients, with a follow-up from 4 to 10 years of age, the predominance of language phonological defects in contrast with a relatively good comprehension ability, bringing out the idea that in this syndrome, the language output is more impaired than the comprehension.

In a prospective study on five patients with Dravet syndrome, with a follow-up between the ages of 24 and 42 months, Chieffo et al. (2011b) have evaluated visual functions, including subcortical abilities (fixation and following) and the cortical ones (acuity, ocular motricity and fixation shift). They have observed (in four of five patients) an early visual function impairment, appearing even before the neuropsychological slowing and persisting during the course of the syndrome (Chieffo et al. 2011a). This is in line with the results of the oculomotor dysfunction reported by Nabbout et al. (2013).

In another prospective study on five patients with Dravet syndrome, Ricci et al. (2015) have observed a persistent deterioration of the visual functions, from the basic to more complex visuomotor functions.

The origin of the impairment of visual and executive functions was hypothesized to be related to the dysfunction of some cerebral regions and circuitry, which are usually known to be involved in the maturation and expression of these abilities.

The cerebellar hypothesis (Chieffo et al. 2011a; 2011b) has already been supported by experimental studies (Kalume et al. 2007). This dysfunction could be compatible with the dysexecutive syndrome, the language disorder and the early visual impairment, in addition to the neurological sign of ataxia frequently observed.

The possible disruption in the maturation of the frontal lobe was also reported as responsible for the dysexecutive syndrome and the language output disorder (Villeneuve et al. 2014).

Chieffo et al. (2011a) have proposed to relate verbal dysfunction to a possible disruption in the auditory dorsal stream, an important auditory–motor integration circuit that plays a role in speech development (Hickok and Poeppel 2007).

Finally, a possible vulnerability of the visual dorsal pathway involved in the processing of spatial information could be responsible for the deficit in visual functions (Ricci et al. 2015).

Prognostic factors

Several prognostic factors for cognitive outcome have been evaluated (Wolff et al. 2006; Ragona et al. 2011; Brunklaus et al. 2012; Nabbout et al. 2013; Takayama et al. 2014). Cognitive outcome was correlated to many variables of this syndrome: age at onset, occurrence of different seizures' types, status epilepticus, number of SEs, EEG backgound activity, EEG abnormalities in the first year or at follow-up and motor disorders (ataxia, spasticity), but still there are no clear and concordant results.

Wolff et al. (2006) studied the correlation between neuropsychological data and clinical data (age at testing, personal and family history, age at onset of epilepsy, seizure type and seizure frequency), EEG data and AEDs, in 12 patients with Dravet syndrome aged from 11 months to 16 years. Because of the limited number of patients, a statistical analysis was not possible. However, they observed a possible correlation between the frequency of seizures (more than five per month) and the course of intellectual deterioration.

In 2011, Ragona et al. (2011) performed a retrospective multicentre study on 26 patients (age ranging from 12mo to 5y). They reported the early appearance of myoclonus and/or absences as a negative factor in the global outcome.

In a large survey study on 241 patients with Dravet syndrome with *SCN1A* mutation (age ranging from 6mo to 42y), Brunklaus et al. (2012) found a correlation between a worse developmental outcome and the presence of a motor disorder (hypotonia, ataxia, spasticity, dyskinesia), abnormal interictal EEG findings in the first year of life, status epilepticus and the early onset of focal seizures (<24mo). However, different seizure precipitants (fever, illness, vaccination, hot bath), photosensitivity and MRI abnormalities had no significant effect on developmental outcome.

Takayama et al. (2014) confirmed the observation that the epilepsy phenotype has a prognostic value. In a series on 64 patients, divided into typical and atypical Dravet syndrome (according to the presence or absence of myoclonic and atypical absence seizures), they found a positive correlation between a more severe intellectual outcome with typical Dravet syndrome and in patients with a higher generalised tonic–clonic seizure frequency (daily to weekly). Furthermore, the presence of an occipital alpha rhythm on EEG seemed to be associated with a milder intellectual disability, as already observed by Akiyama et al. (2010).

Nabbout et al. (2013), on a population of 67 patients with Dravet syndrome aged 1 year 10 months to 24 years, found that only myoclonus and focal seizures were associated with a lower DQ/IQ. They failed to find any significant correlation between DQ/IQ and other seizure types and frequency, status epilepticus, photosensitivity and treatment onset.

The correlations between the *SCN1A* mutation and the cognitive outcome are contradictory. In one retrospective study, the mutation giving rise to a truncated protein (nonsense and frameshift mutations) was significantly correlated to an earlier age of seizure onset and of a worse cognitive outcome compared with missense mutations (Marini et al. 2007). This was not reported by another large study where mutation types (truncation vs missense) did not correlate to the outcome (Brunklaus et al. 2012). Nabbout et al. (2013) also reported a less favourable outcome in patients with *SCN1A* mutation compared to patients without the mutation. They showed that epilepsy phenotype was less severe in the first group, suggesting the role on the outcome of the genetic abnormality per se (Nabbout et al. 2013).

Cognitive effects of AEDs often used in Dravet syndrome

Patients with Dravet syndrome receive often AED polytherapy. AEDs may potentially influence cognitive functions, especially in case of polytherapy and high blood levels (Meador

2010; Bromley et al. 2011; Ijff and Aldenkamp 2013). The impact of AEDs on cognition is to be considered in addition to the impact of the mutation per se and of seizure recurrence in order to rationalize the risk-to-benefit ratio. Specific cognitive effects of AEDs are reported, and for AEDs mostly used in Dravet syndrome, the following should be emphasized:

- *Topiramate*: It can negatively affect the executive functions and the verbal fluency (Kockelmann et al. 2003; Witt et al. 2013). In addition, severe anorexia in some patients leading to weight loss can worsen the side effects of topiramate and other AEDs used on cognition by increasing the blood levels.
- *Levetiracetam*: It can have negative effects on mood (irritability, aggression and depression) (Helmstaedter and Witt 2008). This possible side effect should be monitored mainly in adolescents when oppositial behaviour becomes prominent.
- *Valproate* (*VPA*): Aggression, agitation, disturbance in attention, abnormal behaviour, psychomotor hyperactivity and learning disorder have been primarily observed in the paediatric population treated with VPA (Anderson et al. 2015). It has also been proved that school-aged children exposed to VPA in utero experience significantly poorer cognitive development than control children (Baker et al. 2015). The use of VPA can also cause gastrointestinal discomfort, weigh gain, hair loss, tremor and sedation (Keränen and Sivenius 1983). A severe impairment of cognition can occur in cases of VPA encephalopathy, a rare side effect reported with this drug secondary to hyperammonemia (Ijff and Aldenkamp 2013).
- *Benzodiazepines*: They can induce sedation, or otherwise a paradoxical excitement and agitation (Klehm et al. 2014; Lader 2014). They are known to carry risks of dependence, withdrawal and negative side effects. Among them, the most frequent are drowsiness, increased reaction time, ataxia and motor incoordination (Johnson and Streltzer 2013). Long-term treatment with benzodiazepines has been described as causing impairment in several cognitive domains, such as visuospatial ability, speed of processing and verbal learning (Stewart 2005).
- *Stiripentol*: At high doses, it can cause drowsiness and slowing of mental function. Most adverse events are related to a significant increase in the plasma concentrations of VPA, CLB and Nor-CLB after adding STP, and disappear when the co-medication dose is decreased (Chiron and Dulac 2011). The daily dioses of these AEDs should be decreased almost by one-third when associated with STP (Chiron and Dulac 2011).

Pathophysiological mechanisms

The co-occurrence of high-frequency and difficult-to-treat seizures with cognitive and behavioural abnormalities during the second year of life might suggest that epilepsy plays an important role in determining the cognitive and behavioural outcome. However, there is weak evidence showing a direct and exclusive effect of the epileptic activity on cognitive functions. The underlying mechanisms of neuropsychiatric comorbidities are not yet fully unravelled.

Although SCN1A mutant mice have already been reported as a model for the epileptic aspects of Dravet syndrome (Yu et al. 2006; Ogiwara et al. 2007), the mechanisms responsible for cognitive deficit and autism spectrum behaviours have been less investigated. Two recent studies by Han et al. (2012) and Ito et al. (2013) showed that mice heterozygous for nonsense *SCN1A* mutation can represent per se a good model for the neuropsychiatric comorbidities observed in Dravet syndrome patients. Both studies reported that $SCN1A^{+/-}$ mice present hyperactivity, low sociability, stereotyped behaviours and poor spatial learning abilities. They added that these cognitive and behavioural deficits are linked to a decreased inhibitory GABAergic neurotransmission. Furthermore, in order to confirm this hypothesis, Han et al. (2012) have proven that a single low-dose clonazepam injection reversed the behavioural deficits in their mice model.

The deletion of Nav1.1 channels induces a reduction of action potential firing in GABAergic interneurons of the neocortex and hippocampus, leading to an imbalance between excitatory and inhibitory transmission (Yu et al. 2006; Kalume et al. 2007). There is now increasing evidence that this dysfunction of GABAergic signalling is associated with autism spectrum disorders (Rubenstein and Merzenich 2003; Yizhar et al. 2011), and genome-wide association studies have identified the 2q24.3 region (where the SCN1A gene is located) as an autism susceptibility locus (Pescucci et al. 2007; Ramoz et al. 2008).

In both studies, the role of epilepsy in autism was not studied. Han et al. (2012) observed that cognitive deficit and autism-related behaviours were reversible by clonazepam at the time of training. They concluded that these comorbidities in Dravet syndrome mice are not caused by recurrent seizure-induced excitotoxicity, but instead are caused by SCN1A haploinsufficiency and the resulting reduction of GABAergic transmission.

Ito et al. (2013) realised their behavioural tests after the peak period of spontaneous seizures between the eight and the tenth postnatal week, and none of the mice in their study showed seizures during the behavioural tests.

Conclusion

The cognitive outcome in patients with Dravet syndrome seems to result from complex interaction between seizures, AED effects and the underlying genetic defect. This should be considered when evaluating future therapies for this syndrome.

REFERENCES

Akiyama M, Kobayashi K, Yoshinga H and Ohtsuka Y (2010) A long-term follow-up study of Dravet syndrome up to adulthood. *Epilepsia* 51: 1043–1052.

Anderson M, Egunsola O, Cherrill J et al. (2015) A prospective study of adverse drug reactions to antiepileptic drugs in children. *BMJ Open* 5: e008298. doi:10.1136/bmjopen-2015-008298.

Baker GA, Bromley RL, Briggs M et al. (2015) Liverpool and Manchester Neurodevelopment Group. IQ at 6 years after in utero exposure to antiepileptic drugs: A controlled cohort study. *Neurology* 84: 382–390. doi:10.1212/WNL.0000000000001182.

Berg AT, Berkovic SF, Brodie MJ et al. (2010) Revised terminology and concepts for organization of seizures and epilepsies: Report of the ILAE commission on classification and terminology, 2005–2009. *Epilepsia* 51: 676–85. doi:10.1111/j.1528-1167.2010.02522.x.

Bromley RL, Leeman BA, Baker GA and Meador KJ (2011) Cognitive and neurodevelopmental effects of antiepileptic drugs. *Epilepsy Behav* 22: 9–16. doi:10.1016/j.yebeh.2011.04.009.

Brunklaus A, Ellis R, Reavey E, Forbes GH and Zuberi SM (2012) Prognostic, clinical and demographic features in SCN1A mutation-positive Dravet syndrome. *Brain* 135: 2329–2336. doi:10.1093/brain/aws151.

Bureau M and Dalla Bernardina B (2011) Electroencephalographic characteristics of Dravet syndrome. *Epilepsia* 52: 13–23. doi:10.1111/j.1528-1167.2011.02996.

Buoni S, Orrico A, Galli L et al. (2006) SCN1A 2528del(G) novel truncating mutation with benign outcome of severe myoclonic epilepsy of infancy. *Neurology* 66: 606–607.

Commission on Classification and Terminology of the International League Against Epilepsy (1989) Proposal for revised classification of epilepsies and epileptic syndromes. *Epilepsia* 30: 389–399.

Caraballo RH and Fejerman N (2006) Dravet syndrome: A study of 53 patients. *Epilepsy Res* 70: S231–S238.

Caraballo RH, Flesler S, Pasteris C et al. (2013) Myoclonic epilepsy in infancy: An electroclinical study and long-term follow-up of 38 patients. *Epilepsia* 54: 1605–1612. doi:10.1111/epi.12321.

Cassé-Perrot C, Wolf M and Dravet C (2001) Neuropsychological aspects of severe myoclonic epilepsy in infancy. In Jambaqué I, Lassonde M and Dulac O, editors. *Neuropsychology of Childhood Epilepsy* (pp. 131–140). Kluwer Academic/Plenum Publishers, New York.

Chieffo D, Battaglia D, Lettori D et al. (2011a) Neuropsychological development in children with Dravet syndrome. *Epilepsy Res* 95: 86–93. doi:10.1016/j.eplepsyres.2011.03.005.

Chieffo D, Ricci D, Baranello G et al. (2011b) Early development in Dravet syndrome: Visual function impairment precedes cognitive decline. *Epilepsy Res* 93: 73–79. doi:10.1016/j.eplepsyres.2010.10.015.

Chiron C and Dulac O (2011) The pharmacologic treatment of Dravet syndrome. *Epilepsia* 52: 72–75. doi:10.1111/j.1528-1167.2011.03007.x.

Depienne C, Trouillard O, Saint-Martin C et al. (2009) Spectrum of SCN1A gene mutations associated with Dravet syndrome: Analysis of 333 patients. *J Med Genet* 46:183–191. doi:10.1136/jmg.2008.062323.

Dravet C (1978) Les epilepsies graves de l'enfant. *Vie Med* 8: 543–548.

Dravet C, Bureau M and Oguni H (2002) Severe myoclonic epilepsy in infancy (Dravet Syndrome). In: Roger J, Bureau M, Dravet C et al., editors. *Epileptic Syndromes in Infancy, Childhood and Adolescence* (pp. 75–88). John Libbey Eurotext, Montrouge, France.

Dravet C, Bureau M, Oguni H, Fukuyama Y and Cokar O (2005a) Severe myoclonic epilepsy in infancy (Dravet Syndrome). In Roger J, Bureau M, Dravet C et al., editors. *Epileptic Syndromes in Infancy, Childhood and Adolescence* (4th ed., pp. 89–113). John Libbey Eurotext, Montrouge, France.

Dravet C, Bureau M, Oguni H, Fukuyama Y and Cokar O (2005b) Severe myoclonic epilepsy in infancy: Dravet Syndrome. In Delgado-Escueta AV, Guerrini R, Medina MT et al., editors. *Advances in Neurology, Myoclonic Epilepsies* (Vol. 95, pp. 71–102). Lippincott Williams and Wilkins, Philadelphia, PA.

Dravet C and Guerrini R (2011) Dravet syndrome clinical and EEG description. In: Dravet C, Guerrini R, editors. *Dravet Syndrome* (pp. 16–17). John Libbey Eurotext, Montrouge, France.

Genton P, Velizarova R and Dravet C (2011) Dravet syndrome: The long-term outcome. *Epilepsia* 52: 44–49. doi:10.1111/j.1528-1167.2011.03001.x.

Giovanardi-Rossi PR, Santucci M, Gobbi G et al. (1991) Long-term follow-up of severe myoclonic epilepsy in infancy. In: Fukuyama Y, Kamoshita S, Ohtsuka C, Susuki Y, editors. *Modern Perspectives of Child Neurology* (pp. 205–213). Asahi Daily News, Tokyo.

Guzzetta F (2011) Cognitive and behavioural characteristics of children with Dravet syndrome: An overview. *Epilepsia* 52: 35–38. doi:10.1111/j.1528-1167.2011.02999.x.

Han S, Tai C, Westenbroek RE et al. (2012) Autistic-like behaviour in Scn1a+/- mice and rescue by enhanced GABA-mediated neurotrasmission. *Nature* 489: 385–390. doi:10.1038/nature11356.

Helmstaedter C and Witt JA (2008) The effects of levetiracetam on cognition: A non-interventional surveillance study. *Epilepsy Behav* 13: 642–649. doi:10.1016/j.yebeh.2008.07.012.

Hickok G and Poeppel D (2007) The cortical organization of speech processing. *Nat Rev Neurosci* 8: 393–402.

Ito S, Ogiwara I, Yamada K et al. (2013) Mouse with Nav1.1 haploinsufficiency, a model for Dravet syndrome, exhibits lowered sociability and learning impairment. *Neurobiol Dis* 49: 29–40. doi:10.1016/j.nbd.2012.08.003.

Ijff DM and Aldenkamp AP (2013) Cognitive side-effects of antiepileptic drugs in children. *Handb Clin Neurol* 111: 707–718. doi:10.1016/B978-0-444-52891-9.00073-7.

Johnson B and Streltzer J (2013) Risk associated with long-term benzodiazepine use. *Am Fam Physician* 88: 224–226.

Joose D (1997) Brunet-Lézine révisé : Échelle de développement psychomoteur de la Première enfance, Issy-les-Moulineaux (BP 67, 92133) : Éd. et applications psychologiques.

Kalume F, Yu FH, Westenbroek RE, Scheuer T and Catterall WA (2007) Reduced sodium current in Purkinje neurons from Nav1.1 mutant mice: implications for ataxia in severe myoclonic epilepsy in infancy. *J Neurosci* 27: 11065–11074.

Keränen T and Sivenius J (1983) Side effects of carbamazepine, valproate and clonazepam during long-term treatment of epilepsy. *Acta Neurol Scand Suppl* 97: 69–80.

Klehm J, Thome-Souza S, Sánchez Fernández I et al. (2014) Clobazam: Effect on frequency of seizures and safety profile in different subgroups of children with epilepsy. *Pediatr Neurol* 51: 60–66. doi:10.1016/j.pediatrneurol.2014.01.025.

Kockelmann E, Elger CE and Helmstaedter C (2003) Significant improvement in frontal lobe associated neuropsychological functions after withdrawal of topiramate in epilepsy patients. *Epilepsy Res* 54: 171–178.

Lader M (2014) Benzodiazepine harm: How can it be reduced? *Br J Clin Pharmacol* 77: 295–301. doi: 10.1111/j.1365-2125.2012.04418.x.

Li BM, Liu XR, Yi YH et al. (2011) Autism in Dravet syndrome: Prevalence, features and relationship to the clinical characteristics of epilepsy and mental retardation. *Epilepsy Behav* 21: 291–295. doi:10.1016/j.yebeh.2011.04.060.

Marini C, Mei D, Temudo AR et al. (2007) Idiopathic epilepsies with seizures precipitated by fever and SCN1A abnormalities. *Epilepsia* 48: 1678–1685.

Marini C, Scheffer IE, Nabbout R et al. (2011) The genetics of Dravet syndrome. *Epilepsia* 52: 24–29. doi:10.1111/j.1528-1167.2011.02997.x.

Meador KJ (2010) Cognitive effects of epilepsy and of antiepileptic medications. In: Wyllie E, Cascino G, Gidal B, Goodkin H, editors. *The Treatment of Epilepsy: Principles & Practice* (5th ed., pp. 1028–1036). Lippincott Williams & Wilkins, Philadelphia, PA.

Nabbout R and Dulac O (2003) Epilepstic encephalopathies: A brief overview. *J Clin Neurophysiol* 20: 393–397.

Nabbout R, Chemaly N, Chipaux M et al. (2013) Encephalopathy in children with Dravet syndrome is not a pure consequence of epilepsy. *Orphanet J Rare Dis* 8: 176. doi:10.1186/1750-1172-8-176.

Ogiwara I, Miyamoto H, Morita N et al. (2007) Nav1.1 localizes to axons of parvalbumin-positive inhibitory interneurons: A circuit basis for epileptic seizures in mice carrying an Scn1a gene mutation. *J Neurosci* 27: 5903–5914.

Pescucci C, Caselli R, Grosso S et al. (2007) 2q24-q31 deletion: Report of a case and review of the literature. *Eur J Med Genet* 50: 21–32. Review.

Ragona F, Brazzo D, De Giorgi I et al. (2010) Dravet syndrome: Early clinical manifestations and cognitive outcome in 37 Italian patients. *Brain Dev* 32: 71–77. doi:10.1016/j.braindev.2009.09.014.

Ragona F, Granata T, Dalla Bernardina B et al. (2011) Cognitive development in Dravet syndrome: A retrospective, multicenter study of 26 patients. *Epilepsia* 52: 386–392. doi:10.1111/j.1528-1167.2010.02925.x.

Ramoz N, Cai G, Reichert JG, Silverman JM and Buxbaum JD (2008) Ananalysis of candidate autism loci on chromosome 2q24-q33: Evidence for association to the STK39 gene. *Am J Med Genet B Neuropsychiatr Genet* 147B: 1152–1158. doi: 10.1002/ajmg.b.30739.

Ricci D, Chieffo D, Battaglia D et al. (2015) A prospective longitudinal study on visuo-cognitive development in Dravet syndrome: Is there a 'dorsal stream vulnerability'? *Epilepsy Res* 109: 57–64. doi: 10.1016/j.eplepsyres.2014.10.009.

Rubenstein JL and Merzenich MM (2003) Model of autism: Increased ratio of excitation/inhibition in key neural system. *Genes Brain Behav* 2: 255–267. Review.

Scheffer I and Dravet C (2014) Transition to adult life in the monogenic epilepsies. *Epilepsia* 55: 12–15. doi:10.1111/epi.12707.

Stewart SA (2005) The effects of benzodiazepines on cognition. *J Clin Psychiatry* 66: 9–13.

Takayama R, Fujiwara T, Shigematsu H et al. (2014) Long-term course of Dravet syndrome: A study from an epilepsy center in Japan. *Epilepsia* 55: 528–538. doi:10.1111/epi.12532.

Villeneuve N, Laguitton V, Viellard M et al. (2014) Cognitive and adaptive evaluation of 21 patients with Dravet syndrome. *Epilepsy Behav* 31: 143–148. doi:10.1016/j.yebeh.2013.11.021.

Wang PJ, Fan PC, Lee WT et al. (1996) Severe myoclonic epilepsy in infancy: Evolution of electroencephalographic and clinical features. *Acta Paed Sin* 37: 428–432.

Witt JA, Elger CE and Helmstaedter C (2013) Impaired verbal fluency under topiramate-evidence for synergistic negative effects of epilepsy, topiramate, and polytherapy. *Eur J Neurol* 20: 130–137. doi:10.1111/j.1468-1331.2012.03814.x.

149

Wolff M, Casse-Perrot C and Dravet C (2006) Severe myoclonic epilepsy of infants (Dravet Syndrome): Natural history and neuropsychological findings. *Epilepsia* 47: 45–48.

Yakoub M, Dulac O, Jambaque I, Chiron C and Plouin P (1992) Early diagnosis of severe myoclonic epilepsy in infancy. *Brain Dev* 14: 299–303.

Yizhar O, Fenno LE, Prigge M et al. (2011) Neocortical excitation/inhibition balance in information processing and social dysfunction. *Nature* 477: 171–178. doi:10.1038/nature10360.

Yu FH, Mantegazza M, Westenbroek RE et al. (2006) Reduced sodium current GABAergic interneurons in a mouse model of severe myoclonic epilepsy in infancy. *Nat Neurosci* 9: 1142–1149.

13
THE EPILEPTIC SYNDROMES WITH CONTINUOUS SPIKES AND WAVES DURING SLOW-WAVE SLEEP

Patrick Van Bogaert and Xavier De Tiège

Introduction

In 1957, Landau and Kleffner (1957) reported children with normal early language development who became aphasic after the onset of epileptic seizures and had bilateral temporal interictal epileptiform discharges (IEDs) on EEG (Landau and Kleffner 1957). The authors suspected that persistent convulsive discharges resulted in the functional ablation of brain areas concerned with linguistic communication. The language disturbance was further characterized as auditory verbal agnosia, that is, the inability to decode phonemes despite intact peripheral hearing mechanisms, leading to a severe expressive and receptive verbal deficit (Rapin et al. 1977). Observations of language regression without clinical seizures were further reported (Deonna 1991; Paquie et al. 1992; Soprano et al.1994; Tassinari et al. 2002). Longitudinal follow-up of these children showed that the seizures as well as the EEG abnormalities remit at adolescence (Paquie et al. 1992). The Landau–Kleffner syndrome (LKS) was recognized by the International League Against Epilepsy (ILAE) as synonymous with acquired epileptic aphasia to be classified among the epilepsies and syndromes of childhood undetermined whether focal or generalized.

Electrical status epilepticus during slow sleep (ESES) was proposed by Tassinari et al. in 1971 for a particular EEG pattern characterized by diffuse spike-waves occurring during at least 85% of slow sleep and persisting on three or more records over a period of at least 1 month (Patry et al. 1971). Most children with ESES had refractory seizures and global cognitive regression leading to severe intellectual disability. However, some of them had more selective language-related impairment identical to that observed in LKS. Moreover, the evolution of the epilepsy showed remission at adolescence even if most patients had persistent and sometimes severe neuropsychological sequels.

Despite the clear overlap between ESES and LKS, the ILAE proposed in a first step to classify ESES separately under the name "epilepsy with continuous spikes and waves during slow-wave sleep (CSWS)," but recognized these two syndromes as epileptic encephalopathies, that is, epilepsies in which the epileptiform abnormalities may contribute to progressive neurological dysfunction (Engel 2001).

Subsequently, observations of children with CSWS presenting other types of cognitive deterioration than aphasia or dementia were reported. These included autism and more selective cognitive impairments such as frontal lobe dysfunction, apraxia and hemineglect, pseudo-bulbar palsy, visual agnosia, and learning arrest (Roulet Perez et al. 1993; De Tiege et al. 2004).

The ILAE now consider that there is insufficient evidence for mechanistic differences between LKS and CSWS to warrant considering them separate syndromes, and proposed the term of "epileptic encephalopathy with CSWS including LKS" for this particular childhood epileptic syndrome (Engel 2006).

Definition of epileptic encephalopathy with CSWS

There is now a large consensus to consider epileptic encephalopathy with CSWS as a spectrum of epileptic conditions defined by (1) an onset in childhood (3y to 10y); (2) the occurrence of cognitive or behavioral impairments that appear or worsen after the epilepsy onset; and (3) the presence of abundant IEDs during sleep, which tend to be more frequent, with increased amplitude and diffusion over the whole scalp during non-rapid eye movement sleep than during the awake state. LKS is a particular presentation in which acquired aphasia is the core symptom. Seizures are not a mandatory feature. When they occur, seizures have variable semiology (focal seizures without consciousness impairment, secondary generalized tonic–clonic seizures, focal negative myoclonia, atypical absences) but, unlike in Lennox–Gastaut syndrome, tonic seizures are usually not encountered (Galanopoulou et al. 2000; Tassinari et al. 2000).

However, what is less consensual are the frontiers with classic benign epilepsy with centrotemporal spikes (BECTS), and particularly the minimal EEG and clinical criteria needed to pose the diagnosis of epileptic encephalopathy with CSWS, because these two conditions overlap. This overlap was already pointed out by Aicardi and Chevrie (1982) who reported children who had an epileptic syndrome resembling BECTS but with atypical features such as frequent brief seizures (atypical absences, focal myoclonia), cognitive impairment, and CSWS. Authors now speak about atypical BECTS when daily seizures, CSWS, and neuropsychological impairment occur in a child diagnosed with BECTS (Fejerman 2009; Fujii et al. 2010). Observations of classic BECTS cases evolving to an epileptic encephalopathy with CSWS, sometimes precipitated by the use of some antiepileptic drugs (AEDs) (Tassinari et al. 2000; Saltik et al. 2005), and of CSWS and BECTS cases coexisting within the same family (De Tiege 2006), further outline this overlap. It should be too simplistic to state that it is the presence of CSWS and cognitive deficits that will distinguish BECTS from epileptic encephalopathy with CSWS. Indeed, if a pattern of CSWS was found in the course of the disease in all patients with LKS reported in some series (Dulac et al. 1983; Hirsch et al. 1990; Paquier et al. 1992; Massa et al. 2000; Robinson et al. 2001), it was found only in a minority of patients in another series (McVicar et al. 2005). More recently, three patients with LKS with initial normal sleep EEG were reported, the diagnosis being made after several weeks or months based on the demonstration of IEDs during sleep, including CSWS in two of them (Van Bogaert et al. 2013). Also, some data suggest that it is not only the IED percentage but also their increased amplitude and diffusion during sleep that is detrimental to normal brain function (Aeby et al. 2005; De Tiege et al. 2008). This is evidence that the EEG criteria of CSWS criteria as proposed by the Tassinari's group (Patry et al. 1971) are too restrictive to define the syndrome.

Also, the minimal cognitive impairment needed to make a diagnosis of epileptic encephalopathy with CSWS is a subject of controversy. Indeed, numerous studies have reported an unexpected high rate of cognitive difficulties in the language, attentional, and memory domains in children with classic BECTS, which were associated with IED severity at the acute phase of the disease and resolved with the normalization of the EEG (Deonna 2000; Baglietto et al. 2001; Verrotti et al. 2014).

In conclusion, it is widely accepted that BECTS and epileptic encephalopathy with CSWS are the edges of a spectrum in which the most frequent and diffused IEDs during sleep seem to result in the more severe behavioral and cognitive deficits (Stephani and Carlsson 2006; Kramer et al. 2009; Moeller et al. 2013). The nosological limits between these two conditions are thus somewhat arbitrary.

Aetiology

Epileptic encephalopathy with CSWS is one of the childhood focal epileptic syndromes. According to the terminology revised in 2010 (Berg et al. 2010), the underlying aetiology allows classifying patients within one of the following three subgroups: structural/metabolic, genetic, and unknown. The subgroup of unknown aetiology is the most important, representing more than half of the patients. Patients with structural brain lesions identified on magnetic resonance imaging (MRI) are in the structural/metabolic subgroup and represent approximately 20% of the cases. Lesions are usually antenatal cortical malformations (polymicrogyria) or ante/perinatal cortical destructive lesions, but may also be purely subcortical, the association between thalamic perinatal injury and CSWS being well recognized (Guerrini et al. 1998; Guzzetta et al. 2005). These cases have usually preexisting signs of cerebral palsy. Within this subgroup are also patients with preexisting motor and cognitive deficiencies related to chromosomal anomalies (15q deletion for instance) or genetic syndromes such as Rett syndrome (Van Bogaert et al. 2006). In the genetic subgroup are patients with a demonstrated genetic mutation, but those with mutations associated with structural brain lesions (tubulin genes for instances) and those with chromosomal deletions and preexisting psychomotor delay do not belong to this subgroup. Up to now, there is only one gene demonstrated as pathogenic in the genetic subgroup. This gene is called *GRIN2A*. Mutations of *GRIN2A* have been identified by three independent research groups (Carvill et al. 2013, Lesca et al. 2013, and Lemke et al. 2013). Patients with *GRIN2A* mutations represented about 10% to 20% of cohorts of patients with epileptic encephalopathy with CSWS and normal MRI. Phenotypes are LKS or atypical BECTS, but some patients have a typical BECTS phenotype, further underlying the overlap between these two epileptic syndromes. *GRIN2A* encodes the *N*-methyl-D-aspartate (NMDA) glutamate receptor a2 subunit, GluN2A. Patients have either inherited or *de novo* mutations, which affect NMDA receptor function.

Pathophysiology of cognitive regression

Epileptic encephalopathy with CSWS is one of the best illustrations of the concept of epileptic encephalopathy, that is, conditions in which epileptiform abnormalities may

153

contribute to progressive cognitive dysfunction, so that early effective intervention may improve developmental outcome (Engel 2006; Berg et al. 2010). Indeed, clinical improvement is evident and sometimes impressive when treatment results in EEG normalization, even in lesion-related cases (Guerrini et al. 1998; Aeby et al. 2005; Guzzetta et al. 2005; Buzatu et al. 2009; Peltola et al. 2011).

It should be noted that complete normalization of the sleep EEG is not always mandatory to obtain clinical improvement. Indeed, besides the percentage of spike–wave complexes during non-rapid eye movement sleep, the diffusion of the epileptic activity over the whole scalp is also important to consider, as children with diffuse CSWS may show spectacular clinical improvement under treatment even if a focus of spikes persists during a high percentage of sleep time (Aeby et al. 2005; Buzatu et al. 2009).

The initial hypothesis of a "functional ablation" of eloquent cortical areas by the "persistent convulsive discharge" to explain the neuropsychological impairment, as proposed more than half a century ago by Landau and Kleffner (1957), remains the most largely accepted hypothesis. However, some observations are not fully explained by this theory. First, the temporal association between CSWS on EEG and neurological regression is not always strict (Rapin et al. 1977; Hirsch et al. 1990; Van Bogaert et al. 2013). This suggests that other factors, for example, autoimmune factors as suggested by the response to corticosteroids (see the Treatment section below), could impact on language and cognition in some patients. Second, if some authors found strict association between the pattern of neuropsychological impairment and the location of interictal focus, others did not. Indeed, patients showing clinical frontal dysfunction but a parietal epileptic focus have been reported (De Tiege et al. 2004). This discrepancy can be explained regarding the pathophysiological model that emerged from positron emission tomography with [18F]-fluorodeoxyglucose (FDG-PET) data obtained at the awake state in children at the active phase of the disease as well as at remission. Those studies demonstrated that the acute phase of CSWS is characterized by a metabolic pattern associating regional increase(s) and decrease(s) in glucose metabolism in distinct brain areas, with heterogeneous location of the abnormalities across patients (Fig 13.1) (De Tiege et al. 2004; De Tiege et al. 2008). The combination of magnetoencephalography and FDG-PET demonstrated that focal hypermetabolism was related to the onset or the propagation sites of spike–wave discharges, whereas hypometabolic areas were not involved in the epileptic network as such (De Tiege et al. 2013). At the group level, hypometabolism occurred in regions that belong to the default network (prefrontal and posterior cingulate cortices, parahippocampal gyrus and precuneus) (Ligot et al. 2014). The pathophysiological model proposed to explain these findings is based on the "surrounding and remote inhibition theory," which suggests the existence of epilepsy-induced inhibition of neurons that surround or are remote from the hypermetabolic epileptic focus and connected with it via cortico-cortical or polysynaptic pathways (Bruehl and Witte1995; Schwartz and Bonhoeffer 2001). The validity of this model in epileptic encephalopathy with CSWS is supported by (1) the evidence of altered effective connectivity between hyper- and hypometabolic areas, suggesting that the level of metabolic activity in hypometabolic areas is related to the epilepsy-induced metabolic changes in the hypermetabolic ones (De Tiege et al. 2004; De Tiege et al. 2008; Ligot et al. 2014) and (2) the complete or almost complete parallel regression of hypermetabolic and hypometabolic abnormalities at recovery from CSWS (De Tiege et al. 2008).

Interestingly, patients investigated by FDG-PET during sleep showed regional metabolism alterations that were similar to the wake state (Maquet et al. 1990). Furthermore, EEG combined with functional MRI (EEG-fMRI) investigations demonstrated similar types of findings but were directly linked to CSWS activity, that is, IED-related increases in perfusion at the site of the epileptic focus, were associated with decreases in perfusion in distinct connected brain areas, including nodes of the default mode network (De Tiege et al. 2007; Siniatchkin et al. 2010). Thus, patients with CSWS show during sleep profound metabolic and EEG disturbances that could alter the physiological roles of sleep. One of the physiological functions of sleep is to promote memory consolidation (see Urbain et al. 2013, for review). One study showed impaired consolidation of a declarative memory task during sleep in two children with epileptic encephalopathy and CSWS, and normalization of overnight memory performance after successful treatment of CSWS with hydrocortisone in one of them, suggesting that CSWS could impair the mechanisms of sleep-related brain plasticity (Urbain et al. 2011). An epilepsy-related disruption of synaptic homeostasis processes that take place during sleep is suggested in children with CSWS by a study showing the absence of the expected decrease in the slope of slow waves during sleep (Bolsterli et al. 2011).

In summary, behavioral and functional neuroimaging data suggest sustained epilepsy-related perturbations of neurophysiological processes through the sleep–wake cycle at the acute phase of CSWS. They also incite to attribute the neurological regression not only to neuronal impairment at the epileptic focus site but also to epilepsy-induced inhibition of distant connected brain areas.

Treatment

In the absence of any published controlled study on the use of AED in epileptic encephalopathy with CSWS, treatment relies on expert-based consensus guidelines and uncontrolled published series. The evaluation of a drug effect is probably more difficult in this epileptic syndrome than in others because (1) clinical and EEG fluctuations with time without any change of treatment are frequently observed and (2) the goals of the treatment are not only to abolish the seizures with minimal side effects but also to obtain neuropsychological improvement by decreasing IEDs during sleep.

Valproate is classically proposed as the first choice drug, either in monotherapy or in association with a benzodiazepine (usually clobazam), but this relies on relatively old series, including few patients (Van Bogaert et al. 2006; Lagae 2009). Data concerning the effect of benzodiazepines on the EEG are more convincing. De Negri et al. (1995) reported a remission of CSWS in 9 out of 15 patients with a 1-month intrarectal diazepam treatment; among these 9 patients, 7 showed an improvement in their neuropsychological evaluation after 6 months. A more recent study reported a reduction of approximately 35% of the interictal epileptiform activity 24 hours after the administration of high-dose diazepam (Sanchez Fernandez et al. 2012). Among the other old drugs, there is a consensus stating that carbamazepine, phenobarbital, and diphantoin are usually inefficacious and may even worsen the EEG and clinical conditions of children with CSWS. On the other hand, etho-suximide and sulthiame are the old drugs that may be helpful in reducing CSWS (Lagae 2009; Fejerman et al. 2012).

Concerning the new AEDs, studies suggest that levetiracetam add-on treatment is effective in about half of the patients (Aeby et al. 2005; Wang et al. 2008; Kramer et al. 2009; Atkins and Nikanorova 2011).

Corticosteroids are probably more efficacious and result in more long-lasting effects than classic AEDs. In a series of 30 patients, high-dose diazepam was efficacious in 37%, all the children showing temporary response only, whereas response to steroids was obtained in 65% (Kramer et al. 2009). The larger series on the effects of corticosteroids in epileptic encephalopathy with CSWS published so far included 44 patients (Buzatu et al. 2009). Most of them were treated with hydrocortisone starting at 5mg/kg/day with a maintenance dose of 2mg/kg/day until the end of a full year's treatment. More than 75% of the patients responded to this regimen within the first 3 months, with normalization of the EEG in about half of them. As relapse occurred in 14 patients, 20 patients (45.4%) were long-term responders. Positive response to steroids was associated with higher IQ and shorter CSWS duration. Patients with LKS were all long-term responders in this series. The prolonged use of hydrocortisone resulted in the usual complications, including a cushingoid appearance in all patients, but life-threatening side effects were not observed. Seven patients discontinued the treatment prematurely because of the side effects. Thus, efficacy of corticosteroids must be balanced by their side effects, and this study supports the fact that they should be introduced relatively early in children showing severe regression (Buzatu et al. 2009). The mechanisms of action of corticosteroids are poorly understood. An immunosuppressive effect is possible, but a direct action on epilepsy through the modulation of various neurotransmitter systems, as hypothesized in West syndrome, seems more likely (Hrachovy 1997).

Among the other therapeutic modalities, the benefits of intravenous immunoglobulins were not confirmed in a recent series (Arts et al. 2009). Data on the use of vagus nerve stimulation and ketogenic diet are too scarce to draw conclusions (Lagae 2009).

Resective surgery in patients with cortical lesions was found to be effective on both seizures and cognition; in particular when CSWS is associated with hemiplegia, hemispherotomy may show spectacular cognitive improvement because CSWS is likely to be a secondary generalization of the epileptic activity from the damaged hemisphere (Kallay et al. 2009; Loddenkemper et al. 2009; Peltola et al. 2011).

Concerning palliative surgical procedures, callosotomy and multiple subpial transections may be considered. Callosotomy was found useful in one series (Peltola et al. 2011). Multiple subpial transections have to be considered in refractory cases of LKS. This technique has indeed shown benefits only in patients with a pure verbal auditive agnosia, and not in other phenotypes of CSWS epilepsy (Grote et al. 1999; Irwin et al. 2001). Good candidates are patients with severe persisting aphasia in whom a unilateral perisylvian epileptic origin is suggested on the basis of the non-invasive presurgical evaluation (Cross and Neville 2009). Magnetoencephalography is particularly useful in this regard (Paetau 2009). Improvement of language after surgery was reported in the majority of patients, but was most likely to be seen years, rather than months, after surgery, which raises the question of the natural evolution to recovery (Grote et al. 1999).

Long-term outcome

Long-term outcome for seizures is good in epileptic encephalopathy with CSWS, persisting seizures at adulthood occurring in a minority of patients, even in those with lesion-related epilepsy (Guerrini et al. 1998; Praline et al. 2003; Guzzetta et al. 2005).

Therefore, the main concern in epileptic encephalopathy with CSWS is the cognitive outcome. Long-term studies show persistent cognitive deficits in most patients (Liukkonen et al. 2010; Seegmuller et al. 2012; Pera et al. 2013). Excluding the underlying aetiology, available literature supports that the main variables impacting long-term cognitive outcome are the duration of CSWS or of regression, and the type and severity of cognitive regression at the acute phase of the disease.

The authors have related either the duration of CSWS or the duration of regression with long-term outcome, but these two time periods could not be identical. Indeed, sleep EEG abnormalities may fluctuate from day to day in the early stage of regression, even leading to normal EEG records (Van Bogaert et al. 2013). Therefore, the duration of regression seems more appropriate to be considered in studies designed to identify the dependent factors of cognitive outcome. This has also the advantage to include patients for whom sleep EEG data at early regression are not available.

Long duration of CSWS or regression was found to be predictive of a poor cognitive outcome in several studies (Paquier et al. 1992; Robinson et al. 2001; Veggiotti et al. 2002; Scholtes et al. 2005; Kramer et al. 2009; Liukkonen et al. 2010; Seegmuller et al. 2012; Pera et al. 2013). In some studies, this factor reached statistical significance. In a series of 18 patients with LKS followed for a mean duration of 67 months, long duration of CSWS was associated with outcome, no child with CSWS lasting longer than 36 months having normal outcome (Robinson et al. 2001). In a series of 30 patients with epileptic encephalopathies with CSWS of various aetiologies, including lesion-related cases, followed at a mean of 6.6 years, the duration of CSWS correlated significantly with residual intellectual deficit (Kramer et al. 2009). Long duration of CSWS was statistically associated with bad cognitive outcome in a recent series of 10 patients with different types of cognitive regression and normal MRI followed at long term (Seegmuller et al. 2012).

The type and severity of cognitive regression at the acute phase of the disease also need to be considered. Several studies showed persistence of neuropsychological dysfunctions particularly to each syndrome at long term, so that patients with prolonged global intellectual regression had the worst outcome, whereas those with more specific deficits recovered best (Praline et al. 2003; Debiais et al. 2007; Seegmuller et al. 2012). Concerning more specifically LKS, patients usually keep language difficulties at adulthood, but the disability is highly variable, depending on the response to treatment (Paquier et al. 1992; Praline et al. 2003; Deonna et al. 2009; Van Bogaert et al. 2013). Persistent impairment in verbal short-term memory was demonstrated in patients after recovery from LKS using functional imaging: compared to controls, patients showed decreased activation for an immediate serial

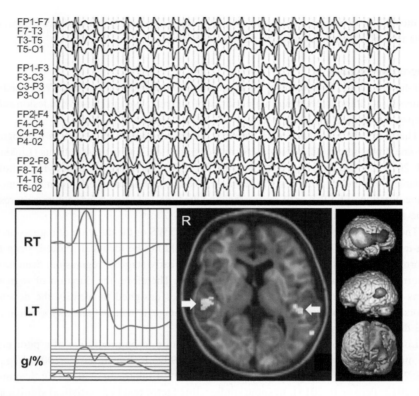

Fig. 13.1. Patient aged 8 years studied at the acute phase of LKS. *Top*: Non-rapid eye movement sleep EEG sample showing high-amplitude and diffuse CSWS with focalization over the right and left temporal regions. *Bottom, left*: The right and left temporal source waveforms identified by MEG for one typical epileptiform discharge occurring during CSWS. The abscissa corresponds to the time in ms (time steps: 10ms) and the ordinate corresponds to the dipole amplitude in nAm. The source waveforms clearly show the onset at the level of the right temporal (RT; maximal amplitude: 660nAm) source with rapid propagation (~20ms) toward the left temporal (LT; maximal amplitude: 602nAm) source. *Middle*: Results of the coregistration in the same three-dimensional space of the DICOM MRI image containing representative MEG equivalent current dipoles with the raw FDG-PET data. Both temporal MEG sources are localized at the superior temporal gyrus within hypermetabolic brain areas. *Right*: Statistical parametric mapping (SPM) analysis of the patient's FDG-PET data showing a significant bilateral increase in metabolism predominating over the superior temporal gyri (top and middle). Significant decrease in metabolism observed over the prefrontal cortex with a left hemisphere predominance (bottom). For viewing purpose, SPM maps are thresholded at $p < 0.001$ uncorrected. (From De Tiege et al., *Epilepsy Res*, 105, 316–325, 2013.) CSWS, continuous spikes and waves during slow-wave sleep; FDG-PET, [18F]-fluorodeoxyglucose; MEG, magnetoencephalography. A colour version of this figure can be seen in the plate section at the end of the book.

recall task in those posterior superior temporal gyri that were involved in the epileptic focus during the active phase of the disease (Majerus et al. 2003).

In atypical BECTS, where cognitive regression may be discrete, long-term outcome may be favorable: a study followed 12 patients until the ages of 6–14 years and showed that long duration of negative motor seizure period was associated with low IQ, four patients having IQ less than 70 (Fujii et al. 2010). Another study found full cognitive recovery in two of the five patients with atypical BECTS (Tovia et al. 2011).

Rehabilitation

Rehabilitation is a very important part of the treatment. In patients with LKS with preserved nonverbal skills, learning of visual forms of language including sign language is useful as they can successfully be learned at different ages and do not interfere with oral language recovery. Still, sign language could facilitate recovery by stimulating functionally connected core language networks (Deonna et al. 2009).

REFERENCES

Aeby A, Poznanski N, Verheulpen D, Wetzburger C and Van Bogaert P (2005) Levetiracetam efficacy in epileptic syndromes with continuous spikes and waves during slow sleep: Experience in 12 cases. *Epilepsia* 46: 1937–1942.

Aicardi J and Chevrie JJ (1982) Atypical benign partial epilepsy of childhood. *Dev Med Child Neurol* 24: 281–292.

Arts WF, Aarsen FK, Scheltens-de Boer M and Catsman-Berrevoets CE (2009) Landau–Kleffner syndrome and CSWS syndrome: Treatment with intravenous immunoglobulins. *Epilepsia* 50: 55–58.

Atkins M and Nikanorova M (2011) A prospective study of levetiracetam efficacy in epileptic syndromes with continuous spikes-waves during slow sleep. *Seizure* 20: 635–639.

Baglietto MG, Battaglia FM, Nobili L et al. (2001) Neuropsychological disorders related to interictal epileptic discharges during sleep in benign epilepsy of childhood with centrotemporal or Rolandic spikes. *Dev Med Child Neurol* 43: 407–412.

Berg AT, Berkovic SF, Brodie MJ et al. (2010) Revised terminology and concepts for organization of seizures and epilepsies: Report of the ILAE commission on classification and terminology, 2005–2009. *Epilepsia* 51: 676–685.

Bolsterli BK, Schmitt B, Bast T et al. (2011) Impaired slow wave sleep downscaling in encephalopathy with status epilepticus during sleep (ESES). *Clin Neurophysiol* 122: 1779–1787.

Bruehl C and Witte OW (1995) Cellular activity underlying altered brain metabolism during focal epileptic activity. *Ann Neurol* 38: 414–420.

Buzatu M, Bulteau C, Altuzarra C, Dulac O and Van Bogaert P (2009) Corticosteroids as treatment of epileptic syndromes with continuous spike-waves during slow-wave sleep. *Epilepsia* 50: 68–72.

Carvill GL, Regan BM, Yendle SC et al. (2013) GRIN2A mutations cause epilepsy-aphasia spectrum disorders. *Nat Genet* 45: 1073–1076.

Cross JH and Neville BG (2009) The surgical treatment of Landau–Kleffner syndrome. *Epilepsia* 50: 63–67.

De Negri M, Baglietto MG, Battaglia FM et al. (1995) Treatment of electrical status epilepticus by short diazepam (DZP) cycles after DZP rectal bolus test. *Brain Dev* 17: 330–333.

De Tiege X, Goldman S, Laureys S et al. (2004) Regional cerebral glucose metabolism in epilepsies with continuous spikes and waves during sleep. *Neurology* 63: 853–857.

De Tiege X, Goldman S, Verheulpen D et al. (2006) Coexistence of idiopathic rolandic epilepsy and CSWS in two families. *Epilepsia* 47: 1723–1727.

De Tiege X, Harrison S, Laufs H et al. (2007) Impact of interictal epileptic activity on normal brain function in epileptic encephalopathy: An electroencephalography-functional magnetic resonance imaging study. *Epilepsy Behav* 11: 460–465.

De Tiege X, Ligot N, Goldman S et al. (2008) Metabolic evidence for remote inhibition in epilepsies with continuous spike-waves during sleep. *Neuroimage* 40: 802–810.

De Tiege X, Trotta N, Op de Beeck M et al. (2013) Neurophysiological activity underlying altered brain metabolism in epileptic encephalopathies with CSWS. *Epilepsy Res* 105: 316–325.

Debiais S, Tuller L, Barthez MA et al. (2007) Epilepsy and language development: The continuous spike-waves during slow sleep syndrome. *Epilepsia* 48: 1104–1110.

Deonna T, Prelaz-Girod AC, Mayor-Dubois C and Roulet-Perez E (2009) Sign language in Landau–Kleffner syndrome. *Epilepsia* 50: 77–82.

Deonna T, Zesiger P, Davidoff V et al. (2000) Benign partial epilepsy of childhood: A longitudinal neuro-psychological and EEG study of cognitive function. *Dev Med Child Neurol* 42: 595–603.

Deonna TW (1991) Acquired epileptiform aphasia in children (Landau–Kleffner syndrome). *J Clin Neuro-physiol* 8: 288–298.

Dulac O, Billard C and Arthuis M (1983) Electroclinical and developmental aspects of epilepsy in the aphasia-epilepsy syndrome. *Arch Fr Pediatr* 40: 299–308.

Engel J Jr. (2001) A proposed diagnostic scheme for people with epileptic seizures and with epilepsy: Report of the ILAE task fon classification and terminology. *Epilepsia* 42: 796–803.

Engel J Jr. (2006) Report of the ILAE classification core group. *Epilepsia* 47: 1558–1568.

Fejerman N (2009) Atypical rolandic epilepsy. *Epilepsia* 50: 9–12.

Fejerman N, Caraballo R, Cersosimo R et al. (2012) Sulthiame add-on therapy in children with focal epi-lepsies associated with encephalopathy related to electrical status epilepticus during slow sleep (ESES). *Epilepsia* 53: 1156–1161.

Fujii A, Oguni H, Hirano Y and Osawa M (2010) Atypical benign partial epilepsy: Recognition can prevent pseudocatastrophe. *Pediatr Neurol* 43: 411–419.

Galanopoulou AS, Bojko A, Lado F and Moshe SL (2000) The spectrum of neuropsychiatric abnormalities associated with electrical status epilepticus in sleep. *Brain Dev* 22: 279–295.

Grote CL, Van Slyke P and Hoeppner JA (1999) Language outcome following multiple subpial transection for Landau–Kleffner syndrome. *Brain* 122: 561–566.

Guerrini R, Genton P, Bureau M et al. (1998) Multilobar polymicrogyria, intractable drop attack seizures, and sleep- related electrical status epilepticus. *Neurology* 51: 504–512.

Guzzetta F, Battaglia D, Veredice C et al. (2005) Early thalamic injury associated with epilepsy and continu-ous spike-wave during slow sleep. *Epilepsia* 46: 889–900.

Hirsch E, Marescaux C, Maquet P et al. (1990) Landau–Kleffner syndrome: A clinical and EEG study of five cases. *Epilepsia* 31: 756–767.

Hrachovy R (1997) ACTH and Steroids. In: Engel JJ and Pedley T editors. *Epilepsy: A Comprehensive Textbook* (pp. 1463–1473). Lippincott-Raven Publishers, Philadelphia, PA.

Irwin K, Birch V, Lees J et al. (2001) Multiple subpial transection in Landau–Kleffner syndrome. *Dev Med Child Neurol* 43: 248–252.

Kallay C, Mayor-Dubois C, Maeder-Ingvar M et al. (2009) Reversible acquired epileptic frontal syndrome and CSWS suppression in a child with congenital hemiparesis treated by hemispherotomy. *Eur J Pae-diatr Neurol* 13: 430–438.

Kramer U, Sagi L, Goldberg-Stern H et al. (2009) Clinical spectrum and medical treatment of children with electrical status epilepticus in sleep (ESES). *Epilepsia* 50: 1517–1524.

Lagae L (2009) Rational treatment options with AEDs and ketogenic diet in Landau–Kleffner syndrome: Still waiting after all these years. *Epilepsia* 50: 59–62.

Landau WM and Kleffner FR (1957) Syndrome of acquired aphasia with convulsive disorder in children. *Neurology* 7: 523–530.

Lemke JR, Lal D, Reinthaler EM et al. (2013) Mutations in GRIN2A cause idiopathic focal epilepsy with rolandic spikes. *Nat Genet* 45: 1067–1072.

Lesca G, Rudolf G, Bruneau N et al. (2013) GRIN2A mutations in acquired epileptic aphasia and related childhood focal epilepsies and encephalopathies with speech and language dysfunction. *Nat Genet* 45: 1061–1066.

Ligot N, Archambaud F, Trotta N et al. (2014) Default mode network hypometabolism in epileptic encepha-lopathies with CSWS. *Epilepsy Res* 108: 861–871.

Liukkonen E, Kantola-Sorsa E, Paetau R et al. (2010) Long-term outcome of 32 children with encephalopa-thy with status epilepticus during sleep, or ESES syndrome. *Epilepsia* 51: 2023–2032.

Loddenkemper T, Cosmo G, Kotagal P et al. (2009) Epilepsy surgery in children with electrical status epi-lepticus in sleep. *Neurosurgery* 64: 328–337.

Majerus S, Laureys S, Collette F et al. (2003) Phonological short-term memory networks following recovery from Landau and Kleffner syndrome. *Hum Brain Mapp* 19: 133–144.

Maquet P, Hirsch E, Dive D et al. (1990) Cerebral glucose utilization during sleep in Landau–Kleffner syndrome: A PET study. *Epilepsia* 31: 778–83.

Massa R, de Saint-Martin A, Hirsch E et al. (2000) Landau–Kleffner syndrome: Sleep EEG characteristics at onset. *Neurophysiol Clin* 111: S87–S93.

McVicar KA, Ballaban-Gil K, Rapin I, Moshe SL and Shinnar S (2005) Epileptiform EEG abnormalities in children with language regression. *Neurology* 65: 129–131.

Moeller F, Moehring J, Ick I et al. (2013) EEG-fMRI in atypical benign partial epilepsy. *Epilepsia* 54: e103–e108.

Paetau R (2009) Magnetoencephalography in Landau–Kleffner syndrome. *Epilepsia* 50: 51–54.

Paquier PF, Van Dongen HR and Loonen CB (1992) The Landau–Kleffner syndrome or "acquired aphasia with convulsive disorder." Long-term follow-up of six children and a review of the recent literature. *Arch Neurol* 49: 354–359.

Patry G, Lyagoubi S and Tassinari CA (1971) Subclinical "electrical status epilepticus" induced by sleep in children. A clinical and electroencephalographic study of six cases. *Arch Neurol* 24: 242–252.

Peltola ME, Liukkonen E, Granstrom ML et al. (2011) The effect of surgery in encephalopathy with electrical status epilepticus during sleep. *Epilepsia* 52: 602–609.

Pera MC, Brazzo D, Altieri N, Balottin U and Veggiotti P (2013) Long-term evolution of neuropsychological competences in encephalopathy with status epilepticus during sleep: A variable prognosis. *Epilepsia* 54: 77–85.

Praline J, Hommet C, Barthez MA et al. (2003) Outcome at adulthood of the continuous spike-waves during slow sleep and Landau–Kleffner syndromes. *Epilepsia* 44: 1434–1440.

Rapin I, Mattis S, Rowan AJ and Golden GG (1977) Verbal auditory agnosia in children. *Dev Med Child Neurol* 19: 197–207.

Robinson RO, Baird G, Robinson G and Simonoff E (2001) Landau–Kleffner syndrome: Course and correlates with outcome. *Dev Med Child Neurol* 43: 243–247.

Roulet Perez E, Davidoff V, Despland PA and Deonna T (1993) Mental and behavioural deterioration of children with epilepsy and CSWS: Acquired epileptic frontal syndrome. *Dev Med Child Neurol* 35: 661–674.

Saltik S, Uluduz D, Cokar O, Demirbilek V and Dervent A (2005) A clinical and EEG study on idiopathic partial epilepsies with evolution into ESES spectrum disorders. *Epilepsia* 46: 524–533.

Sanchez Fernandez I, Hadjiloizou S, Eksioglu Y et al. (2012) Short-term response of sleep-potentiated spiking to high-dose diazepam in electric status epilepticus during sleep. *Pediatr Neurol* 46: 312–318.

Scholtes FB, Hendriks MP and Renier WO (2005) Cognitive deterioration and electrical status epilepticus during slow sleep. *Epilepsy Behav* 6: 167–173.

Schwartz TH and Bonhoeffer T (2001) In vivo optical mapping of epileptic foci and surround inhibition in ferret cerebral cortex. *Nat Med* 7: 1063–1067.

Seegmuller C, Deonna T, Dubois CM et al. (2012) Long-term outcome after cognitive and behavioral regression in nonlesional epilepsy with continuous spike-waves during slow-wave sleep. *Epilepsia* 53: 1067–1076.

Siniatchkin M, Groening K, Moehring J et al. (2010) Neuronal networks in children with continuous spikes and waves during slow sleep. *Brain* 133: 2798–2813.

Soprano AM, Garcia EF, Caraballo R and Fejerman N (1994) Acquired epileptic aphasia: Neuropsychologic follow-up of 12 patients. *Pediatr Neurol* 11: 230–235.

Stephani U and Carlsson G (2006) The spectrum from BCECTS to LKS: The rolandic EEG trait-impact on cognition. *Epilepsia* 47: 67–70.

Tassinari CA, Rubboli G, Volpi L et al. (2000) Encephalopathy with electrical status epilepticus during slow sleep or ESES syndrome including the acquired aphasia. *Clin Neurophysiol* 111: S94–S102.

Tassinari CA, Rubboli G, Volpi L, Billard C and Bureau M (2002) Etat de mal électrique épileptique pendant le sommeil lent (ESES ou POCS) incluant l'aphasie épileptique acquise (syndrome de Landau–Kleffner). In: Roger J, Bureau M, Dravet C et al., editors. *Les syndromes épileptiques de l'enfant et de l'adolescent* (3rd ed., pp. 265–283). John Libbey, Eastleigh.

Tovia E, Goldberg-Stern H, Ben Zeev B et al. 2011 The prevalence of atypical presentations and comorbidities of benign childhood epilepsy with centrotemporal spikes. *Epilepsia* 52: 1483–1488.

Urbain C, Di Vincenzo T, Peigneux P and Van Bogaert P (2011) Is sleep-related consolidation impaired in focal idiopathic epilepsies of childhood? A pilot study. *Epilepsy Behav* 22: 380–384.

Urbain C, Galer S, Van Bogaert P and Peigneux P (2013) Pathophysiology of sleep-dependent memory consolidation processes in children. *Int J Psychophysiol* 89: 273–283.

Van Bogaert P, Aeby A, De Borchgrave V et al. (2006) The epileptic syndromes with continuous spikes and waves during slow sleep: Definition and management guidelines. *Acta Neurol Belg* 106: 52–60.

Van Bogaert P, King MD, Paquier P et al. (2013) Acquired auditory agnosia in childhood and normal sleep electroencephalography subsequently diagnosed as Landau–Kleffner syndrome: A report of three cases. *Dev Med Child Neurol* 55: 575–579.

Veggiotti P, Termine C, Granocchio E et al. (2002) Long-term neuropsychological follow-up and nosological considerations in five patients with continuous spikes and waves during slow sleep. *Epileptic Disord* 4: 243–249.

Verrotti A, Filippini M, Matricardi S, Agostinelli MF and Gobbi G (2014) Memory impairment and benign epilepsy with centrotemporal spike (BECTS): A growing suspicion. *Brain Cogn* 84: 123–131.

Wang SB, Weng WC, Fan PC and Lee WT (2008) Levetiracetam in continuous spike waves during slow-wave sleep syndrome. *Pediatr Neurol* 39: 85–90.

14
GLOBAL PROGNOSIS AND NEUROPSYCHOLOGICAL OUTCOME OF LENNOX–GASTAUT SYNDROME

Alexis Arzimanoglou, Eleni Panagiotakaki and Alia Ramirez Camacho

Lennox–Gastaut syndrome (LGS) is a severe and chronic epileptic encephalopathy with onset in early childhood. Following the medical thesis of Dr. Charlotte Dravet (1965), Gastaut et al. (1966) described in *Epilepsia* a childhood-onset epilepsy type characterized by the progressive appearance of several types of seizures (including tonic seizures particularly during sleep), associated with EEG tracings to an interictal pattern of diffuse spike–wave complexes and 10Hz discharges often translating tonic events during slow sleep and neurodevelopmental regression. Several publications followed and LGS was adopted by the International League Against Epilepsy Classification Commission in 1989. However, the nosological uncertainty surrounding the syndrome persisted and the term LGS is, even today, applied rather loosely.

There are a number of reasons for the nosological uncertainty, some of which are as follows:

- The core seizures (i.e. tonic, atonic and atypical absences) are not always present at onset, but appear progressively within the first 2–3 years of evolution.
- The interictal EEG pattern of slow spike–wave complexes that is associated with LGS is not pathognomonic.
- Although a constant feature, neurodevelopmental regression is of variable degree. It is certainly influenced by a number of parameters, especially seizure frequency and severity.

The main factor contributing to the nosological uncertainties is probably related to the aetiological heterogeneity. Indeed, the syndrome has been described in association with a great variety of brain pathologies, including focal or multifocal abnormalities of cortical development, acquired destructive lesions, metabolic and/or genetic disorders and tuberous sclerosis and also in MRI-negative patients. Arzimanoglou et al. (2009) published a comprehensive review of the clinical and EEG characteristics of LGS and a critical review of currently available optimal treatment attitudes, based on the opinion of a panel of experts.

It was suggested that LGS is a nonspecific response of the 1- to 7-year-old brain to diffuse, or occasionally localized, damage (Aicardi 1973). Blume (2001) discussed the pathogenesis of LGS and suggested that the occurrence of factors enhancing excitability during a vulnerable period of cortical and thalamic development, when the child's nervous system is still immature, may permanently imprint a bilateral diffuse epileptogenic system. Frontal lesions may be particularly apt to produce the picture of LGS (Bancaud and Talairach 1992).

Also taking this into consideration, we believe that LGS should be perceived as an age-dependent electroclinical pattern rather than an epilepsy disease proper. Such an electroclinical pattern (syndrome) can be found in a variety of distinct diseases such as tuberous sclerosis complex or Sturge-Weber syndrome, as well as in association with developmental abnormalities of the brain, both extended or relatively focal. In fact, it is the conjunction of certain clinical and EEG features that allow the diagnosis of LGS in patients with a variety of underlying neurological disorders (Arzimanoglou et al. 2004).

Issues related to prognosis

A comprehensive debate on prognosis should imply that we are dealing with a well-defined entity and that prospective data are available on the natural evolution of the disease for a statistically significant number of patients, rigorously corresponding to predefined criteria. The number of parameters to be considered when evaluating complex epilepsies, such as LGS, makes prospective large-scale studies very difficult to realize, not only because of the rarity of the syndrome but also because one would need to integrate the potential role of different aetiologies, the presence of various types of seizures with an onset at various phases of the disorder and at different ages, and the use of a number of antiepileptic drugs (AEDs) (order of prescription, which combination(s), at what dose(s), for which type(s) of seizures, etc.). The reasons include (1) the long-term evolution and prognosis were poorly investigated and (2) the reports on large numbers of patients remain relatively few (Chevrie and Aicardi 1972; Yagi 1996; Heiskala 1997).

Short-term mortality has been estimated to be 4.2% to 7% of those affected, in part as a result of tonic status. Up to 10% of children with LGS die prior to age 11 years (Beaumanoir et al. 1988; Rai et al. 1988).

Most of the published data on the prognosis of LGS come from *retrospective series*. The inherent risk with such studies is to include patients not on the basis of the hypothesized diagnosis at onset but after some years of evolution, influenced by what is already considered being the syndrome's evolution.

PROGNOSIS OF EPILEPTIC SEIZURES IN LGS

Patients with tonic seizures, episodes of non-convulsive or tonic status epilepticus, and rapid discharges during sleep are most likely as adults to manifest the same seizure types. Beaumanoir (1981) studied a group of 103 patients followed up for a mean of 19.7 years and divided it into 2 subgroups:

1. Patients with a typical picture including tonic seizures, non-convulsive or tonic status, and 10-Hz discharges during slow sleep, and who continued to exhibit an unchanged pattern at the end of follow-up in three of four of cases

2. Patients with less typical features, often following the occurrence of initial focal seizures, who mainly evolved to a picture of focal epilepsy or of multifocal seizures and who often lost the characteristics of the LGS

In the second group, with a better outcome, LGS seemed to represent only an age-related mode of expression of a focal epilepsy with temporary diffusion of the EEG abnormalities.

Similar results have been reported (Yagi 1996) on the persistence of tonic seizures in typical patients. Furthermore, in typical cases, the clinical pattern changes with age. Between 15 and 20 years old, the overall seizure frequency usually diminishes. Atypical absences and drop attacks may become rare, but all other types of seizures, including tonic seizures at sleep, persist. In older patients, tonic seizures during sleep are probably under-reported.

Prognosis may also be different in the group of patients who develop atonic and/or tonic seizures in the course of focal epilepsies (Pazzaglia et al. 1985; Roger et al. 1987). Gastaut and Zifkin (1988) drew similar conclusions in their study of 40 patients. In all studies, the occurrence of tonic and atonic attacks was associated with the appearance in the EEG records of *bilateral fast or slow spike–wave complexes and/or bursts of 10-Hz recruiting rhythm*, especially during sleep. Such secondary diffusion of initially focal epilepsy may be very difficult to distinguish it from classic LGS. In fact, most of such cases fulfil all or most of the criteria for the syndrome, of which they may constitute a subgroup and should not be regarded as a different entity. Their practical interest is that they may be due to localized lesions that could conceivably be amenable to surgical treatment. It is, indeed, possible that many cases of LGS are due to undetectable focal lesions or regions of dysfunction.

Prognosis is difficult to establish for patients presenting at onset only with myoclonic-astatic seizures. Most of them will have a long-term evolution that differs from the typical evolution of LGS. However, some patients will later also present tonic seizures and/or bursts of rapid rhythms during sleep, thus fulfilling the criteria for LGS diagnosis (Kaminska et al. 1999; Arzimanoglou et al. 2009; Kaminska and Oguni 2013).

PROGNOSIS AND THE ROLE OF AEDs
Regarding overall efficacy, the vast majority of patients with LGS remain intractable to AEDs or to other treatment options such as ketogenic diet or vagal nerve stimulation.

Undoubtedly, a small number of patients experience a reduction in seizure frequency, particularly when appropriately treated from onset with large-spectrum drugs such as valproate or lamotrigine, alone or in combination. For a greater proportion of patients, drop attacks could be controlled, thus influencing the quality of life. However, none of the new or old AEDs has brought a meaningful change in the overall prognosis of the syndrome (Arzimanoglou et al. 2009). For the very few patients that rapidly became seizure free, we do not dispose of any controlled data on the evolution of the other components of the syndrome, such as intellectual disability and behavioural problems.

Partly, this is due to the inappropriate methodology of drug trials, often the result of requests from the regulatory agencies that do not consider the particularities of these epilepsies. Indeed, when the inclusion criteria request an established diagnosis of LGS, the trials are performed too late in the course of the disorder, when drug resistance and cognitive impairment are already well established. Consequently, the only parameter that can be evaluated is not global outcome but an eventual reduction of one or more types of seizures very late in the course of a highly disabling disorder.

Clinical experience of centres dealing with a large number of rare and complex epilepsies suggests a decrease in the number of patients with the full electroclinical picture of LGS. In the absence of biological markers and prospective studies with inclusion at onset, it is difficult to interpret this observational impression. Part of the explanation could be related to the availability of a larger number of large-spectrum AEDs; an increase in the capacity of centres of expertise to suspect, earlier in the course, an evolution towards LGS; a more appropriate use of certain AEDs early in the course of the disorder; an increase in the number of children with underlying pathologies such as tuberous sclerosis or Sturge-Weber syndrome, operated on, whenever possible, early in the course of the disease and despite the presence of diffuse multifocal EEG abnormalities; and avoidance of polytherapy, that usually has an aggravating effect.

Intellectual disability and behavioural problems: characteristics and prognosis
Intellectual disability is reported to be present before the onset of the seizures in 20%–60% of patients with LGS (Chevrie and Aicardi 1972; Beaumanoir and Blume 2005). By analogy with infantile spasms, such cases were called secondary or symptomatic. They are often associated with an underlying neurological disorder (structural and/or genetic) and neuroimaging abnormalities. Psychomotor impairment tends to be particularly severe. In primary patients, initial cognitive and neurological development is normal, and cognitive deterioration is all the more striking when the onset is at several years of age.

Five years after onset, the proportion of patients with intellectual disability increases to 75%–93% (Chevrie and Aicardi 1972; Furune et al. 1986; Livingston 1988). The degree of intellectual disability is often severe: Chevrie and Aicardi (1972) found that 55% of their patients had IQs less than 50, and this was the case of 48% of Gastaut's patients (Gastaut et al. 1973). Even in the rare patients with normal IQ, there is extreme slowness in ideation and action. Intellectual disability is often accompanied by disturbances of behaviour and personality. Frank psychotic behaviour is common.

Progressive diminution of IQ scores in LGS has initially been attributed to lack of new learning rather than loss of previously acquired skills (Gastaut et al. 1973). However, clinical evidence of marked *deterioration* is present in many children, especially in those who had had long periods of previous normal development, and it is difficult to escape the impression of a degenerative central nervous system disease. There is, however, no other evidence for such disorders, the process of deterioration is self-limited and there is a temporal correlation between the presence of intense paroxysmal activity and deterioration. Indeed, deterioration may well result from the epileptic activity itself, including the interictal EEG pattern. However, it has been suggested that IQ scores remain constant during remissions and exacerbations of the syndrome, whereas studies of motor reaction time, verbal latencies, and percentage of correctness in simple cognitive tasks are definitely related to the patients' current clinical status (Erba and Cavazzuti 1977).

In a retrospective study, Hoffmann-Riem et al. (2000) reported on the course of the disease, EEG tracings and intellectual function in 101 patients. Tonic seizures and diffuse slow spike–wave complexes in the interictal EEG were necessary for the diagnosis of LGS. The mean age at onset of tonic seizures was 5.2 years (range: 2y–14y) and the mean age of the patients at the moment of the study was 17 years (range: 5y–34y) with an average observation period of 16 years (range: 4y–31y). Note that epilepsy started with tonic seizures allowing the classification as LGS from the onset in only 6% of patients. Overall, only 4% of the patients became seizure free. Neurological dysfunction was a common feature (24% presented with signs of severe encephalopathy with ataxia and pyramidal signs; inability to walk was registered in 21%; inability to speak in 38%; disturbed motor coordination in 52%). Cognitive impairment, which legitimately did not belong to the inclusion criteria, was evaluated as severe (IQ <35) in 57 (56%) and mild or moderate (IQ >35) in 44 (43%) patients. Multivariate analysis revealed four independent risk factors significantly correlated with severe intellectual disability. These were listed in decreasing order of importance: non-convulsive status epilepticus (NCSE) (odds ratio [OR] 25.2), a previous diagnosis of West syndrome (OR 11.6), a symptomatic aetiology (OR 9.5) and an early age at onset (OR 4.7) of epilepsy. The results of this study confirmed the existing data concerning the role of factors such as aetiology and age at onset in intellectual deterioration in LGS patients and brought evidence to suggest that, within the setting of this syndrome, NCSE may also play a major role. Similar assumptions on the role of NCSE were advanced by Doose and Völzke (1989) to explain the development of dementia in some patients with 'myoclonic-astatic epilepsy'.

However, episodes of status may only be another expression of the severity of an unknown process responsible for both the loss of cognitive abilities and the epileptic activity, and no relation has been found in other studies (Aicardi and Levy Gomes 1988) between cognitive level at the end of follow-up and the occurrence of overt episodes of status. Moreover, a relationship could exist between 'bad periods' that may represent minimal status and deterioration. Many patients with the LGS develop abnormalities of behaviour that include autistic features or hyperkinetic syndrome. Even patients with relatively normal intelligence are usually extremely slow in all their cognitive processes.

LONG-TERM PROGNOSIS

Beaumanoir (1981) reported on the long-term evolution of patients with LGS, underlining the fact that most of those with typical symptoms will continue to present a similar clinical picture.

According to Ohtahara and Yamatogi (1990), three groups can be delineated depending on the course: patients in the first group (42 of their 89 patients) continue to display a typical electroclinical picture of LGS; those in the second group (19 patients) develop other types of EEG discharges, mainly focal ones; and those in the third group (28 patients) present with multiple independent spike foci following the typical EEG features. Patients in the second group fared better than those of the other groups, and only 40.5% of them had intellectual disability. Patients who developed multiple independent spike foci had intellectual disability in 47.4% of cases but continued to present 'minor' seizures in 60% of cases. Patients in the first group more often belonged to the symptomatic type of LGS and more frequently had experienced infantile spasms than those in the other groups.

Long-term prognosis of LGS in 72 patients followed up for more than 10 years was also reported (Oguni et al. 1996). Patients were included who had more than two types of seizures, including generalized tonic seizures, and presenting diffuse EEG slow spike–wave complexes with or without rapid rhythm during sleep. The mean age at onset of epilepsy was 2 years 4 months (range: 1mo–14y). The diagnosis was first made in the age range from 2 to 15 years with a peak occurrence at 5 years. LGS of unknown aetiology was diagnosed in 21 patients and symptomatic in 51, of whom 24 had previously had West syndrome (West plus group). In the last examination, the mean age was 21 ± 5 years in the cryptogenic group and 23 ± 5 years in the symptomatic group. The follow-up period was 17 ± 4 years in the former and 17 ± 5 in the latter. At the end of follow-up, 33% of patients with unknown aetiology and 55% with symptomatic LGS had lost the characteristics of LGS. In the group with non-identified aetiology, epilepsy was classified as follows: LGS in 14 (67%) patients, nonspecific symptomatic generalized epilepsy in 5 (24%) patients lacking diffuse slow spike–wave complexes or multiple seizure types, localization-related epilepsy in 1 patient and no more seizures in 1 patient. In the symptomatic group, the diagnosis remained that of LGS in 23 (45%) patients but was considered nonspecific symptomatic generalized in 14 (27%), severe epilepsy with multiple independent spike foci in 8 (16%), localization-related epilepsy in 4 (8%) and no more seizures in only 2 patients. More than 60% of the patients had daily or weekly seizures, of which generalized tonic seizures were the most frequent. An IQ score decrease of at least 15 points was demonstrated in 9 of the 11 patients with cryptogenic LGS who were able to retake the test and in 7 of the 9 patients with symptomatic LGS. Deterioration of gait over several years was a prominent feature in 12 patients, and, according to the authors (Oguni et al 1996), it seemed to be due largely to progression of the epileptic encephalopathy caused by repeated seizures.

Ohtsuka et al. (1990) reported the clinical and EEG features of 89 patients with LGS followed up for more than 5 years and concluded that only 31 (34.8%) still had the characteristic LGS features at the time of last observation. Of those, 28 had progressed to severe epilepsy with multiple independent spike foci. Similar results, confirming that the characteristic LGS features disappear with age in 30% to 50% of the cases, were also reported by Beaumanoir (1981). Cryptogenic LGS appears to have a more homogeneous clinical picture because evolution to other syndromes is seen less often (Yagi 1996).

Yagi (1996) also reported on the evolution of LGS in 102 patients observed for an average of 16 years (range: 10y–20y). The mean age at onset of epilepsy was 4.3 years (range: 2mo–18y). All patients included had more than one type of seizure, but, this being a retrospective study, the authors do not state that all had tonic seizures at early stages. Twenty-two patients had evolved from West syndrome to LGS, 36 began as unspecific epilepsies, either generalized or localization-related, and 44 began primarily with the electroclinical characteristics of LGS. At the end of the study, 8 have been completely seizure free for more than 1 year and the remaining 94 patients still had seizures. Nearly all of the 94 had tonic seizures (52 as the only type of seizures from which 17 in sleep). The characteristic clinical symptoms and EEG discharges continued in one-third of the patients. At the end of the survey, 5 patients were students at a special school for the disabled, and of the remaining 97 patients, 12 were working normally, 1 was a housewife, 7 were working part-time, 19 were under custodial care at home, 29 were working at either work centres or industrial training centres, 21 were institutionalized for care, 6 were hospitalized for treatment of seizures and 2 died during the survey.

Aicardi and Levy Gomes (1988) studied 10 patients with a possible mild variant of the syndrome. All had a normal neurological examination, a relatively late onset (43mo) and a predominance of absence attacks over tonic seizures. They had relatively normal background EEG tracings and a positive response to hyperpnoea, and typical 3-Hz absences were sometimes observed early in their course. Such cases were reminiscent of the so-called 'intermediate petit mal' (Hoffmann-Riem et al. 2000). However, complete separation of a subgroup was not possible because all patients fulfilled the strict criteria for LGS and because several patients with regular LGS exhibited similar features.

Conclusion

LGS is one of the severest forms of childhood epilepsy. From an aetiological point of view, LGS is highly heterogeneous. In the absence of biological markers, early diagnosis may prove to be difficult, particularly in children who do not at onset present with infantile epileptic spasms. Consequently, both global prognosis and individual neuropsychological outcome are difficult to predict. The electroclinical patterns observed undoubtedly contribute to this complexity of the issue, but another major component is the underlying neurological disorder. Due to intellectual and/or neurological deficits, only very few patients are ultimately able to live independent lives. Approximately 80% will continue to have seizures and will have to remain on AEDs.

Despite discrepancies and methodological biases, nearly all known general predictors for a bad prognosis are present, at a variable degree: neurological and cognitive deficit prior to the onset of epileptic seizures; progressive appearance of several types of seizures, often high drug-resistant; a relatively early age of onset; prolonged episodes of NCSE; and a progressive course, apparently not significantly affected by currently available anti-seizure agents.

The proportion of severely impaired patients can be estimated as high as 72% for secondary cases and up to 22% for primary cases. Cases of LGS following infantile spasms evolve significantly worse, whereas patients in whom myoclonic seizures and atypical absences are prominent may do significantly better. The evidence that the electroclinical expression of LGS often changes with age raises the question of whether the fundamental pathophysiology differs in patients in whom the underlying LGS evolves into other epilepsy syndromes compared with those patients retaining all of the LGS characteristics.

REFERENCES

Aicardi J (1973) The problem of the Lennox syndrome. *Dev Med Child Neurol* 15: 77–81.

Aicardi J and Levy Gomes A (1988) The Lennox–Gastaut syndrome: Clinical and electroencephalographic features. In: Niedermeyer E and Degen D, editors. *The Lennox–Gastaut Syndrome* (pp. 25–46). Alan R. Liss, New York.

Arzimanoglou A, French J, Blume WT et al. (2009) Lennox–Gastaut syndrome: A consensus approach on diagnosis, assessment, management, and trial methodology. *Lancet Neurol* 8: 82–93. doi:10.1016/S1474-4422(08)70292-8.

Arzimanoglou A, Guerrini R and Aicardi J (2004) *Aicardi's Epilepsy in Children*, LWW, Philadelphia, PA.

Bancaud J and Talairach J (1992) Semiology of frontal lobe epilepsy seizures in man. In: Chauvel P, Delgado–Escueta AV, Halgren E and Bancaud J, editors. *Frontal Lobe Seizures and Epilepsies* (pp. 3–58). Raven Press, New York.

Beaumanoir A (1981) Les limites nosologiques du syndrome de Lennox–Gastaut. *Rev EEG Neurophysiol Clin* 11: 468–473.

Beaumanoir A and Blume W (2005) The Lennox–Gastaut syndrome. In: Roger J, Bureau M, Dravet C et al., editors. *Epileptic Syndromes in Infancy, Childhood and Adolescence* (4th ed., pp. 125–148). John Libbey Eurotext, France.

Beaumanoir A, Foletti G, Magistris M and Volanschi D (1988) Status epilepticus in the Lennox–Gastaut syndrome. In: Niedermeyer E and Degen R, editors. *The Lennox–Gastaut Syndrome* (pp. 283–299). Alan R. Liss, New York.

Blume WT (2001) Pathogenesis of Lennox–Gastaut syndrome: Considerations and hypotheses. *Epileptic Disord* 3: 183–196.

Chevrie JJ and Aicardi J (1972) Childhood epileptic encephalopathy with slow-spike wave: A statistical study of 80 cases. *Epilepsia* 13: 259–271.

Doose H and Völzke E (1989) Petit mal status in early childhood and dementia. *NeuroPédiatrie* 10: 10–14.

Dravet C (1965) *Encéphalopathie épileptique de l'enfant avec pointe-onde lente diffuse*. Thèse. Marseille.

Erba G and Cavazzuti V (1977) Ictal and interictal response latency in Lennox–Gastaut syndrome. *Electroencephalogr Clin Neurophysiol* 42: 717.

Furune S, Watanabe K, Negoro T et al. (1986) Long-term prognosis and clinicoelectroencephalographic evolution of Lennox–Gastaut syndrome. *Brain Dysfunct* 1: 146–153.

Gastaut H and Zifkin BG (1988) Secondary bilateral synchrony and Lennox–Gastaut syndrome. In: Niedermeyer E and Degen R, editors. *The Lennox–Gastaut Syndrome* (pp. 221–242). Alan R. Liss, New York.

Gastaut H, Dravet C, Loubier D et al. (1973) Evolution clinique et pronostic du syndrome de Lennox–Gastaut. In: Lugaresi E, Pazzaglia P and Tassinari CA, editors. *Evolution and Prognosis of Epilepsies* (pp. 133–154). Aulo Goggi, Bologna.

Gastaut H, Roger J, Soulayrol R et al. (1966) Childhood epileptic encephalopathy with diffuse slow spike-waves (otherwise known as 'petit mal variant') or Lennox syndrome. *Epilepsia* 7: 139–179.

Heiskala H (1997) Community-based study of Lennox–Gastaut syndrome. *Epilepsia* 38: 526–531.

Hoffmann-Riem M, Diener W, Benninger C et al. (2000) Nonconvulsive status epilepticus—A possible cause of mental retardation in patients with Lennox–Gastaut syndrome. *Neuropediatrics* 31: 169–174.

Kaminska A, Ickowicz A, Plouin P et al. (1999) Delineation of cryptogenic Lennox–Gastaut syndrome and myoclonic astatic epilepsy using multiple correspondence analysis. *Epilepsy Res* 36: 15–29.

Kaminska A and Oguni H (2013) Lennox–Gastaut syndrome and epilepsy with myoclonic-astatic seizures. In: O. Dulac, M. Lassonde and Sarnat HB, editors. *Handbook of Clinical Neurology*, Vol. 111 (3rd series): *Pediatric Neurology* (pp. 641–652). Elsevier, Amsterdam.

Livingston JH (1988) The Lennox–Gastaut syndrome. *Dev Med Child Neurol* 30: 536–540.

Oguni H, Hayashi K and Osawa M (1996) Long-term prognosis of Lennox–Gastaut syndrome. *Epilepsia* 37: 44–47.

Ohtahara S and Yamatogi Y (1990) Evolution of seizures and EEG abnormalities in childhood onset epilepsy. In: Wada JA and Ellingson RJ, editors. *Clinical Neurophysiology of Epilepsy. EEG Handbook* (revised series, Vol. 4, pp. 457–477). Elsevier, Amsterdam.

Ohtsuka Y, Amano R, Mizukawa M and Ohtahara S (1990) Long-term prognosis of the Lennox–Gastaut syndrome. *Jpn J Psychiatry Neurol* 44: 257–268.

Pazzaglia P, D'Alessandro R, Ambrosetto G and Lugaresi E (1985) Drop attacks: An ominous change in the evaluation of partial epilepsy. *Neurology* 35: 1725–1730.

Rai PV, Fulop T and Ercal S (1988) Clinical course of Lennox–Gastaut syndrome in institutionalized adult patients, In: Niedermeyer E and Degen R, editors. *The Lennox–Gastaut Syndrome* (pp. 409–418). Alan R. Liss, New York.

Roger J, Rémy C, Bureau M et al. (1987) Le syndrome de Lennox–Gastaut chez l'adulte. *Rev Neurol* (Paris) 143: 401–405.

Yagi K (1996) Evolution of Lennox–Gastaut syndrome: A long-term longitudinal study. *Epilepsia* 37: 48–51.

15
COGNITIVE AND BEHAVIOURAL OUTCOMES AFTER EPILEPSY SURGERY IN CHILDREN

Monique MJ van Schooneveld, Kees PJ Braun and J Helen Cross

Introduction

Almost 30% of children with epilepsy continue to have troublesome seizures despite trying antiepileptic drugs (AEDs). For children with lesional focal epilepsy, uncontrolled by medical treatment (i.e. failure of, or disabling side effects from, two or three appropriate drugs), epilepsy surgery has increasingly become an important treatment option over the past 30 years (Ryvlin et al. 2014; Pestana Knight et al. 2015; Lamberink et al. 2015). It is now considered possible to offer surgery much earlier in the course of the epilepsy and to younger children. Furthermore, developmental delay is no longer a contraindication for epilepsy surgery (Cross et al. 2006; 2013; Ryvlin et al. 2014).

The most frequently used surgical techniques intended to abolish seizures and cure the epilepsy are functional hemispherectomy (hemispherotomy) and resective surgery. Hemispherectomy, a disconnection of one-half of the brain with limited resection, is indicated when seizures originate from, and the underlying pathology affects, an entire cerebral hemisphere. Children who may benefit from this procedure usually have a preexisting hemiparesis as a result of the severe contralateral hemispheric pathology, which has mostly been present from birth. A focal, tailored, resection or lobectomy is considered when the area of the brain thought to be responsible for the seizures is well circumscribed or confined to a single lobe. This in the majority of cases concerns the temporal lobe. Increasingly, however, children undergo epilepsy surgery for extratemporal lobe epilepsy. Resection or disconnection of more than one lobe is called multi-lobar or subhemispheric surgery. Additional types of surgery that are not intended to cure epilepsy but to improve seizure status (the so-called palliative procedures) are multiple subpial transections and corpus callosotomy. These techniques will not be discussed here in detail.

The beneficial effect of paediatric epilepsy surgery on seizure control in carefully selected candidates has been well established (Spencer and Huh 2008; Ryvlin et al. 2014). People with pharmacoresistant epilepsy, however, often have additional developmental problems, due to the underlying epileptogenic pathology, the frequent seizures themselves or the chronic use of (in most cases) multiple AEDs (Lah 2004), particularly in infancy and early childhood. Both the anticipated seizure freedom and the expected improvement of postoperative cognitive development contribute to the final decision to accept or reject a candidate for epilepsy surgery (Perry and Duchowny 2013).

Early surgical intervention—thus a shorter duration of active epilepsy—has been reported to correlate with a higher chance of reaching seizure freedom (Englot et al. 2013a, 2013b; Lamberink et al. 2015). It is not unexpected that early intervention also reduces the eventual severity of cognitive impairment. In addition, given the known cognitive side effects of AEDs (Park and Kwon 2008; Mula and Trimble 2009) and the improvement of cognitive function after discontinuation of AEDs in non-surgical cohorts (Aldenkamp et al. 1998; Hessen et al. 2006; Lossius et al. 2008), AED withdrawal, which is possible after anticipated curative surgery, increases the probability of postoperative cognitive improvement. In fact, it has convincingly been demonstrated that AED reduction improves postoperative intelligence and other domains of cognitive outcome (Skirrow et al. 2011; Meekes et al. 2013; van Schooneveld et al. 2013; Boshuisen et al. 2015). Therefore, the ultimate goal of epilepsy surgery in children should be not only to achieve freedom from seizures and enable AED discontinuation, but also to improve developmental capacities (Shields 2000; Cross 2002; van Schooneveld and Braun 2013). Postoperative outcome after childhood epilepsy surgery is therefore preferably expressed in terms of seizure freedom; cognitive outcome can be considered an equally important outcome measure (Spencer and Huh 2008; Ryvlin et al. 2014). Age-appropriate neuropsychological assessments are a mandatory aspect of the pre- and postsurgical evaluation (Cross et al. 2006).

This chapter provides an overview of what is known about neuropsychological assessment and cognitive outcome and its predictors after hemidisconnective or resective epilepsy surgery in children. Because presurgical cognitive functioning significantly correlates with postsurgical cognitive outcome, we included a section about cognitive (dys)function and its determinants in children with epilepsy, prior to surgical treatment. We summarize the current knowledge about different domains of cognitive outcome after surgery. As children with complex epilepsy and ongoing seizures have high rates of associated behaviour disorders (Davies et al. 2003), particularly those with focal epilepsy that are candidates for epilepsy surgery (McLellan et al. 2005; Colonnelli et al. 2012), a section on behaviour is also included.

Neuropsychological assessment

The purpose of the assessment is to evaluate cognitive, behavioural and emotional consequences of the epilepsy and its treatment. It should preferably encompass all the domains of cognitive development: intelligence, memory and learning, language, visual spatial skills, processing speed, attention and executive functions (Lassonde et al. 2000; Battaglia et al. 2006). The neuropsychological assessment of infants and children, however, is complicated for a number of reasons. Given the extensive neurodevelopmental trajectory that children undergo, different periods of development require different skills, and not all cognitive functions can be reliably assessed in early childhood. Furthermore, there is a high incidence of cognitive disability in paediatric epilepsy surgery candidates. Accordingly, the test battery varies depending on the child's age and skill level. Different tests used at different ages and varying levels of cognitive functioning are difficult to compare and hamper accurate longitudinal monitoring of functions over time. Intelligence—or in younger children indices of general cognitive development—is the most common measure of cognitive outcome after paediatric epilepsy surgery (Lah 2004). Less research has addressed specific cognitive functions, such as memory, language, visual spatial skills, attention, and executive functions after surgery in children. Assessments should be performed at regular intervals, before and at least once after surgery. In most studies, postsurgical follow-up intervals are limited to either 1 or 2 years, with only few reports describing the long-term cognitive outcome, or more than 5 years after paediatric epilepsy (Tellez-Zenteno et al. 2007; D'Argenzio et al. 2011; Skirrow et al. 2011; Viggedal et al. 2012; van Schooneveld et al. 2016). A more extensive follow-up may be required to establish the full developmental impact of surgery, as it has been suggested that epilepsy surgery, ending a shorter or longer time of severe epilepsy, needs an unusually long time to manifest cognitive improvement or recovery (Freitag and Tuxhorn 2005; Skirrow et al. 2011).

Although non-invasive tests—such as functional magnetic resonance imaging (fMRI) (Wang et al. 2012)—are increasingly used to lateralize or localize language functions, in children who are too young, impaired or uncooperative to reliably undergo fMRI, the neuropsychologist is invaluable in testing the child during the intracarotid amybarbital—the so-called Wada—test (anesthetizing one hemisphere), by presenting test material that the child has to recognize, name or read, as well as by testing comprehension of simple questions (Jansen et al. 2002). In contrast to speech lateralization, the assessment of memory function during the Wada test is less successful in children (Jones-Gotman et al. 2010). Other invasive procedures, such as functional mapping by means of cortical stimulation during intracranial monitoring with subdural grid or depth electrodes or during awake surgery, may be indicated to localize eloquent areas in relation to the epileptogenic zone, when alternative and non-invasive methods are inconclusive or when the epileptogenic focus lies in close proximity to what is believed to be functional cortex. The neuropsychologist has a critical role in testing eloquent functions during the cortical stimulations.

In the neuropsychological follow-up of epilepsy surgery patients, there are a large variety of tests in use. To compare the results of neuropsychological assessments in multicenter cohorts, there is a need for standardized core neuropsychological test batteries, which can be used across epilepsy surgical centers. However, although a core battery of tests can be valuable, a flexible battery with additional tests tailored to the clinical reference questions and the individual needs is especially important in the assessment of children, as tests need to be age sensitive and appropriate for the child's development (Wilson et al. 2015).

Presurgical cognitive functioning in childhood epilepsy

Subnormal cognitive function (intelligence quotient [IQ] <80) is apparent in approximately 25% of all children with newly diagnosed epilepsy (Berg et al. 2008). Younger age at onset of epilepsy, a lesional cause, epileptic encephalopathy, and continuing AEDs have been reported to independently predict suboptimal cognitive functioning (Berg et al. 2008). Intellectual abilities may be particularly vulnerable to seizure-related disturbances during the period of rapid development in early childhood (Bjørnaes et al. 2001). In a group of children aged less than 3 years with refractory focal epilepsy due to cortical malformations, 89% had a presurgical IQ less than 85, with 64% of the children having impairments in the severe range (IQ <50) (Ramantani et al. 2013). Abnormal IQ levels, or even severe intellectual disability (IQ <50), have also been reported in children with temporal lobe epilepsy who present as candidates for surgical resection (Cormack et al. 2007; de Koning et al. 2009; Skirrow et al. 2011). Children with refractory extratemporal epilepsy, with lesions in frontal, parietal or occipital lobes, also frequently have preoperative learning impairments (D'Argenzio et al. 2011). Many studies have shown that 74%–88% of childhood hemispherectomy candidates have a severe cognitive delay (Devlin et al. 2003; Jonas et al. 2004; Boshuisen et al. 2010). Furthermore, case histories of infants and children who have undergone hemispherectomy have revealed that cognitive development had arrested or even regressed following the onset of epilepsy in 82% of these patients (van Schooneveld et al. 2011).

Infants and young children with frequent seizures are particularly at risk of developing a so-called epileptic encephalopathy, by definition implying that developmental arrest or regression can at least partially be attributed to the ongoing severe epileptic activity, and not merely to the underlying epileptogenic pathology (Berg et al. 2010). At a young age, an encephalopathic course may occur in association with any cause of epilepsy (Berg et al. 2010).

Postsurgical cognitive function in paediatric epilepsy
Cognitive profiles have most often been reported following temporal lobe resection or hemispherectomy. Studies on cognitive outcome after frontal, parietal or occipital resections are rather scarce, often including only small groups of children.

GENERAL MEASURES OF INTELLIGENCE AND DEVELOPMENT
In the relevant literature, cognitive functioning is usually defined as intelligence or development, with cognitive improvement being expressed as an increase of Mental Developmental Index (MDI) of 5 to 15, developmental quotient (DQ), or IQ points or as a shift from one to another predefined category of cognitive function, such as from below average to low average. Viewing case by case, a significant number of children (61% of the hemispherectomized and 70% of those who underwent a focal resection) have an almost unchanged cognitive level or remain in their presurgical category of functioning (for review, see van Schooneveld and Braun 2013). This would imply a maintained cognitive trajectory, because if children preserve their presurgical MDI/DQ/IQ level, they must continuously acquire new skills and knowledge over time, as IQ is measured relative to normal peers and is corrected for increasing age. However, many young children, particularly those who undergo hemispherectomy, are severely delayed, both before and after surgery. Test scores of these children usually lie in the lower end of the score distribution (MDI or IQ values < 55), where it is known that instruments do not measure accurately. This problem of inaccurate measurement in the lower tail of the scale distribution has consequences for longitudinal assessment, as some increase in raw scores of a developmental or intelligence test may go unnoticed after converting into standard scores. In those patients, a subtle progression of cognitive function can probably not be quantified and expressed in formal MDI, DQ or IQ scores.

The frequency of cognitive improvement may therefore be underestimated in these often low-functioning children. Measurement of cognitive age, however, unveils and quantifies change. Even children with a 'catastrophic' course of their epilepsy, who had a very poor developmental progress with ongoing seizures, resume cognitive development after hemispherectomy, which was reflected by clear increases in cognitive age (Schooneveld et al. 2011). When pooling results from several studies, in only a minority of children, the standardized MDI, DQ or IQ values decreased significantly after epilepsy surgery: 10% of the hemispherectomy group and 11% of the focal resection group (van Schooneveld and Braun 2013). A decrease in IQ value may indicate a true loss of skills, but in children, it is possible that the conversion from raw to standard scores results in a lower IQ value, even in the presence of some positive development. Catch-up of development is noticed at least 2 times more frequently (20%–30%) after hemispherectomy or focal epilepsy surgery than a decrease of a similar amount of MDI/DQ/IQ points (van Schooneveld and Braun 2013). To truly appreciate the meaning of an unchanged or decreased MDI/DQ/IQ value, individual developmental trajectories should be assessed.

Multiple and often mutually dependent variables influence eventual intelligence or developmental outcome and change after paediatric surgery. Here, we report on the clinically most important presurgical, surgical, and postsurgical variables that may influence general cognitive outcome or change after epilepsy surgery in childhood. Children with developmental pathology who undergo hemispherectomy have relatively lower preoperative IQ/DQ scores but have most to gain from surgery, with higher chances of postsurgical cognitive improvement compared to those with acquired pathology (Pulsifer et al. 2004; Jonas et al. 2004). Actual achievement, however, is limited, possibly related to a more diffuse or bilateral nature of the underlying pathology. This is substantiated by the finding that a disturbed structural integrity of the remaining hemisphere, as defined by the presence of contralateral MRI abnormalities, affects cognitive functioning after hemispherectomy, both in terms of eventual IQ as the chance of significant IQ increases (Boshuisen et al. 2010).

Younger age at onset of epilepsy predicted poor IQ scores after extratemporal resections (D'Argenzio et al. 2011) and, more generally, after epilepsy surgery below the age of 15 years (Matsuzaka et al. 2001), but was not related to postoperative cognitive improvement. Shorter duration of epilepsy has been reported to predict both good (Jonas et al. 2004) and poor (Boshuisen et al. 2010) outcomes after hemispherectomy. It was related to good outcome in a cohort of children who underwent extratemporal surgery (D'Argenzio et al. 2011) and to more gain in IQ scores after surgery in preschool children (Freitag and Tuxhorn 2005). Younger age at surgery predicted poor eventual outcome after hemispherectomy, (Boshuisen et al. 2010) but was also associated with a larger positive change in cognitive scores after epilepsy surgery in infants and children (Bourgeois et al. 2007; Loddenkemper et al. 2007). These findings confirm several hypotheses and assumptions that are part of everyday clinical thinking and decision making. Early-onset epilepsy reflects severe epileptogenic pathology that, by itself, restricts future cognitive abilities. When hemispherectomy is indicated at very young age, the epileptic encephalopathy is severe, development has arrested or regressed, and surgical treatment can induce more pronounced cognitive improvement, although eventual cognitive function is limited. A shorter duration of active epilepsy limits the potentially irreversible effects of ongoing seizures and AEDs on brain function. This problem is independent of the underlying pathology. A higher presurgical level of cognitive functioning is significantly related to higher postsurgical cognition scores (Jonas et al. 2004; Loddenkemper et al. 2007, D'Argenzio et al. 2011), although cognitive improvement occurs less often (Loddenkemper et al. 2007), and IQ changes after temporal resection are only seen as late as 6 or more years after surgery (Skirrow et al. 2011). In general, children at the low end of the IQ spectrum improve more than those with a higher presurgical IQ/DQ level (Bjørnaes et al. 2001; Miranda and Smith 2001; Freitag and Tuxhorn 2005; Spencer and Huh 2008).

Side of surgery has not been found to be related to eventual cognitive outcomes or to changes in general cognitive outcome levels postoperatively. Postsurgery seizure control is associated with higher DQ/IQ scores after hemispherectomy (Pulsifer et al. 2003; Jonas et al. 2004) and with improvement in DQ/IQ and verbal IQ scores after paediatric epilepsy surgery in general (Miranda and Smith 2001; Bourgeois et al. 2007; Lee et al. 2010). However, several studies have not been able to establish a relation between postoperative seizure freedom and cognitive improvement (Westerveld et al. 2000; Pulsifer et al. 2003; Freitag and Tuxhorn 2005; Korkman et al. 2005; Boshuisen et al. 2010; Skirrow et al. 2011). In other words, complete seizure freedom seems not to be a prerequisite for cognitive improvement after epilepsy surgery in childhood.

Cessation of antiepileptic medication was first shown to be an important and independent predictor of IQ change in a cohort of children who underwent temporal lobe surgery (Skirrow et al. 2011). Very recently, a large study on postoperative IQ and IQ change in 301 children who were operated on in 11 European centers has convincingly demonstrated that start of AED withdrawal and complete discontinuation of AEDs independently predicted higher IQ and more gain in IQ after having accounted for possible confounders. The more drugs reduced, the better the cognitive outcome (Boshuisen et al. 2015).

Parental education, a variable that includes both environmental and genetic aspects, proved to be significantly associated with postoperative IQ increase. Children of higher educated parents had on average a larger increase in IQ after surgery and a higher postsurgical—but not presurgical—IQ, compared to children whose parents had completed at most lower secondary education (Meekes et al. 2015). The lack of association between parental education and presurgical IQ is more interesting in light of the recent finding that IQ in children with new-onset epilepsy is not correlated with parental IQ (Walker et al. 2012). These results suggest that the child after surgery, freed from the disruptive effects of seizures and finally also from the adverse effects of AEDs, may again develop in accordance with what would be expected on the education of his or her parents.

MEMORY

Memory and learning are vulnerable in children with refractory epilepsy (Smith et al. 2011; Cormack et al. 2012), and impairments have been reported with any type of epilepsy, particularly temporal lobe epilepsy. Although the left hippocampus is crucial for verbal memory, visual memory is subserved by a wider network, which includes the areas in the frontal, parietal, and temporal lobes of both hemispheres (Postma et al. 2008).

Hemispherectomy is often performed in young and low-functioning children in whom measurement of memory with standardized tests is not possible. In older children with Rasmussen encephalitis, memory scores were found to be sub-average, both before and after the hemispherectomy (Devlin et al. 2003; Pulsifer et al. 2003).

After temporal lobectomy in childhood, unchanged or improved verbal and visual memory has been reported more frequently than a decline (Lah 2004). Material-specific memory deficits, however, have been noted 1 year after temporal lobe resection in children, with those undergoing left-sided resections having worse verbal memory measures (Jambaqué et al. 2007) than predicted on the basis of their presurgical performance (Meekes et al. 2013). These findings reflect a particular vulnerability of verbal memory after left temporal surgery, also in children. Nevertheless, there is evidence suggesting that plasticity is more pronounced in childhood, because verbal memory declines after left temporal lobe resection has been reported to recover rapidly in children (Gleissner et al. 2005; Viggedal et al. 2012). A recent study (Skirrow et al. 2015) showed no significant pre- to postoperative decrements in memory associated with temporal surgery. In contrast, gains in verbal episodic memory (memory for events) were seen after right temporal lobe surgery, and visual episodic memory improved after left temporal lobe surgery, indicating a functional release in the unoperated temporal lobe after seizure reduction or cessation. In the study of Skirrow et al. (2015), better verbal memory at follow-up was linked to greater postsurgical residual hippocampal volumes, most robustly in left surgical participants, and better semantic memory (memory for facts and concepts) at follow-up was associated with smaller resection volumes and greater temporal pole integrity after left temporal surgery. Results were independent of postsurgical intellectual function and language lateralization (Skirrow et al. 2015).

In children with parietal lobe epilepsy, preoperative memory disturbances have been reported, which did not improve after surgery (Gleissner et al. 2008). Memory improves slightly after frontal lobe resection in childhood, with no consistent difference between seizure-free patients and those with continuing seizures (Lendt et al. 2002). No change or minor improvements of visual memory are noted after frontal lobe surgery in childhood (Lendt et al. 2002).

LANGUAGE

Speech and language are predominantly represented in the left hemisphere in typically developing children. Early-onset epilepsy, due to large structural epileptogenic lesions with lateralization to the left hemisphere, however, will often result in relocalization of language to the right hemisphere. Consequently after hemispherectomy in children with early acquired or large developmental lesions, language functions are remarkably preserved, even after left hemispherectomy (Devlin et al. 2003; Pulsifer et al. 2004; Thomas et al. 2010), within the limits of memory and intellectual abilities (Liégeois et al. 2008). It is much more difficult in more circumscribed pathology, when language functions may still reside in the affected hemisphere, or when there may be bilateral representation, to decide whether resection or hemispherectomy can be performed without loss of function, necessitating presurgical functional investigations. Children who have undergone right hemispherectomy after postnatally acquired pathology are likely to show age-appropriate language functions, whereas those with pre/perinatal pathology may show language deficits in line with more general intellectual limitations (Liégeois et al. 2008). Mild dysarthria is reported to be persistent after left or right hemispherectomy, irrespective of age at onset of hemiplegia, indicating an incomplete functional reorganization for the control of fine speech motor movements (Liégeois et al. 2010).

The prediction of language function following resective or hemidisconnective surgery is more difficult in older children with later acquired or progressive pathology, such as Rasmussen syndrome. This is an acquired disorder of one cerebral hemisphere, with an onset of focal motor seizures in a previously normal child, progressive hemiparesis, and cognitive decline, with progressive cerebral atrophy of the affected cerebral hemisphere. Although the exact cause is as yet unclear, much evidence has been accumulated to suggest an autoimmune process, probably T-cell mediated (Varadkar et al. 2014). In children with disease affecting the dominant hemisphere, where there has been a period of normal acquired language, the ability to relocalize will depend on the age at onset of the disease and the age of surgery. Children aged less than 5 years at onset are likely to relocalize language to the previously non-dominant hemisphere; older children will relocalize to a varying degree (Boatman et al. 1999; Hertz Pannier et al. 2002). The decision to perform hemispheric surgery in these children will remain an individual one, balancing the obvious benefits from surgery—with high chances of permanent seizure freedom—versus the risks of permanent loss of language function. Fortunately, in the long-term, it is unlikely that such children will be mute; most will achieve conversational speech even with relatively late onset of disease and older age at surgery.

Intractable temporal lobe epilepsy is a significant risk factor for delayed language development. In the majority of children with early-onset refractory temporal lobe epilepsy, language development is already significantly and globally delayed before the operation. Temporal epilepsy surgery does not result in acceleration of language development. If language is still mediated in the operated left hemisphere, development of particular language components may slow down after surgery (de Koning et al. 2009).

VISUOSPATIAL SKILLS

As far as we are aware, cohort studies on visuospatial skills have not yet been performed in children after epilepsy surgery. Performance IQ, sometimes interpreted as a reflection of visuospatial skills, has been reported to remain stable, both after temporal and extra-temporal resection for drug-resistant epilepsy in childhood (Westerveld et al. 2000; Korkman et al. 2005), even in children with IQ scores less than 70 (Bjørnaes et al. 2004). Performances on visuomotor coordination tasks have been reported not to change after hemidisconnection; most of these children performed far below average prior to surgery (Pulsifer et al. 2003).

ATTENTION/EXECUTIVE FUNCTIONING

Data on attention or executive functioning after focal paediatric epilepsy surgery are scarce, and there are no studies that specifically describe attention or executive functioning after hemispherectomy. However, very early—almost immediately—after hemispherectomy in young children with epileptic encephalopathies, parents and clinicians often describe an improved alertness, awareness, attention, and communication, which is difficult to quantify but referred to as 'awakening'.

Improved general attention is noted after frontal lobe surgery, with postoperative changes not being different between seizure-free patients and those who had continuing seizures (Lendt et al. 2002). Impairment of executive functions is already noted in frontal lobe epilepsy patients before surgery, with a slight deterioration of executive functions after the resection in a minority (Chieffo et al. 2011). Impairments in attention and executive function have also been reported in children with parietal lobe epilepsy. After parietal lobe resection, attention improved and executive function remained unchanged (Gleissner et al. 2008). Increased ability to sustain attention and unchanged executive functioning has also been reported after paediatric epilepsy surgery in general (Viggedal et al. 2012). Children and adolescents with left temporal resections took longer than controls to reorient their attention on lexical attention tasks. Children with right temporal resections differed from controls in the number of errors made on a spatial task (Billingsley and Smith 2000).

Behaviour

The rate of behaviour disorders is particularly high in children with temporal lobe epilepsy, with a high proportion having a DSM-IV, diagnosis at any time pre- or postoperatively. In one study of 60 children coming to temporal lobe resection, 72% had at least one diagnosis preoperatively and 72% postoperatively (McLellan et al. 2005). However, some children had more than one diagnosis; some lost diagnoses following surgery and some gained in other diagnoses. In 9 of 57 (16%) children, mental health problems completely resolved postoperatively, whereas in 7 of 57 (12%) children who had been free of psychopathology, a diagnosis evolved postoperatively. What was clear, however, was that no prediction was possible as to who would lose and who would gain such diagnoses. Pervasive developmental disorder occurred in 38% of children (38% preoperatively, 37% postoperatively), attention-deficit–hyperactivity disorder in 27% (23% preoperatively, 23% postoperatively), oppositional defiant disorder/conduct disorder in 27% (23% preoperatively, 23% postoperatively), emotional disorder in 25% (8% preoperatively, 21% postoperatively), disruptive behaviour disorder not otherwise specified in 50% (40% preoperatively, 42% postoperatively), eating disorders in 4%, conversion disorders in 4%, and psychosis in 2% of children (McLellan et al. 2005).

In extratemporal lobe epilepsy coming to surgery, the rate of behaviour disorders is not quite as high as that seen in temporal lobe epilepsy, with DSM-IV, diagnoses seen in 52% at any time, 44% preoperatively and 45% postoperatively (Colonnelli et al. 2012). In a group of 71 children coming to extratemporal resection, attention-deficit–hyperactivity disorder occurred at some point in 10% of children (6% preoperatively, 10% postoperatively), oppositional defiant disorder/conduct disorder in 14% of children (13% preoperatively, 14 % postoperatively), emotional disorder in 17% of children (14% preoperatively, 17% postoperatively), autism spectrum disorder (ASD) in 14% of children (13% preoperatively, 14% postoperatively), other major disorders in 4% of children (3% preoperatively, 4% postoperatively), and disruptive behaviour disorder not otherwise specified in 28% of children (20% preoperatively, 14% postoperatively). Within the category that was best described as disruptive behaviour disorder, a significant number (from the whole sample, 13% preoperatively and 9% postoperatively) had a profile which was similar to 'frontal lobe behaviour' described in adults. Their behaviour was characterized by one or more of disinhibition, emotional liability, unpredictability, lack of motivation, and overactivity/underactivity (Colonnelli et al. 2012). Although behaviour disorder has to be recognized as common among the resective surgical population, parents have to be counselled about the fact that any change, particularly improvement, cannot be predicted or expected from surgery. Further, individual assessment has to be made according to the cognitive level of the child; there is no reason why behavioural interventions should work any differently in such children to those without epilepsy and should be treated accordingly.

Hemispherectomy was performed historically for infantile hemiplegia associated with epilepsy and behaviour disorder. In this group, there has been a more consistent report of improvement. Wilson (1970) originally described 50 patients of whom 80% had behavioural problems and 94% had a normalization of behaviour following surgery. Pulsifer reported a series of 71 patients with hemispherectomy in whom the Child Behaviour Checklist was used to assess behaviour, 53 of whom underwent follow-up at a mean of 5.4 years postoperatively (Pulsifer et al 2004). The overall scores were not consistent with clinical problems, but on the subscales highlighting attention and thought problems, the scores were consistent with a clinically significant problem, which improved after surgery.

Overall however, on assessment of behaviour, it may be the subjective opinion of parents that determines whether a disorder is reported, and the degree to which it is a problem that they may feel requires intervention. Further, a more 'awake' child following cessation of seizures may be perceived to be more disruptive. In one study utilizing the Strengths and Difficulties Questionnaire preoperatively to up to 8 years postoperatively in a small group of children undergoing resective surgery for epilepsy, the total difficulties score gradually improved with time, whereas the impact score improved significantly postoperatively but not further thereafter (Hannan et al. 2009). Parental expectation appeared to change over time postoperatively and influenced the degree of behavioural difficulty reported.

Conclusion

The earlier the onset of epilepsy, the more severely cognitive development of the child is affected. Furthermore, the longer the duration of epilepsy, the poorer the postoperative cognitive outcome will be. This stresses the point of early intervention in order to preserve cognitive function, which is particularly crucial in young children with epileptic encephalopathy and developmental arrest or regression. The consequences of epilepsy, in particular the impairment of cognition, are often as serious as having the seizure disorder itself (Aldenkamp et al. 2004) and may have even more impact on daily living, school performance (Schouten et al. 2002; Dunn et al. 2010), and quality of life (Sherman et al. 2006) than the seizures themselves. When deciding whether to proceed with epilepsy surgery, parents are concerned about the potential cognitive effects on their child. Queries of parents are, among others, whether surgery is another threat for the development of the child or

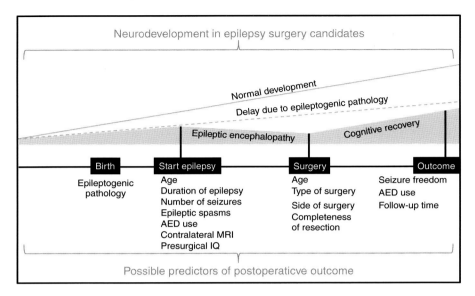

Fig. 15.1. Neurodevelopment in epilepsy surgery candidates and possible predictors of postoperative outcome. (Adapted from van Schooneveld MM and Braun KP, *Brain Dev*, 35, 721–729, 2013.) AED, antiepileptic drug; MRI, magnetic resonance imaging; IQ, intelligence quotient.

may hold the potential to improve cognition. The influence of surgery itself on the course of the child's neurocognitive development will be reflected by the differences between post- and preoperative cognitive function scores. Parents are also keen to know the likely influence on behaviour, particularly in light of the high rate of behaviour disorders in surgical candidates. Such needs to be assessed in the context of the presurgical cognitive level of each individual patient. Counselling of parents prior to surgery should be realistic about the cognitive consequences of the intervention: early surgical intervention may halt deterioration and open the possibility for appropriate neurodevelopment relative to the presurgical situation. It is, however, unlikely that surgery results in major improvement of MDI/DQ/IQ or other specific cognitive domains. However, some specific domains of cognitive function, such as verbal and visual memory, may be affected by surgery (Meekes et al. 2013; 2014). Long-term cognitive outcome after epilepsy surgery reflects the sum of many factors, both epilepsy-related and other presurgical variables, surgical factors, as well as postoperative determinants that can each influence long-term cognitive abilities independently (see Fig 15.1).

Some of these can be influenced by the treating physicians and surgical teams, such as the duration from the onset of epilepsy to surgery (the shorter, the better the outcome) (Jonas et al. 2004; Freitag and Tuxhorn 2005, Basheer et al. 2007), and AED withdrawal policies (the more AEDs reduced, the higher the—gain in—IQ) (Boshuisen et al. 2015). Unlike in adults, we have to consider the effects of dysfunction within a developing nervous system, ongoing maturational changes, as well as structural and functional plasticity. There is still a need for neuropsychological evidence, especially in terms of longitudinal data, to better understand why there is in some children a catch-up growth in the long-term and in others a decline. Attention should also be paid to the so-called growing into deficits, the appearance of deficits that could not be researched in younger children because different periods during development require different skills. Whereas up till now cognitive functioning and its impairments, particularly intelligence and development, have been the focus of neuropsychological research effort, other aspects of functioning after epilepsy surgery need to be addressed in more depth. Domains of full human functioning, activities and their limitations, and participation and restrictions therein (World Health Organization 2008) should be analyzed against the background of (impairments in) cognitive functioning, with the ultimate goal to discover barriers that can be remedied and to enhance the quality of life after epilepsy surgery.

REFERENCES

Aldenkamp AP, Alpherts WC, Sandstedt P et al. (1998) Antiepileptic drug-related cognitive complaints in seizure-free children with epilepsy before and after drug discontinuation. *Epilepsia* 39: 1070–1074.

Aldenkamp AP, Baker GA and Meador KJ (2004) The neuropsychology of epilepsy: What are the factors involved? *Epilepsy Behav* 5: S1–S2.

D'Argenzio L, Colonnelli MC, Harrison S et al. (2011) Cognitive outcome after extratemporal epilepsy surgery in childhood. *Epilepsia* 52: 1966–1972.

Basheer SN, Connolly MB, Lautzenhiser A et al. (2007) Hemispheric surgery in children with refractory epilepsy: Seizure outcome, complications, and adaptive function. *Epilepsia* 48: 133–140.

Battaglia D, Chieffo D, Lettori D et al. (2006) Cognitive assessment in epilepsy surgery of children. *Childs Nerv Syst* 22: 744–759.

Berg AT, Langfitt JT, Testa FM et al. (2008) Global cognitive function in children with epilepsy: A community-based study. *Epilepsia* 49: 608–614.

Berg AT, Berkovic SF, Brodie MJ et al. (2010) Revised terminology and concepts for organization of seizures and epilepsies: Report of the ILAE commission on classification and terminology, 2005–2009. *Epilepsia* 51: 676–685.

Billingsley R and Smith ML (2000) with left temporal lobe epilepsy: Relationship to language intelligence profiles in children and adolescents laterality. *Brain Cogn* 43: 44–49.

Bjørnaes H, Stabell K, Henriksen O et al. (2001) The effects of refractory epilepsy on intellectual functioning in children and adults. A longitudinal study. *Seizure* 10: 250–259.

Bjørnaes H, Stabell KE, Heminghyt E et al. (2004) Resective surgery for intractable focal epilepsy in patients with low IQ: Predictors for seizure control and outcome with respect to seizures and neuropsychological and psychosocial functioning. *Epilepsia* 45: 131–139.

Boatman D, Freeman J, Vining E et al. (1999) Language recovery after left hemispherectomy in children with late-onset sieuzres. *Ann Neurol* 46: 579–586.

Boshuisen K, van Schooneveld MMJ, Leijten FSS et al. (2010) Contralateral MRI abnormalities affect seizure and cognitive outcome after hemispherectomy. *Neurology* 75: 1623–1630.

Boshuisen K, van Schooneveld MM, Uiterwaal CS et al. (2015) TimeToStop cognitive outcome study group. Intelligence quotient improves after antiepileptic drug withdrawal following pediatric epilepsy surgery. *Ann Neurol* 78: 104–114.

Bourgeois M, Crimmins DW, de Oliveira RS et al. (2007) Surgical treatment of epilepsy in Sturge-Weber syndrome in children. *J Neurosurg: Pediatr* 106: 20–28.

Cormack F, Cross JH, Isaacs E et al. (2007) The development of intellectual abilities in pediatric temporal lobe epilepsy. *Epilepsia* 48: 201–204.

Cormack F, Vargha-Khadem F, Wood SJ, Cross JH and Baldeweg T (2012) Memory in paediatric temporal lobe epilepsy: Effects of lesion type and side. *Epilepsy Res* 98: 255–259.

Chieffo D, Lettori D, Contaldo I et al. (2011) Surgery of children with frontal lobe lesional epilepsy: Neuropsychological study. *Brain Dev* 33: 310–315.

Colonnelli MC, Cross JH, Davies S et al. (2012) Psychopathology in children before and after surgery for extratemporal lobe epilepsy. *Dev Med Child Neurol* 54: 521–526.

Cross JH (2002) Epilepsy surgery in childhood. *Epilepsia* 43: 65–70.

Cross JH, Jayakar P, Nordli D et al. (2006) Proposed criteria for referral and evaluation of children for epilepsy surgery: Recommendations of the subcommission for pediatric epilepsy surgery. *Epilepsia* 47: 952–959.

Cross JH and Guerrini R (2013) The epileptic encephalopathies. *Handb Clin Neurol* 111: 619–626.

Davies S, Heyman I and Goodman R (2003) A population based survey of mental health problmes in children with epilepsy. *Dev Med Child Neurol* 45: 292–295.

Devlin AM, Cross JH, Harkness W et al. (2003) Clinical outcomes of hemispherectomy for epilepsy in childhood and adolescence. *Brain* 126: 556–566.

Dunn DW, Johnson CS, Perkins SM et al. (2010) Academic problems in children with seizures: Relationships with neuropsychological functioning and family variables during the 3 years after onset. *Epilepsy Behav* 19: 455–461.

Englot DJ, Breshears JD, Sun PP, Chang EF and Auguste KI (2013a) Seizure outcomes after resective surgery for extra-temporal lobe epilepsy in pediatric patients. *J Neurosurg Pediatr* 12: 126–133.

Englot DJ, Rolston JD, Wang DD (2013b) Seizure outcomes after temporal lobectomy in pediatric patients. *J Neurosurg Pediatr* 12: 134–141.

Freitag H and Tuxhorn I (2005) Cognitive function in preschool children after epilepsy surgery: Rationale for early intervention. *Epilepsia* 46: 561–567.

Gleissner U, Kuczaty S, Clusman H et al. (2008) Neuropsychological results in pediatric patients with epilepsy in the parietal cortex. *Epilepsia* 49: 700–704.

Gleissner U, Sassen R, Schramm J, Elger CE and Helmstaedter C (2005) Greater functional recovery after temporal lobe epilepsy surgery in children. *Brain* 128: 2822–2829.

Hannan S, Cross JH, Scott RC, Harkness W and Heyman I (2009) The effects of epilepsy surgery on emotions, behavior, and psychosocial impariment in children and adolescents with drug-resistant epilepsy: A prospective study. *Epilepsy Behav* 15: 318–324.

Hertz-Pannier L, Chuon C, Jambaque I et al. (2002) Late Plasticity for language in a child's non-dominant hemisphere: A pre- and post-surgical fMRI study. *Brain* 125: 361–372.

Hessen E, Lossius MI, Reinvang I and Gjerstad L (2006) Influence of major antiepileptic drugs on attention, reaction time, and speed of information processing: Results from a randomized, double-blind, placebo-controlled withdrawal study of seizure-free epilepsy patients receiving monotherapy. *Epilepsia* 47: 2038–2045.

Jambaqué I, Dellatolas G, Fohlen M et al. (2007) Memory functions following surgery for temporal lobe epilepsy in children. *Neuropsychologia* 45: 2850–2862.

Jansen FE, Jennekens-Schinkel A, Van Huffelen AC et al. (2002) Diagnostic significance of Wada procedure in very young children and children with developmental delay. *Eur J Paediatr Neurol* 6: 315–320.

Jonas R, Nguyen S, Hu B et al. Cerebral hemispherectomy: Hospital course, seizure, developmental, language, and motor outcomes. *Neurology* 62: 1712–1721.

Jones-Gotman M, Smith M Lou, Risse GL et al. (2010) The contribution of neuropsychology to diagnostic assessment in epilepsy. *Epilepsy Behav* 18: 3–12.

de Koning T, Versnel H, Jennekens-Schinkel A et al. (2009) Dutch Collaborative Epilepsy Surgery Programme (DuCESP). Language development before and after temporal surgery in children with intractable epilepsy. *Epilepsia* 50: 2408–2419.

Korkman M, Granström ML, Kantola-Sorsa E et al. (2005) Two-year follow-up of intelligence after pediatric epilepsy surgery. *Pediatric Neurol* 33: 173–178.

Lah S (2004) Neuropsychological outcome following focal cortical removal for intractable epilepsy in children. *Epilepsy Behav* 5: 804–817.

Lamberink HJ, Boshuisen K, van Rijen PC et al. (2015) Changing profiles of pediatric epilepsy surgery candidates over time: A nationwide single-center experience from 1990 to 2011. *Epilepsia* 56: 717–725.

Lassonde M, Sauerwein HC, Jambaqué I, Smith ML and Helmstaedter C (2000) Neuropsychology of childhood epilepsy: Pre- and postsurgical assessment. *Epileptic Disord* 2: 3–13.

Loddenkemper T, Holland KD, Stanford LD et al. (2007) Developmental outcome after epilepsy surgery in infancy. *Pediatrics* 119: 930–935.

Lee YJ, Kang HC, Lee JS et al. (2010) Resective pediatric epilepsy surgery in Lennox-Gastaut syndrome. *Pediatrics* 125: e58–e65.

Lendt M, Gleissner U, Helmstaedter C et al. (2002) Neuropsychological outcome in children after frontal lobe epilepsy surgery. *Epilepsy Behav* 3: 51–59.

Liégeois F, Cross JH, Polkey C, Harkness W and Vargha-Khadem F (2008) Language after hemispherectomy in childhood: contributions from memory and intelligence. *Neuropsychologica* 46: 3101–3107.

Liégeois F, Morgan AT, Stewart LH et al. Speech and oral motor profile after childhood hemispherectomy. *Brain Lang* 114: 126–134.

Lossius MI, Hessen E, Mowinckel P et al. Consequences of antiepileptic drug withdrawal: A randomized, double-blind study (Akershus Study). *Epilepsia* 49: 455–463.

Matsuzaka T, Baba H, Matsuo A et al. (2001) Developmental assessment-based surgical intervention for intractable epilepsies in infants and young children. *Epilepsia* 42: 9–12.

McLellan A, Davies S, Heyman I et al. (2005) Psychopathology in children with epilepsy before and after temporal lobe resection. *Dev Med Child Neurol* 47: 666–672.

Miranda C and Smith ML (2001) Predictors of intelligence after temporal lobectomy in children with epilepsy. *Epilepsy Behav* 2: 13–19.

Meekes J, Braams O, Braun KPJ et al. (2013) Verbal memory after epilepsy surgery in childhood. *Epilepsy Res* 107: 146–155.

Meekes J, Braams O, Braun KPJ et al. Visual memory after epilepsy surgery in children: A standardized regression-based analysis of group and individual outcomes. *Epilepsy Behav* 36: 57–67.

Meekes J, van Schooneveld MM, Braams OB et al. (2015) Parental education predicts change in intelligence quotient after childhood epilepsy surgery. *Epilepsia* 56: 599–607.

Mula M and Trimble MR (2009) Antiepileptic drug-induced cognitive adverse effects. Potential mechanisms and contributing factors. *CNS Drugs* 23: 121–137.

Park SP and Kwon SH (2008) Cognitive effects of antiepileptic drugs. *J Clin Neurol* 4: 99–106.

Perry MS and Duchowny M (2013) Surgical versus medical treatment for refractory epilepsy: Outcomes beyond seizure control. *Epilepsia* 54: 2060–2070.

Pestana Knight EM, Schiltz NK, Bakaki BM et al. (2015) Increasing utilization of pediatric epilepsy surgery in the United States between 1997 and 2009. *Epilepsia* 56: 375–381.

Postma A, Kessels RPC and van Asselen M (2008) How the brain remembers and forgets where things are: The neurocognition of object location memory. *Neurosci Biobehav Rev* 32: 1339–1345.

Pulsifer MB, Brandt J, Salorio CF et al. (2004) The cognitive outcome of hemispherectomy in 71 children. *Epilepsia* 45: 243–254.

Ramantani G, Kadish NE, Strobl K et al. (2013) Seizure and cognitive outcomes of epilepsy surgery in infancy and early childhood. *Eur J Paediatr Neurol* 17: 498–506.

Ryvlin P, Cross JH and Rheims S (2014) Epilepsy surgery in children and adults. *Lancet Neurol* 13: 1114–1126.

Sherman EM, Slick DJ and Eyrl KL (2006) Executive dysfunction is a significant predictor of poor quality of life in children with epilepsy. *Epilepsia* 47: 1936–1942.

Shields WD (2000) Catastrophic epilepsy in childhood. *Epilepsia* 41: 2–6.

Schouten A, Oostrom KJ, Pestman WR et al. (2002) Dutch study group of epilepsy in childhood learning and memory of school children with epilepsy: A prospective controlled longitudinal study. *Dev Med Child Neurol* 44: 803–811.

van Schooneveld MMJ, Jennekens-Schinkel A, van Rijen PC, Braun KPJ and van Nieuwenhuizen O (2011) Hemispherectomy: A basis for mental development in children with epilepsy. *Epileptic Disord* 13: 47–55.

van Schooneveld MM and Braun KP (2013) Cognitive outcome after epilepsy surgery in children. *Brain Dev* 35: 721–729.

van Schooneveld MMJ, Braun KPJ and van Rijen PC (2016) The spectrum of long-term cognitive and functional outcome after hemispherectomy in childhood. *Eur J Pediatr Neurol* 20: 376–384. doi: 10.1016/j.ejpn.2016.01.004.

Skirrow C, Cross JH, Cormack F et al. (2011) Long-term intellectual outcome after temporal lobe surgery in childhood. *Neurology* 76: 1330–1337.

Skirrow C, Cross JH, Harrison S et al. (2015) Temporal lobe surgery in childhood and neuroanatomical predictors of long-term declarative memory outcome. *Brain* 138: 80–93.

Smith ML and Lah S (2011) One declarative memory system or two? The relationship between episodic and semantic memory in children with temporal lobe epilepsy. *Neuropsychologie* 25: 634–644.

Spencer S and Huh L (2008) Outcomes of epilepsy surgery in adults and children. *Lancet Neurol* 7: 525–537.

Téllez-Zenteno JF, Dhar R, Hernandez-Ronquillo L and Wiebe S (2007) Long-term outcomes in epilepsy surgery: Antiepileptic drugs, mortality, cognitive and psychosocial aspects. *Brain* 130: 334–345.

Thomas SG, Daniel RT, Chacko AG, Thomas M and Russell PS (2010) Cognitive changes following surgery in intractable hemispheric and sub-hemispheric pediatric epilepsy. *Childs Nerv Syst* 26: 1067–1073.

van Schooneveld MMJ, van Erp N, Boshuisen K et al. (2013) Withdrawal of antiepileptic drugs improves psychomotor speed after childhood epilepsy surgery. *Epilepsy Res* 107: 200–203.

Varadkar S, Bien CG, Kruse CA et al. (2014) Rasmussen's encephalitis: Clinical features, pathobiology, and treatment advances. *Lancet Neurol* 13: 195–205.

Viggedal G, Kristjansdottir R, Olsson I, Rydenhag B and Uvebrant P et al. (2012) Cognitive development from two to ten years after pediatric epilepsy surgery. *Epilepsy Behav* 25: 2–8.

Walker N, Jackson D, Dabbs K et al. (2012) Is lower IQ in children with epilepsy due to lower parental IQ? A controlled comparison study. *Dev Med Child Neurol* 55: 278–282.

Wang A, Peters RM and de Ribaupierre S (2012) Functional Magnetic resonance imaging for language mapping in temporal lobe epilepsy. *Epilepsy Res Treat* 2012: 1–8. doi:10.1155/2012/198183.

Westerveld M, Sass KJ, Chelune GJ et al. (2000) Temporal lobectomy in children: Cognitive outcome. *J Neurosurg* 92: 24–30.

Wilson PJ (1970) Cerebral hemispherectomy for infantile hemiplegia. A report of 50 cases. *Brain* 93: 147–180.

Wilson SJ, Baxendale S, Barr W et al. (2015) Indications and expectations for neuropsychological assessment in routine epilepsy care; Report of the ILAE Neuropsychological Task Force, Diagnostic Methods Commission, 2013–2017. *Epilepsia* 56: 674–681.

World Health Organization (WHO) (2008) Nederlandse vertaling van de international classification of functioning, disability and health, version Children & Youth. Houten, Bohn Stafleu van Loghum.

INDEX

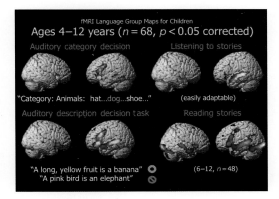

Fig. 5.1. Group activation ($p < 0.05$) from children across four language tasks.

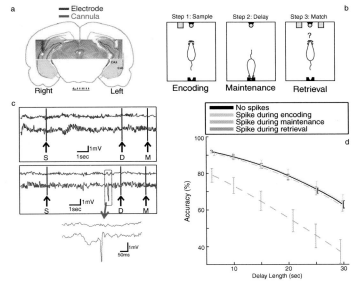

Fig. 6.1. To assess the effects of IISs on memory rats underwent intra-hippocampal pilocarpine injections to induced status epilepticus. (a) Bilateral electrodes are placed in the ventral hippocampus. (b) In the delayed match-to-sample test during the sample step, one of the two levers is randomly presented (right or left) and is pressed by the rat. Then, in the delay step, the rat has to poke its nose into a hole in the opposite wall for a random length of time (6–30s). After this time period has elapsed, the first nose poked into the hole turns off the stimulus light above and extends both the levers. Then, in the match step, the rat has to remember which lever it pressed during the sample phase and press the same lever again to procure a food reward. During the sampling stage, memory is encoded; during the delay phase memory is maintained; and during the match phase, memory is retrieved. Performance is recorded for trials without spikes (c, top trace) and trials with spikes (c, bottom). (d) Among trials in which an IIS occurs during the encoding or maintenance epoch of short-term memory, accuracy does not differ from trials without IIS. However, IISs during the retrieval phase produce a marked decrease in accuracy. Increasing delays produce decreases in accuracy, regardless of IIS epoch timing. (Modified from Kleen JK et al., *Ann Neurol*, 67, 250–257, 2010.)

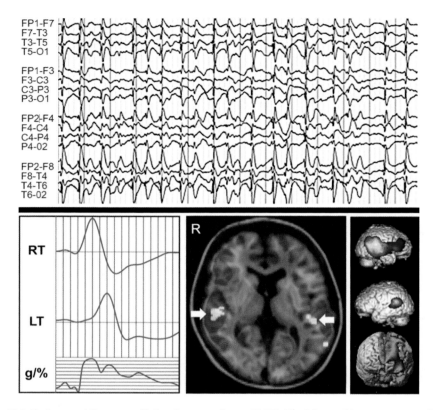

Fig. 13.1. Patient aged 8 years studied at the acute phase of LKS. *Top*: Non-rapid eye movement sleep EEG sample showing high-amplitude and diffuse CSWS with focalization over the right and left temporal regions. *Bottom*, *left*: The right and left temporal source waveforms identified by MEG for one typical epileptiform discharge occurring during CSWS. The abscissa corresponds to the time in ms (time steps: 10ms) and the ordinate corresponds to the dipole amplitude in nAm. The source waveforms clearly show the onset at the level of the right temporal (RT; maximal amplitude: 660nAm) source with rapid propagation (~20ms) toward the left temporal (LT; maximal amplitude: 602nAm) source. *Middle*: Results of the coregistration in the same three-dimensional space of the DICOM MRI image containing representative MEG equivalent current dipoles with the raw FDG-PET data. Both temporal MEG sources are localized at the superior temporal gyrus within hypermetabolic brain areas. *Right*: Statistical parametric mapping (SPM) analysis of the patient's FDG-PET data showing a significant bilateral increase in metabolism predominating over the superior temporal gyri (top and middle). Significant decrease in metabolism observed over the prefrontal cortex with a left hemisphere predominance (bottom). For viewing purpose, SPM maps are thresholded at $p < 0.001$ uncorrected. (From De Tiege et al., *Epilepsy Res*, 105, 316–325, 2013.) CSWS, continuous spikes and waves during slow-wave sleep; FDG-PET, [18F]-fluorodeoxyglucose; MEG, magnetoencephalography.

Recent titles from Mac Keith Press www.mackeith.co.uk

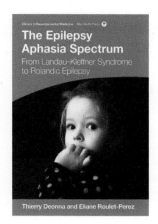

The Epilepsy Aphasia Spectrum: From Landau-Kleffner Syndrome to Rolandic Epilepsy
Thierry Deonna and Elaine Roulet-Perez

Clinics in Developmental Medicine
2017 ▪ 200pp ▪ hardback ▪ 978-1-909962-76-7
£50.00 / €62.94 / $75.00

Landau-Kleffner syndrome (LKS) is a rare childhood epilepsy, now considered to be at the severe end of the 'epilepsy-aphasia spectrum'. This book is aimed at the large range of professionals involved in the diagnosis, therapy and rehabilitation of children on the spectrum. The authors discuss work-up and management strategies and the reader will find chapters on topics such as the link between LKS and developmental language and communication disorders.

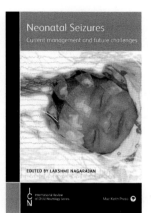

Neonatal Seizures: Current Management and Future Challenges
Lakshmi Nagarajan (Editor)

International Review of Child Neurology Series
2016 ▪ 214pp ▪ hardback ▪ 978-1-909962-67-5
£44.99 / €58.40 / $65.00

This book distils what is known about the many advances in the management of neonatal seizures into one scholarly yet practical text. Chapters cover the neonatal neuron, the use of video EEG in diagnosis, advances in neurophysiology, genetics and neuroprotective strategies, as well as outcomes. This volume will be of use to neonatologists, paediatricians, neurologists and all health professionals involved in the care of neonates experiencing seizures.

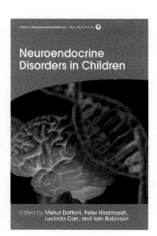

Neuroendocrine Disorders in Children
Mehul Dattani, Peter Hindmarsh, Lucinda Carr and Iain Robinson (Editors)

Clinics in Developmental Medicine
November 2016 ▪ 422pp ▪ hardback ▪ 978-1-909962-50-7
£74.95/ €93.70/ $120.00

Impairments in the interaction between the central nervous system and the endocrine system can lead to a number of disorders in children. These include type 1 diabetes, growth disorders, adrenal thyroid and pituitary problems, Addison's disease and Cushing syndrome, among others. *Neuroendocrine Disorders in Children* provides a comprehensive examination of paediatric and adolescent disorders focusing on the basic science and its clinical relevance.

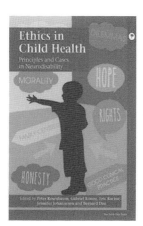

The Management of ADHD in Children and Young People
Val Harpin (Editor)

A practical guide from Mac Keith Press
2017 ▪ 292pp ▪ softback ▪ 978-1-909962-72-9
£34.95 / €43.70 / $64.50

This book is an accessible and practical guide on all aspects of assessment of children and young people with attention-deficit–hyperactivity disorder (ADHD) and how they can be managed successfully. The multi-professional team of authors discusses referral, assessment and diagnosis, psychological management, pharmacological management, and co-existing conditions, as well as ADHD in the school setting. New research on girls with ADHD is also featured. Case scenarios are included that bring these topics to life.

Ethics in Child Health: Principles and Cases in Neurodisability
Peter L. Rosenbaum, Gabriel M. Ronen, Eric Racine, Jenifer Johannesen and Bernard Dan (Editors)

2016 ▪ 396pp ▪ softback ▪ 978-1-909962-63-7
£39.95 / €50.00 / $60.00

This book explores the ethical dimensions of issues that have either been ignored or not recognised. Each chapter is built around an illustrative scenario and discusses how ethical principles can be utilised to inform decision-making. 'Themes for Discussion' at the end of each chapter will help professionals and policy makers put practical ethical thinking at the heart of care.

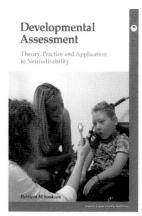

Developmental Assessment: Theory, Practice and Application to Neurodisability
Patricia M. Sonksen

A practical guide from Mac Keith Press
2016 ▪ 384pp ▪ softback ▪ 978-1-909962-56-9
£39.95 / €56.50 / $65.00

This handbook presents a new approach to assessing development in preschool children that can be applied across the developmental spectrum. The reader is taught how to confirm whether development is typical, and if it is not, is signposted to the likely nature and severity of the impairments with a plan of action. The author uses numerous case vignettes from her 40 years' experience to bring to life her approach with clear summary key points and helpful illustrations.